Pediatric Sinusitis and Sinus Surgery

Pediatric Sinusitis and Sinus Surgery

Edited by

Ramzi T. Younis
University of Miami
Miami, Florida, U.S.A.

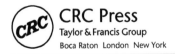

CRC Press
Taylor & Francis Group
Boca Raton London New York

CRC Press is an imprint of the
Taylor & Francis Group, an **informa** business

CRC Press
Taylor & Francis Group
6000 Broken Sound Parkway NW, Suite 300
Boca Raton, FL 33487-2742

First issued in paperback 2019

© 2006 by Taylor & Francis Group, LLC
CRC Press is an imprint of Taylor & Francis Group, an Informa business

No claim to original U.S. Government works

ISBN-13: 978-0-8247-2881-6 (hbk)
ISBN-13: 978-0-367-39205-5 (pbk)

Library of Congress Cataloging-in-Publication Data

Catalog record is available from the Library of Congress

**Visit the Taylor & Francis Web site at
http://www.taylorandfrancis.com**

**and the CRC Press Web site at
http://www.crcpress.com**

This book is dedicated to
My dad—God bless his soul—for the great education he has provided,
my mom for the love and care she planted in me,
my wife, Dina, and my children, Karen, Jessica, and Tamer for their support
encouragement, understanding, and everlasting love

Foreword

The evolution of the specialty of pediatric otolaryngology in the latter half of the twentieth century has been remarkable. Capitalizing on advances in imaging and technology, and the development of drugs that control infection, the care of children with ear, nose, and throat disorders has reduced not only the morbidity caused by disease, but also that caused by its treatment. In no case is this truer than in the treatment of pediatric sinus disease.

Dr. Ramzi Younis and a group of experts in pediatric sinus disease have written the first textbook completely dedicated to this disease. Because of the recent advances in the diagnosis and treatment, it is a disease process that warrants this focused approach and is appropriate for pediatric otolaryngologists and otolaryngologists in general, as well as residents in training, pediatricians, and other primary care specialists. The book begins with developmental anatomy and pathophysiology of sinusitis and quickly moves on to appropriate diagnostic evaluation. One chapter in particular contrasts the nature of adult and pediatric sinusitis, especially in diagnosis and treatment.

This explicit book detailly endoscopic surgical management, along with practical tips regarding surgical anatomy and ways to avoid complications. Other important areas include the use of image-guided surgery and management of comorbidities, such as diseases of tonsils and adenoids, cystic fibrosis, immune deficiency, and allergy.

Pediatric Sinusitis is a pioneering book, the first of its kind dedicated to this disorder. As such, it will be a cornerstone in the field of pediatric otolaryngology and will be extremely useful for rhinologists, sinus surgeons, pediatricians, and other primary care specialists. The authors are internationally recognized and deal with this complex and dynamic disease entity in a clear, concise, and complete way.

Thomas J. Balkany, MD FACS
Chairman, Department of Otolaryngology
University of Miami
Miami, Florida, U.S.A.

Foreword

Pediatric sinusitis is now well recognized as a common malady of children. In years past, the "snotty-nosed kid" was given little attention by the medical community, often leading to unnecessary morbidity and all too frequent minor and serious complications.

In the 1980s, more serious attention began to be paid to this condition by the medical community. Among others, Charles Bluestone, MD, a pediatric otolaryngologist, deserves much credit for focusing our attention to the importance of the proper recognition and evaluation of this condition, as well as the necessity for proper treatment. With the advent of functional sinus surgery, attention to adult sinusitis as well as pediatric sinusitis had a marked awakening. In 1989, we presented the first series showing the feasibility of functional endonasal surgery in pediatric patients. Following this, much more enthusiasm resulted. Rodney Lusk, MD, published his landmark *Pediatric Sinusitis* in 1992. Since its publication, there have been quite significant advancements in this field and many worthwhile publications, but no comprehensive compendium of this knowledge have been provided by the medical community. In this text, Dr. Younis has assembled a cadre of experts to present a contemporary detailed overview of the subject, including basic knowledge and practical application of medical and surgical management of pediatric sinusitis. As a final point, practical advice is given in regard to setting up a sinus center.

Charles Gross, MD
Department of Otolaryngology
UVA Health System
Charlottesville, Virginia, U.S.A.

Foreword

It is indeed my pleasure and privilege to write a foreword for *Pediatric Sinusitis*, an invaluable textbook edited by Professor Ramzi T. Younis. The contributors include some of the finest pediatric sinus surgeons. The topics for each chapter are well-placed and the contents succinctly executed. It will serve as an excellent companion for otolaryngology residents and attendings alike. It will be of much benefit to medical students and paramedical staff, as well as primary care physicians.

Ramzi, I salute you for a job well done.

K. J. Lee, MD, FACS

Preface

Sinusitis is a common disease entity in the pediatric and adult age groups. Pediatric sinusitis is a dynamic complex entity manifesting itself with a variety of signs and symptoms that may be compounded by a multitude of comorbidities. The etiological factors may vary from the most common upper respiratory tract infections and allergy to unusual systemic genetic disorders, such as cystic fibrosis or immune deficiency. The diagnosis and management of pediatric sinusitis requires meticulous attention to details.

Pediatric patients are not young adults; many etiological and inherent factors of pediatric sinusitis may not apply to adults. Even in the pediatric age group, younger patients should be addressed and treated differently than older and adolescent children. Sinusitis may be confused in pre-school-age children more than in adolescents, and adults. In this age group, it may be difficult to differentiate upper respiratory tract infections from allergy or what is commonly known as "day care syndrome," yet these latter factors can easily lead to sinusitis. Additionally, adenoiditis or adenoidal hypertrophy may mimic or cause sinusitis; however, the perspective and management may be similar. Furthermore, whenever treating pediatric sinusitis, our attention should not just be concentrated on sinuses as a variety of other contributing factors should be identified and controlled. These can include, but not be limited to, gastroesophageal reflux, allergy, cystic fibrosis, and immotile cilia syndrome.

In the past, pediatric sinusitis may have been poorly recognized and understood. Currently we face the problem of overdiagnosis and treatment. This is why we need to exhaust our efforts in isolating any "contributory" or etiological factors prior to labeling or treating a child. Diagnosis in children is challenging because we are commonly dealing with a sick, nervous, appre-hendive child who is difficult to examine. Moreover, the history is given by parents or caretakers who have their own perspectives and expectations of the child.

The mainstay of therapy is medical treatment, with antibiotics and nasal steroid spray being the cornerstones. A wide variety of surgical proce-dures have been discussed. Pediatric endoscopic sinus surgery has become the surgical procedure of choice since its introduction in the late 1980s. It had evolved over the years to include additional instrumentation and appli-cations with extremely rewarding and successful results; yet standardized outcomes are not well identified.

In this textbook, the various aspects of pediatric sinusitis are addressed in detail. It is a unique book that covers pediatric sinusitis and sinus surgery in a comprehensive and explicit fashion. The uniqueness of this work is that it comprises a spectrum of factors manifested by scientifically sound subject matter and easy flow of information. It is meticulously tailored and written by world-renowned experts in the field. This book is not directed only to otolaryngologists, but also to medical students, pediatric or primary care residents, and paramedical specialists.

The chapters are easy to read with a wealth of information that is easily accessible. All pertinent aspects of pediatric sinus diseases are discussed. Embryology, anatomy, and physiology along with detailed diagnostic work-up are discussed in the first chapters to allow the reader to understand and visualize a clear image of the sinusitis in children. The complications of sinusitis that are most common in children are then detailed, along with an additional chapter comparing adult versus pediatric sinusitis. Several factors may affect sinusitis in children; hence, each and every factor is critical and has been explicitly detailed in four other chapters that include pediatric sinu-sitis and comorbidities, allergy, immune deficiency, and cystic fibrosis. Sur-gical and medical management are dealt with at length in two other chapters. Emphasis is further made on the delicate and critical role of endo-scopic sinus surgery by detailing the various aspects of pediatric endoscopic sinus surgery. Additional chapters that discuss the role of computer-assisted surgery and new stepwise approaches to endoscopic sinus surgery, along with another chapter on the importance of sphenoid sinus and complica-tions of endoscopic sinus surgery are provided. The critical role of tonsils and adenoids in sinusitis in children is also very well elicited. In addition to all these important features, we felt it prudent to give advice it on how to set up and establish a successful and productive sinus center in the final chapter.

This textbook has been adequately structured to cover the wide spec-trum of sinusitis in children. The content and scope are written to appeal to various subspecialists involved in the management of pediatric sinusitis. This may include pediatricians, immunologists, allergists, infectious disease specialists, intensivists, pulmunologists, and otolaryngologists. The complex and delicate nature of pediatric sinusitis dictates the need of teamwork of specialists along with caretakers. The importance and necessity of multispecialty efforts to tackle sinusitis in children are well portrayed. The chapters are elegantly written in a resourceful and scientific fashion. The uniqueness and universality of this textbook had been unseen earlier. Finally, I would like to thank my publisher for helping me to get this dream into factual reality with special recognition and thanks to my valuable authors. I would like also to extend my sincere and warmest appreciation to my wife and children who have endured tirelessly with me to produce this magnificent book.

Ramzi T. Younis

Contents

Contributors

Frank C. Astor Departments of ENT and Otolaryngology, University of Miami, Miami, Florida, U.S.A.

Fuad M. Baroody Section of Otolaryngology—Head and Neck Surgery, Pritzker School of Medicine, University of Chicago, Chicago, Illinois, U.S.A.

Michael S. Benninger Department of Otolaryngology—Head and Neck Surgery, Henry Ford Hospital, Detroit, Michigan, U.S.A.

Roy R. Casiano Department of Otolaryngology, University of Miami School of Medicine, Miami, Florida, U.S.A.

Raphael Chan Bossier City, Louisiana, U.S.A.

Sam J. Daniel Department of Otolaryngology, McGill University, Montreal, Quebec, Canada

Craig S. Derkay Departments of Otolaryngology—Head and Neck Surgery and Pediatrics, Eastern Virginia Medical School, The Children's Hospital of the King's Daughters, Norfolk, Virginia, U.S.A.

Tina P. Elkins University of Texas, Cypress, Texas, U.S.A.

Joshua A. Gottschall   Department of Otolaryngology—Head and Neck Surgery, Henry Ford Hospital, Detroit, Michigan, U.S.A.

Edward Hepworth   Division of Otolaryngology Head and Neck Surgery, Department of Surgery, University of New Mexico, Albuquerque, New Mexico, U.S.A.

Melissa A. M. Hertler   Division of Otolaryngology Head and Neck Surgery, Department of Surgery, University of New Mexico, Albuquerque, New Mexico, U.S.A.

Sarita Kaza   New York, New York, U.S.A.

Gary Kleiner   Department of Pediatrics and Division of Immunology and Infectious diseases, University of Miami School of Medicine, Miami, Florida, U.S.A.

Rande H. Lazar   Pediatric Otolaryngology Fellowship Program, Le Bonheur Children's Medical Center, Memphis, Tennessee, U.S.A.

Mary LeGrand   KarenZupko & Associates Inc., Chicago, Illinois, U.S.A.

Ron B. Mitchell   Department of Otolaryngology, Virginia Commonwealth University, Richmond, Virginia, U.S.A.

Samantha M. Mucha   Section of Otolaryngology—Head and Neck Surgery, Pritzker School of Medicine, University of Chicago, Chicago, Illinois, U.S.A.

Maria T. Peña   Department of Otolaryngology, Children's Research Institute, Children's National Medical Center, Washington, D.C., U.S.A.

Kevin D. Pereira   Medical Center of Otolaryngology Department, University of Texas, Houston, Texas, U.S.A.

Hassan H. Ramadan   Department of Otolaryngology, Head and Neck Surgery, West Virginia University, Morgantown, West Virginia, U.S.A.

Scott A. Schraff   Department of Otolaryngology—Head and Neck Surgery, Eastern Virginia Medical School, Norfolk, Virginia, U.S.A.

Gavin Setzen   Department of Surgery and Albany ENT and Allergy Services, Albany Medical College, Albany, Newy York, U.S.A.

Michael Setzen   Department of Otolaryngology, North Shore University Hospital, Manhasset, New York, U.S.A.

Ramzi T. Younis   Department of Pediatrics, University of Miami, Miami, Florida, U.S.A.

George H. Zalzal   Department of Otolaryngology, Children's Research Institute, Children's National Medical Center, Washington, D.C., U.S.A.

1

Embryology and Anatomy of the Nose and Paranasal Sinuses

Raphael Chan
Bossier City, Louisiana, U.S.A.

Frank C. Astor
Departments of ENT and Otolaryngology, University of Miami, Miami, Florida, U.S.A.

Ramzi T. Younis
Department of Pediatrics, University of Miami, Miami, Florida, U.S.A.

EMBRYOLOGY OF THE NOSE

At the fourth week of gestation, the stomodeum is formed superiorly by the midline frontonasal process. The maxillary processes of the first branchial arch form the lateral borders.

By the end of the fourth week, nasal placodes, which are bilateral oval-shaped ectodermal thickenings, form on each side of the frontonasal process. The proliferation of mesenchyme around the placode creates the medial and lateral processes and the placodes eventually come to lie in depressions called nasal pits.

The maxillary processes grow toward each other and to the medial nasal processes. The lateral nasal process is separated from the maxillary process by a cleft or furrow, called the nasolacrimal groove.

The medial nasal processes merge with each other and with the maxillary processes during the sixth and seventh weeks. This merging results in the formation of the philtrum, the premaxillary process, and the primitive septum.

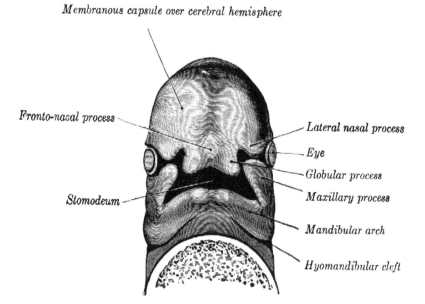

Figure 1 Undersurface of the head of a human embryo about 29 days old. *Source*: From Ref. 1.

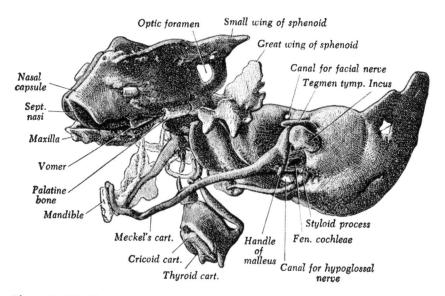

Figure 2 Model of the chondrocranium of a human embryo, 8-cm long. *Source*: From Ref. 1.

The frontonasal process develops into the forehead and the bridge and tip of the nose, while the sides of the nose are derived from the lateral nasal processes.

The primary palate develops from the premaxillary process at the end of the fifth week while the secondary palate develops from the horizontal mesodermal projections from the inner maxillary processes. These are the palatine processes and grow medially, fusing with each other and with the primary palate and nasal septum.

The primitive nasal capsule forms the framework for the development of the bony and cartilaginous structures of the upper face. The cartilaginous nasal capsule is formed from the condensation of mesenchyme during the third fetal month. Later, in-growth of connective tissue divides the structure into the lower lateral and upper lateral and septal cartilage. Most of the posterior capsule ossifies into the portions of the sphenoid bones, ethmoid bone including the ethmoid turbinates, sinus walls, and perpendicular plate. The nasal bone and maxilla form upon its lateral surface. Ossification of the cartilaginous capsule is not complete as cartilaginous segments remain in the anterior nose (Figs. 1, 2).

THE DEVELOPMENTAL ANATOMY OF THE LATERAL NASAL WALL

The progenitor of the inferior turbinate first appears as a swelling just above the palatal shelf in the anterior aspect of the lateral nasal wall at 38–40 days of gestation. This is the maxilloturbinal swelling. Another swelling, the ethmoturbinal, arises at 40–43 days at the junction of the nasal septum and nasal roof. The space between the maxilloturbinal and the ethmoturbinal develops into the future middle meatus. The ethmoturbinal swelling forms the middle, superior, and supreme turbinates. The supreme turbinate is seen by 95–105 days. The supreme turbinate differentiates further after the seventh month, but by puberty, they are usually absorbed, attaining the adult configuration by 12 years of age. The nasoturbinal swelling can be seen at approximately 60 days. This embryologic anlage is representative of the future agger nasi.

A thickened area develops at the junction of the ascending and descending parts of the middle meatus at 40–60 days. This sinks into the lateral nasal wall forming a furrow that is the future infundibulum, and the ridge that develops anterior to it on the nasoturbinal swelling becomes the uncinate process.

Further deepening of the floor of the infundibulum as a pouch forms the precursor of the maxillary sinus by 60–75 days. The frontal recess cells develop medial to the uncinate and between it and the anterior attachment of the middle turbinate at approximately 105 days. The ethmoid bulla forms posterior to the infundibular furrow.

The superior meatus differentiates in a truncated manner; at 110 days, the anterior end develops a superior and inferior arm (like the infundibulum) and a crista (like the bulla). The bony lamellae of the lateral nasal wall consist of the middle, superior, and the supreme turbinates, the ethmoid bulla, and the uncinate. These lamellae are attached to the lamina papyracea and remain constant throughout development, although with differentiation, they may be distorted by pneumatization. The lamellae partition the lateral wall into compartments in which cellular development is organized. The basal lamella of

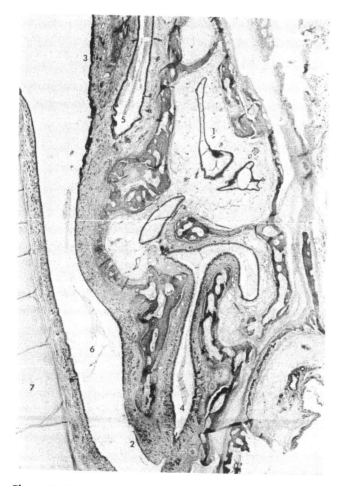

Figure 3 Horizontal section of the left ethmoid bone and the ethmoidal sinuses of a 7-month fetus. 1. ethmoidal sinuses, 2. middle turbinate, 3. superior turbinate, 4. middle meatus, 5. superior meatus, 6. nasal chamber, 7. nasal septum. *Source:* From Ref. 2.

the middle turbinate is the most constant and it divides the anterior from the posterior ethmoid cells (Fig. 3).

THE ETHMOID SINUS

The ethmoid sinuses develop from evagination of the nasal mucosa from the middle, superior, and supreme meatuses. During the first few years of life, the development is rapid and then slows thereafter. The final form is only reached between ages 12 and 14. There is no uniformity in the development of the ethmoid sinus. Each air cell of the ethmoid sinus will communicate with the meatus that it arises from. Cells arising from a different meatus of origin will not communicate with another. Anterior aircells arise from the middle meatus from three areas: the frontal recess, the infundibulum, and the bullar furrow. In almost all individuals, the ethmoid bulla will be pneumatized as a constant feature, while the posterior aircells are present in 96% of cases and the agger nasi in 89% (3).

The adult ethmoid labyrinth has common extensions beyond the ethmoid bone with growth in the supraorbital plate of the frontal bone and infraorbital extensions into the maxilla, which are called Haller cells. The anterior ethmoid cells may encroach on the frontonasal recess or invade the middle turbinate as the chonchal bullosa.

The posterior cells may encroach on the sphenoid sinus or extend into the palatine bone. These posterior ethmoid cells may also extend superiorly and laterally over the orbit as supraorbital cells and could extend as far as the vertical portion of the frontal bone (Table 1).

The roof of the most anterior cells forms the floor of the frontal sinus. Anteriorly, the lacrimal bone with the lacrimal sac is the anterolateral relationship, while the agger nasi relates to the medial surface. The inferior aspect of the ethmoid complex relates to the medial maxillary sinus roof, while the lamina papyracea is the lateral relationship.

The turbinates and meatuses are the medial structures relating to the ethmoid complex.

The posterior cells have a close relationship with the anterolateral surface of the sphenoid sinus.

There may be extensive pneumatization of the posterior ethmoid cells into the body and lesser wing of the sphenoid bone forming ethmosphenoidal cells that become the superior and posterior boundaries of the pterygopalatine fossa. These ethmosphenoidal cells have an intimate relationship with the optic nerve.

Maxillary Sinus

At the tenth week of gestation, an evagination in the lateral wall of the ethmoid infundibulum initiates the formation of the maxillary sinus. By birth, a tubular

Table 1 Measurements of the Ethmoid Sinus Through Different Ages

Age (years)	Group	Cephalocaudal (mm) (height)	Mediolateral (mm) (width)	Ventrodosal (mm) (length)
Newborn	Anterior	5	2	2
	Posterior	5	4	2
1	Anterior	2–8	1.5–6	2–7
	Posterior	2–8	1.5–7	2–9
2	Anterior	3–9	2–6	2–6
	Posterior	5–8	3–4	4–6
5	Anterior	7–8	5–7	5–6
	Posterior	7–8	7–10	6–7
8	Anterior	8–11	7–10	6–7
	Posterior	8–11	7–10	9–16
10	Anterior	9–12	8–12	8–10
	Posterior	9–14	8–12	9–17
14	Anterior	9–16	10	5–23
	Posterior	9–15	14	8–20

Source: From Ref. 4.

sac represents the maxillary sinus. This is 8 mm deep, 4 mm wide, and 4 mm high. The relatively small diameters of fetal and infantile maxillae and the close relationship of the developing teeth to the orbital floor preclude the possibility of a rapid increase in the vertical and lateral diameters of the sinus during the early periods.

By one year of age, the sinus has extended laterally to below the orbit to the infraorbital nerve. Thereafter, it grows rapidly during ages 3 and 4. By age 9, pneumatization has proceeded to the zygomatic process of the maxilla. Inferior growth accelerates after the eruption of the permanent teeth by age 7. At ages 8 and 12, the floor of the maxillary sinus has reached the floor of the nose, and the adult size is reached by age 15.

In early childhood, the general outline of the sinus is rather ovoid, but in later childhood, it is gradually changed into a pyramidal form, which represents the usual adult type. The base is directed toward the nasal fossae and corresponds to the medial wall, while the apex extends into the zygomatic process (5) (Table 2).

The adult maxillary sinus has septations in about 50% of cases, resulting in the sinus having different cavities. During surgery, this may have to be considered.

The maxillary sinus ostium is bounded superiorly by the ethmoid bulla and inferiorly the uncinate process. It opens into the infundibulum. Extensive pneumatization into these structures can cause narrowing of the hiatus semilunaris, with resulting impedance of drainage from the maxillary sinus.

Table 2 Measurements of the Maxillary Sinus Through Different Ages

Age	Ventreodosal (length) (mm)	Cophalocaudal (height) (mm)	Mediolateral (width) (mm)
Newborn	7.0–8.0	4.0–6.0	3.0–4.0
6 months	10.0–10.5	4.0–5.0	4.0–4.5
9 months	11.0–14.0	5.0–5.0	5.0–5.5
1 year	14.0–16.0	6.0–6.5	5.0–5.5
1.5 years	20.0–20.5	8.0–9.0	5.0–6.0
2 years	21.0–22.0	10.0–11.0	6.0–6.5
3 years	22.0–23.0	11.0–12.0	8.0–9.0
6 years	27.0–28.0	16.0–17.0	9.0–10.0
8 years	28.0–29.0	17.0–17.5	17.0–18.0
10 years	30.0–31.0	17.5–18.0	19.0–20.0
12 years	31.0–32.0	18.0–20.0	19.0–20.0
15 years	31.0–32.0	18.0–20.0	19.0–20.0

Source: From Ref. 4.

The accessory maxillary ostium opens directly into the middle meatus and not into the infundibulum, unlike the natural ostium or duplicated ostium. If present, the accessory ostium is usually located posteriorly and often inferiorly to the natural opening. It opens into the medial wall of the maxillary sinus at the membranous segment. This area is bound by mucous membranes on both sides and there are two dehiscences, termed fontanelles. The anterior fontanelle is found anterior and inferior and the posterior fontanelle is found posterior and inferior. Accessory ostia are not common before the 15th year (4). In the fetus and infancy, the walls of the sinuses are still relatively thick. During the development of the sinus cavity, the sinus walls become thinner and thinner, resulting in time with the fontanelle, comprised of the two layers of abutting mucosal membranes. Further attenuation of these areas results in the formation of an opening (Fig. 4).

The maxillary sinus can vary tremendously in size depending on the degree of pneumatization. A poorly developed maxillary sinus may be associated with other anomalies such as cleft palate, choanal atresia, and mandibular facial dysotosis. Unilateral maxillary hypoplasia was noted in 10.4% of cases in the series reported, which is higher than the usually reported incidence of 3% and 6.3%. This was attributed by the authors to better imaging by CT scanning. About 77.8% of their patients with a sinus volume estimate ratio of less than 0.425 had an associated aplasia or hypoplasia of the corresponding uncinate process. The recognition of an anomalous uncinate process has particular significance in patients with maxillary sinus hypoplasia who undergo surgical procedures for chronic sinusitis (6–10). Should this structure be hypoplastic or malformed, the first bony structure encountered in this area during

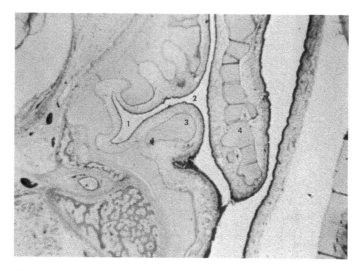

Figure 4 Evagination from the right nasal chamber in the infundibulum of a 4-month fetus. This coronal section is at the site of the ostium of the future maxillary sinus. 1. Maxillary sinus, 2. ostium, 3. uncinate ridge, 4. middle turbinate. *Source*: From Ref. 2.

functional endoscopic surgery (FES) surgery may in fact be the lamina papyracea.

Conversely, with extensive pneumatization, the maxillary sinus is huge. Such pneumatization can occur with the alveolus, frontal, or zygomatic processes, the orbital process of the palatine bone, or even beneath the nasal floor into the palatal recess.

The alveolar process of the maxillary bone forms the floor of the sinus, which is separated from the teeth by cancellous bone. Thinning of the bone may cause the appearance of irregularities on the sinus floor. In severe thinning, the tooth roots are covered only by mucosa in the sinus cavity. The sinus is closely related to the premolars and the first and second molars.

Before age 12, the level of the maxillary sinus is about 4–5 mm above the floor of the nasal cavity. After age 14, the level of the maxillary sinus is about 3–4 mm inferior to the nasal cavity floor. Moreover, the inferior nasal meatus is exceedingly narrow at this time due to the relatively large inferior turbinate (6–10).

This is an important consideration in the introduction of a trocar into the maxillary sinus in the pediatric age group. Endonasal procedures in children should be carried out through the middle meatus.

The infraorbital nerve exits from the infraorbital foramen, which is situated on the anterior wall 0.5 cm below the infraorbital rim. Surgery on the roof of the maxillary sinus places the nerve at risk. Damage to this nerve

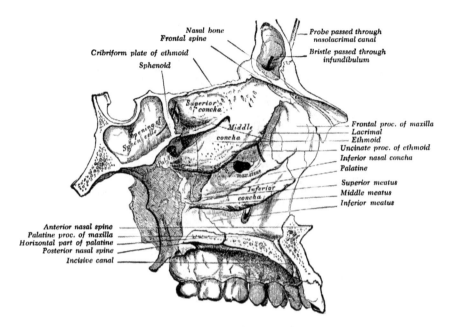

Figure 5 Roof, floor, and lateral wall of left nasal cavity. *Source*: From Ref. 1.

results in paraesthesia to the cheek and upper lip and, if there is subsequent neuroma formation, intractable pain may follow.

The posterior superior dental nerves, which are branches of the maxillary nerve, enter the maxilla through foramina in the posterior wall above the turberosity. They innervate the mucous membrane of the maxillary sinus and the three molars. These nerves lie just below the mucosa of the sinus floor and are at risk of damage during aggressive curettage of the sinus floor.

The anterior superior dental nerves branch off the infraorbital nerve canal midway or at the anterior wall of the sinus. The nerve runs medially to innervate the canine and the two incisors, before reaching the anterior inferior quadrant of the lateral wall of the nose and the adjacent floor before ending at the nasal septum. Surgical approaches through the anterior wall, especially if high and medial, can injure the nerve.

The posterior wall of the maxillary sinus is the anterior border of the pterygopalatine fossa. In the fossa, the maxillary artery has branches that accompany the branches of the pterygopalatine ganglion. The greater palatine artery runs inferiorly in the greater palatine canal behind the posterior wall of the sinus (Figs. 5,6). In the creation of nasoantral windows, the removal of this posterior wall can be a source of bleeding when the artery is encountered.

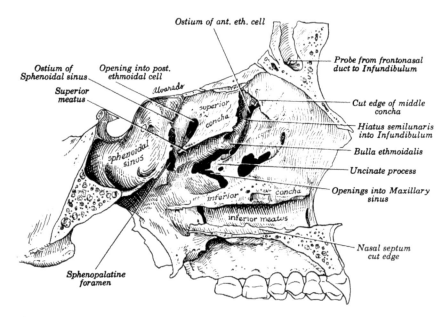

Figure 6 Lateral wall of nasal cavity with middle turbinate removed to show middle meatus. *Source*: From Ref. 1.

Sphenoid Sinus

The sphenoid sinus develops from the primordium at 3 months of gestation. This primordium is an ovoid recess within the posterior end of the cartilaginous nasal capsule. At birth, this sphenoid sinus primordium grows inferiorly and posteriorly, while ossifying during development. The primordial sinus cavity may be several millimeters in diameter. The primordium invades the sphenoid bone at 3–4 years and pneumatization of the sphenoid sinus begins (6–10).

The initial growth is posterolateral, with gradual thinning of the lateral walls, and developing a relationship with the ophthalmic and maxillary nerves by then, thus taking on a clinical significance.

By ages 6–7, the vidian canal is closely related to the floor of the sinus. Growth of the sphenoid sinus proceeds fairly uniformly at the rate of about 1.4 mm per year in children ages 3–15 (6–11).

If the sphenoid sinus primordium should fuse with the sphenoid bone, then pneumatization will not take place by this route. The sphenoid sinus will then either be undeveloped or the posterior ethmoids will invade the sphenoid bone.

There are three forms of sphenoid sinuses that denote the extent of pneumatization that relates to the sella turcica (12).

1. *Conchal*: This is the most rudimentary and uncommon form seen often in the preteen years. Pneumatization does not extend into the sphenoid bone. A thick bony septum separates left and right sinuses. It is small and separated from the sella turcica by a cancellous wall, 10 mm thick. This type may persist in 3% of adults.
2. *Presellar*: The sphenoid is pneumatized to the vertical plane of the sella turcica and not beyond. The anterior wall of the sella turcica does not bulge into the sphenoid sinus. This is seen throughout childhood and in 11% of adults.
3. *Sellar*: This is the most common type in 86% of adults on one side and bilaterally in 59%. The pneumatization extends beyond the floor of the sella turcica. On average, the anterior wall of the sella turcica is only 0.5 mm thick. This wall invariably bulges into the sphenoid sinus; sometimes the sellar floor bulges into this sinus.

In a well-pneumatized sphenoid sinus, the optic nerve and carotid artery canals form projecting impressions into the sinus cavity and are at risk during sphenoid surgery. In 22% of specimens examined, there is clinical dehiscence of the internal carotid canal (13). In 4%, the optic canal is dehiscent.

The entire sphenoid bone may be pneumatized and there may be extension into the lesser and greater wings, the basiocciput, the superior medial orbit, and the orbital process of the palatine bone (Figs. 5,6). Total absence of both sphenoid sinuses occurs in about 1% of cases.

The interior of the sphenoid sinus demonstrates a wide variation of recesses and septae. The intersinus septum may be in the midline, S-shaped, C-shaped, or asymmetrically located posteriorly, or even lying semi-horizontally. An absent septum suggests an agenesis; with a compensatory pneumatization by the other side, resulting in an anomalous single sphenoid sinus ostium instead of two. The sphenoid ostia may vary in size and location in the same individual, but they will always open into the sphenoethmoid recess.

Frontal Sinus

At the fourth fetal month, the ventrocephalic region of the middle meatus begins to extend anteriorly and superiorly into the region of the fetal frontal recess. This recess consists of thick cartilaginous areas that are level with the lateral nasal walls. At birth, this region forms small folds and furrows. The anterior ethmoid cells develop from this same region (6–10).

The development of the frontal sinus can arise from different potential routes (3):

1. Direct extension from the frontonasal recess, resulting in a wide communication between the frontal sinus and nasal cavity, anterior and superior to the hiatus semilunaris

2. From anterior ethmoid cells within the furrows or pits extending into the frontal bone
3. From an aircell in the anterior region of the ethmoid infundibulum
4. An extension of the ethmoid infundibulum
5. A combination of any of these routes, and producing more than one frontal sinus on the same side. These supernumerary frontal sinuses each drain separately into the nose by their own ostia and can be a challenging task for the surgeon.

The frontal sinus begins to extend superiorly into the vertical plate of the frontal bone by age 2; by age 3, the sinus has reached above the level of the nasion. In 50% of cases, the frontal sinus is at the level of the orbital roof by the eighth year. Further growth is then more rapid and the mature size is reached by puberty.

The drainage channel of the frontal sinus may not appear as a solitary structure or as a single duct. The drainage may be in the form of multiple openings. Expanding anterior ethmoidal cells of the frontal recess may distort and displace the drainage channel, which presents as a serpentine and inconstant course upward toward the frontal sinus. Early investigators described the outflow of the frontal sinus more often to drain medial and anterior to the uncinate process (Figs. 5,6). Recent studies suggest that the frontal sinus opens more frequently into the infundibulum (14).

The relationship between the ethmoid infundibulum and the skull base, especially the frontal recess, depends on the uncinates process (15). Superiorly, the ethmoid infundibulum may end blindly in the terminal recess or recessus terminalis if the uncinate process bends laterally and inserts into the lamina papyracea. If the uncinate process reaches the skull base or fuses with the middle turbinate medially, the ethmoid infundibulum may pass into the frontal recess superiorly (Figs. 5,6). Any approach to the sinus endonasally can be performed through the agger nasi cells, which are quite large in size, constant in occurrence, and lie at an accessible location in the middle meatus (16).

The anterior ethmoid cells may balloon into the floor of the frontal sinus floor. These frontal bullae may be mistaken for the frontal sinus cavity in external approaches to the frontal sinus. This occurs in 20% of cases.

The frontal sinus is hypoplastic in 30% of skulls examined. The frontal sinus may have extensive horizontal growth with minimal vertical development. This occurs bilaterally in 4% and unilaterally in 10% (17). This may be mistaken for agenesis of the frontal sinus.

The entire frontal bone can be pneumatized with extensions into the greater and lesser wings of the sphenoid, the parietal bone, maxilla, and temporal bones.

Extreme sinus development is associated with osteogenesis imperfecta tarda, Turner syndrome, Klinefelter syndrome, and acromegaly. Small sinuses are associated with Down syndrome, Apert syndrome, Treacher Collins syndrome, and pituitary dwarfism. The horizontal plate is invaded by supraorbital cells in 20% of skulls. They are found within the medial third of the orbital roof. These cells can extend posteriorly to the optic foramen.

REFERENCES

1. Gray H. Anatomy of the Human Body. 29th ed. Philadelphia: Lea & Febiger, 1973.
2. Ritter FN. The Paranasal Sinuses: Anatomy and Surgical Technique. 1st ed. St. Louis: The C. V. Mosby Company, 1973.
3. Van Alyea OE. Nasal sinuses. In: Anatomic and Clinical Consideration. 2nd ed. Baltimore: Williams and Wilkins, 1951.
4. Schaffer JP. The Nose, Paranasal Sinuses, Nasolacrimal Passage Ways and Olfactory Organs in Man. 1st ed. Philadelphia: Blakiston, 1920.
5. Davis WB. Development and Anatomy of the Nasal Accessory Sinuses in Man. 1st ed. Philadelphia and London: WB Saunders, 1914.
6. Moore KL. The Developing Human. 4th ed. Philadelphia: WB Saunders, 1988.
7. Anon JB, Rontal M, Zinreich SJ. Embryology and anatomy of the paranasal sinus. In: Bluestone DC, Stool SE, Kenna MA, eds. Pediatric Otolaryngology. Philadelphia: WB Saunders, 1996:719–734.
8. Vaidya AM, Fairbanks DNF, Stankiewicz JA. Embryology and anatomy of the nose and paranasal sinuses. In: de Souza C, Stankiewicz J, Pellitteri KP, eds. Pediatric Otorhinolaryngology Head and Neck Surgery. Vol. 1. San Diego, London: Singular Publishing Group Inc., 1999:315–326.
9. Bolger W, Woodruff WW, Moorehead J, Parsons DS. Maxillary sinus hypoplasia: classification and description of associated uncinate process hypoplasia. Otolaryngol Head Neck Surg 1990; 103:759–765.
10. Skillern RH. The Accessory Sinus of the Nose. 4th ed. Philadelphia and London: JP Lippincott, 1923.
11. Hinck VC, Hopkins CE. Concerning growth of the sphenoid sinus. Arch Otolaryngol 1965; 82:62–66.
12. Hamberger C, Hammer G, Norlen G, Sjogren B. Transantrosphenoidal hypophysectomy. Arch Otolaryngol 1961; 74:2–8.
13. Kennedy D, Roth M. Functional endoscopic sinus surgery. In: Ballenger JJ, Snow JB Jr, eds. Otolaryngology, Head and Neck Surgery. Williams and Wilkins, 1996:173–180.
14. Lee D, Brody R, Har-El G. Frontal sinus outflow anatomy. Am J Rhinol 1997; 11(4):283–285.
15. Stammberger H, Kennedy D, Bolger W. Paranasal sinus: anatomic terminology and nomenclature. Ann Otol Rhinol Laryngol 1995; 104(167):7–16.
16. Wormald PJ. The agger nasi cells: the key to understanding the anatomy of the frontal recess. Otolaryngol Head Neck Surg 2003; 129(5):497–507.
17. Dixon FW. Clinical significance of anatomical arrangements of paranasal sinus. Ann Otol Rhinol Laryngol 1958; 67:736–741.

2

Pathophysiology and Etiology of Pediatric Rhinosinusitis

Melissa A. M. Hertler

*Division of Otolaryngology Head and Neck Surgery, Department of Surgery,
University of New Mexico, New Mexico, U.S.A.*

Ron B. Mitchell

*Department of Otolaryngology, Virginia Commonwealth University,
Richmond, Virginia, U.S.A.*

Rande H. Lazar

*Pediatric Otolaryngology Fellowship Program, Le Bonheur Children's Medical
Center, Memphis, Tennessee, U.S.A.*

INTRODUCTION

Rhinosinusitis is a disease state that affects the nasal passages and the paranasal sinuses. During the initial 7 to 10 days of the disease process, acute rhinosinusitis is difficult to distinguish from a simple upper respiratory infection. Acute rhinosinusitis becomes evident when the signs and symptoms persist beyond 10 days. Chronic rhinosinusitis is a disease state that persists for longer than 12 weeks. Chronic rhinosinusitis may be exacerbated by acute rhinosinusitis (1). Rhinosinusitis can be further divided into a subacute form with duration of symptoms intermediate between acute and chronic disease (2). Clinically, rhinosinusitis is indistinguishable from rhinitis. Although isolated rhinitis may occur, isolated sinusitis is rare (1,3).

The paranasal sinuses are air-filled spaces within the skull bones. Their function may include provision of vocal resonance and sound projection, humidification of inspired air, and regulation of intranasal pressure and mucus production. They may also have a function in decreasing the total weight of the head (4). The paranasal sinuses develop as diverticula from the lateral nasal wall, extending into the maxilla, ethmoid, frontal, and sphenoid bones. The maxillary sinuses are present at birth and exhibit a two-phased growth spurt, between birth and 3 years and again from 7 to 12 years of age. The ethmoid sinuses are present at birth, but are fluid-filled. Pneumatization occurs prior to age 12. The frontal sinuses are present, but not visible on imaging at birth, and become fully pneumatized by 20 years of age. The sphenoids develop as an invagination of the sphenoethmoidal recess. Pneumatization begins at approximately age seven and continues to adulthood.

The drainage of the paranasal sinuses into the nasal cavity is as follows: the maxillary sinuses and the anterior ethmoid air cells drain into the ipsilateral middle meatus, the posterior ethmoid air cells and the sphenoid sinuses drain into the ipsilateral superior meatus, and the frontal sinuses drain into the ipsilateral frontal recess. In contrast to the middle meatus, the ostiomeatal complex (OMC) is not a discrete anatomic location that can be defined (Fig. 1). Instead, it is a functional entity composed of the infundibulum, hiatus semilunaris, frontal recess, anterior ethmoid cells, ethmoid bulla, and the anterior wall of the middle turbinate. It represents the drainage and ventilation pathway of the frontal, maxillary, and anterior ethmoid cells (5).

A definition of anatomic normalcy of the nose and sinuses is evolving. Anatomic variations between the two sides of the paranasal sinuses in the

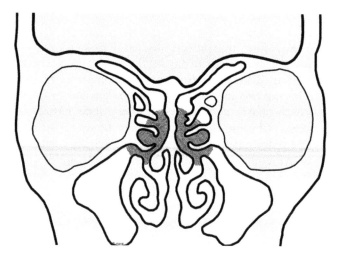

Figure 1   The ostiomeatal complex.

same patient are frequently seen and are rarely abnormal. Abnormal structures such as Haller or Onodi cells or concha bullosa may or may not lead to a pathologic condition (4).

PATHOPHYSIOLOGY

For the paranasal sinuses to function effectively, the ostia must be patent, the mucociliary clearance mechanism must be adequate, and the secretions must be of normal consistency and makeup (6). Any number of factors can adversely affect this system and cause thickening of the mucosal layer, epithelial dysfunction, obstruction of the ostia, retention of secretions, and ultimately, rhinosinusitis.

Anatomic or acquired obstruction of the ostia appears to be the primary factor in initiation of rhinosinusitis (3,6). Obstruction of the OMC may be incited by local, regional, or systemic factors. Locally, obstruction may be caused by anatomic obstruction, such as septal deviation, polyps, choanal atresia, or concha bullosa. Viral infections, allergic or non-allergic inflammation, or foreign bodies may cause edema. Obstruction of the natural sinus ostia can result in mucosal damage and ciliary dysfunction. This can lead to mucous stasis, bacterial invasion from the upper respiratory tract, and subsequent infection (6).

The mucociliary system consists of ciliated stratified or pseudostratified columnar epithelium, with goblet cells that produce mucous. Drainage of the

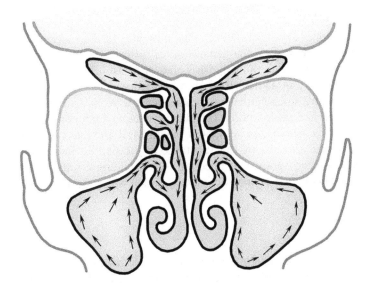

Figure 2 Direction of mucociliary flow in the paranasal sinuses.

paranasal sinuses is dependent on the effectiveness of the mucociliary clearance mechanism (Fig. 2). The ostia is not necessarily located in the lowest region of the sinus, and adequate drainage may not occur with gravity alone. Mucociliary clearance occurs due to the direction and speed of the beating cilia upon the epithelium. In the maxillary and frontal sinuses, this occurs in a spiral or circular manner, while in the sphenoid and ethmoid cells this is more directly toward the ostia. Smooth mucociliary flow is considered to be about 0.8 cm/min, while mucostasis is less than 0.3 cm/min.

A normal mucous blanket is the third aspect essential to the maintenance of mucociliary clearance and healthy paranasal sinuses. The blanket of mucous contains mast cells, neutrophils, eosinophils, lysozymes, and immunoglobulin A (IgA) and is renewed every 10 to 15 minutes. Multiple intrinsic and extrinsic properties can affect the mucociliary clearance mechanism. Intrinsic factors include ciliary dyskinesias that are abnormalities of ciliary form or function, alterations in local nitric oxide production, and cystic fibrosis (CF) which alters the consistency of mucous. Extrinsic factors include exposure to environmental irritants such as tobacco smoke and certain chemicals, as well as infection with viral upper respiratory pathogens. Braverman et al. used mucosal biopsies from the paranasal sinus to study the effect of temperature on ciliary beat frequency. In vitro, beat frequency was significantly decreased at a temperature of 22°C compared to 35°C (7).

Infection of paranasal sinus epithelial cells with viruses that cause common upper respiratory infections (URIs) has been shown to induce the production of several cytokines. The altered production of inflammatory mediators by paranasal sinus epithelial cells may incite cellular inflammation, whereby inducing increased vascular permeability and subsequent epithelial edema and ciliary dysfunction. This may also lead to alteration in the mucus composition, with the generation of an increased volume of more viscous secretions. Acute rhinosinusitis may then result from obstruction of the ostiomeatal unit as described above (8–10).

Healthy paranasal sinus epithelium generates nitric oxide in relatively large quantities under normal conditions (11). Under inflammatory conditions, altered production of nitric oxide may inhibit the antiviral and bacteriostatic protection mechanisms afforded by this substance in the sinuses, facilitating bacterial colonization and subsequent infection (4). In addition, nitric oxide has been implicated in epithelial ciliary activity regulation within the paranasal sinuses (12).

ETIOLOGY

The high incidence of rhinosinusitis in children with allergic disease, asthma, CF, nasal polyposis (NP), immune deficiency, ciliary dysfunction, and gastroesophageal reflux disease (GERD) is well documented. Other factors that have been studied in association with pediatric rhinosinusitis include upper respiratory tract infections, nasal and paranasal sinus anatomic abnormalities or variations, adenotonsillar hypertrophy, and environmental exposures.

Allergy and Asthma

The presence of allergies is an important factor in the development of rhinosinusitis in children. Up to 15% of children have seasonal or perennial allergic rhinitis by the age of 16 (5). In children with rhinosinusitis, more than 80% have a family history of allergy (13). An association between allergy and pediatric rhinosinusitis is seen 25–70% of the time (5). Radiographic changes including mucosal edema or sinus opacification are noted in 78% of children with a positive allergen challenge, but in only 16% after a negative challenge (14). In addition, over half of all pediatric patients with chronic rhinosinusitis will test positive to allergy tests (15). Almost half of pediatric patients undergoing functional endoscopic sinus surgery (FESS) in one large series had positive allergy testing. Of the pediatric patients in whom FESS failed to relieve symptoms, all also tested positive for allergies (16).

There are a number of mechanisms that are thought to be important in predisposing children with allergies to rhinosinusitis. The association of allergy with eosinophilia may make the mucosa of atopic patients more vulnerable to infection through the action of major basic protein (MBP) (5). In vitro studies show a direct toxic effect of MBP on the sinus mucosa as well as inhibition of ciliary function. These effects were more pronounced in the mucosa of allergic children (17).

The association of asthma and rhinosinusitis is also well documented. More than 25% of children referred for allergy evaluation with chronic respiratory symptoms had chronic asthma (18). Of the children with chronic asthma, over one-third had clinical signs as well as CT scan findings consistent with chronic rhinosinusitis. Conversely, acute rhinosinusitis is a predisposing factor for asthma exacerbations. Manning et al. showed that the majority of asthmatic children undergoing FESS demonstrated a reduction in hospitalization and missed school days postoperatively. They also had a significant improvement in asthma and sinusitis symptom scores (19). Palmer et al. also showed a reduction in postoperative steroid requirement and antibiotic usage in asthmatic children undergoing FESS (20).

Cystic Fibrosis

Cystic fibrosis (CF) is the most common life-limiting recessive disorder in the Caucasian population, affecting one in 3200 white newborns in the United States (21). The carrier rate among Caucasians is 1:20, in African Americans 1:30,000, and in Asians 1:90,000 (22). CF is a result of one of many identified mutations of the CF gene, on the 7q31 chromosome, which encodes the CF transmembrane regulator protein (CFTR). Defects of this protein cause abnormal ion transport across the exocrine gland apical cell membrane, resulting in reduced chloride ion permeability. This change in permeability affects the water content of the secretions of the exocrine glands. This can profoundly affect the viscosity of mucous in CF patients, leading to breakdown of the otherwise normal mucociliary clearance mechanism, mucostasis, and blockage of the sinus ostia. This ultimately leads to recurrent and chronic rhinosinusitis in these children (22).

Cuyler and Monoghan evaluated the incidence of rhinosinusitis in 10 children (age range 3–19 years) with CF referred to a pediatric otolaryngology clinic for assessment of nasal and sinus disease (23). Rhinosinusitis, diagnosed by a coronal CT scan, was seen in all these patients despite a normal intranasal examination. These authors also showed that children with CF benefited in the short-term from symptom relief following FESS. Long-term benefits remain unknown. Gentile and Isaacson found two distinct patterns of sinus disease in children with CF. NP was seen in the majority of children while chronic rhinosinusitis was seen in the minority of children. FESS provided marked and lasting improvement in both subgroups of children (24).

Jones et al. evaluated the effect of FESS on CF patient satisfaction and subjective improvement in symptoms (25). The response to surgery was overwhelmingly positive, with improvement in nasal congestion, purulent nasal discharge, and postnasal drainage in the vast majority of children. Also, all patients reported that they would undergo the procedure again with benefits outweighing the temporary postoperative discomfort.

Nasal Polyposis

Nasal polyposis (NP) is characterized by chronic inflammation of the nasal and sinus mucosa, resulting in multifocal edematous transformation of the mucosa with formation of polyps. Polyps are generally translucent-to-white edematous mucosal growths that are wide-based or pedunculated (Fig. 3). Symptoms of polyposis include nasal obstruction, rhinorrhea, anosmia, facial pain, and mouth breathing, as well as signs and symptoms of chronic rhinosinusitis. Unilateral polyps are rare and should instigate evaluation for antral choanal polyps and those polypoidal lesions associated with malignant or congenital tumors such as menigoencephaloceles and intranasal gliomas. Children with NP should be screened for CF and asthma, which are the most common associated conditions.

Triglia and Nicollas evaluated 46 children with NP for comorbidities (26). Asthma was found in five children (10%) and CF was found in 27 children (58.6%). Other studies place the incidence of NP in CF children between 6.7% and 48% (23,26). Allergy was associated with 21.7% of patients with CF, and 33.3% of patients without CF. Allergy is clearly an important factor in many children with NP.

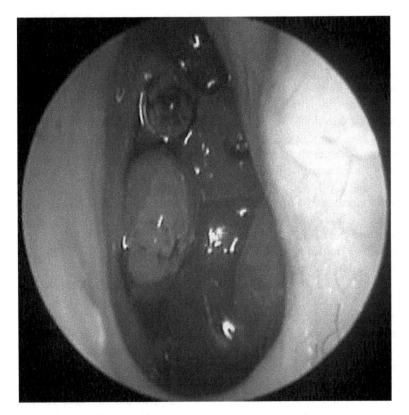

Figure 3 Nasal polyposis.

In children with symptomatic NP, medical management should be attempted prior to a surgical polypectomy. Short-term recurrence rate is as high as 87% after polypectomy alone (27–29). A much lower recurrence rate, as low as 10%, is reported following FESS and medical treatment in children (28).

Immunologic Defects

Recurrent chronic rhinosinusitis with or without otitis media may be the first and only indication of underlying immunodeficiency (30). The most common immunodeficiencies seen in childhood include common variable immunodeficiency, immunoglobulin G (IgG) subclass deficiency, selective antibody deficiency, IgA deficiency, and complement component C4 deficiency. Frequent bacterial infections with frequent URIs should increase suspicion of immunodeficiency. A patient with an undiagnosed immunodeficiency is typically always taking antibiotics, with recurrence of illness as soon as the antibiotics are discontinued.

Children with more severe immunodeficiency syndromes suffer from recurrent pneumonias, meningitis, cellulitis, candidiasis, chronic diarrhea, and failure to thrive. The diagnosis is usually made earlier in life. Chronic rhinosinusitis is not generally a presenting illness of T-cell defects, such as severe combined immunodeficiency disease, neutrophil dysfunction, or human immunodeficiency virus (HIV) infection. These generally present with more severe bacterial infections, or more typically with fungal infections. If rhino-sinusitis is a problem in these patients, it is generally not a prominent feature.

Immunologic evaluation is recommended in children with frequent episodes of rhinosinusitis (more than three per year), failure of appropriate medical management, such as a return of symptoms less than one month after discontinuation of antibiotic therapy, or recurrence of sinus disease after surgery (30). Immunologic evaluation should be considered after an allergy evaluation and treatment is completed. Shapiro et al. evaluated 61 children with chronic rhinosinusitis for immunologic defects (31). About 55% were found to have either low immunoglobulin levels (total IgG, IgG sub-classes, or IgA) or were hyporesponsive to bacterial polysaccharide vaccines. Interestingly, allergic disease, identified by high IgE levels and/or positive prick tests, was found concurrently in 40% of the children in this study.

Immunoglobulin class and subclass deficiencies as well as hyporespon-siveness to certain polysaccharide antigens, typified by suboptimal response to vaccinations to *Hemophilus influenzae* type B, have been found in patients with chronic and recurrent URIs including rhinosinusitis (31–33). This relative decrease in responsiveness to certain antigens may account for the preponderance of infections with *H. influenzae, Streptococcus pneumoniae,* and *Moraxella catarrhalis* observed in these patients.

Immunoglobulin studies should include subclass quantification for serum IgG, IgM, IgA, and IgE. For patients over two years of age, antibody respon-siveness to pneumococcal polysaccharide and unconjugated *H. influenzae* type B polysaccharide should be evaluated to identify patients with selective antibody deficiencies, alone or in association with IgG subclass deficiencies (30).Serum complement components C3 and C4, as well as total hemolytic complement (CH50), should be measured. In patients with low levels of two or more immunoglobulin classes, both B- and T-lymphocyte population analysis should be performed to discriminate between X-linked agammaglo-bulinemia, which lacks B cells, and common variable immunodeficiency in which B cells are often present (30). Another entity, transient hypogammaglo-bulinemia of infancy, can be distinguished with T- and B-cell analysis, as these patients have low levels of two or more classes of immunoglobulins but have normal B- and T-cell populations and make antibody to tetanus toxoid. This is unlike X-linked agammaglobulinemia and common variable immunodeficiency, in which patients cannot mount an antibody response to tetanus toxoid (30).

The treatment of immunodeficiency may include long-term antibiotics and intravenous gammaglobulin therapy (IVIG). Many of these patients may improve with time, but it is yet unclear whether antibody hyporesponsiveness or hypogammaglobulinemia is a transient or a permanent phenomenon.

Primary Ciliary Dyskinesia

Primary ciliary dyskinesia is a rare disorder involving structural or functional abnormalities of cilia that may be isolated or occur as a component of Kartagener's syndrome. The structural abnormalities can be demonstrated by electron microscopy of respiratory epithelial biopsies, and include abnormalities of the normal $9 + 2$ microtubular structure of cilia, or a more subtle finding of decreased total dynein arm count (34). Normal ciliary architecture may be found, but functional abnormalities may exist, as seen with decreased beat frequency of the cilia (35). Recurrent or chronic rhinosinusitis may be seen in these patients in conjunction with other upper and lower respiratory tract infections secondary to decreased mucociliary clearance.

Gastroesophageal Reflux Disease

Gastroesophageal reflux is nearly universal and physiologic in children. When the frequency or duration is severe enough to induce symptoms or histological changes of chronic inflammation, it becomes pathologic and is labeled GERD. Gastropharyngeal or laryngopharyngeal reflux (LPR) and gastronasal reflux (GNR) are now recognized entities, measured objectively using double-lumen or dual pH probe testing (36,37). GERD has been shown to play an important causative role in acute and chronic inflammatory conditions of the airway, as well as leading to complications of choanal atresia repair (38–40).

The association of GERD and rhinosinusitis is well recognized. Phipps et al. evaluated 30 children with rhinosinusitis using a 24-hour dual pH probe (36). Of the 30 children, 63% were found to have GERD. The prevalence of GERD in the general pediatric population is 5%. About 32% of the children with GERD also had measurable reflux into the nasopharynx. About 79% of the children with GERD had an improvement in the signs and symptoms of rhinosinusitis after medical treatment for GERD.

Bothwell et al. studied 28 children with chronic rhinosinusitis who were considered for FESS (41). They were all referred for pH probe studies and subsequently underwent medical treatment for GERD. After 24 months, 89% of these patients had avoided sinus surgery because of improvement or resolution of symptoms. These results suggest that adequate treatment for GERD dramatically reduces the need for FESS in children. The researchers postulated that GERD causes nasal inflammation and resultant edema, predisposing children to chronic rhinosinusitis. It is reasonable to therefore recommend that GERD be evaluated and treated in all children with refractory rhinosinusitis in which FESS is being considered.

Upper Respiratory Infections

Children average between six and eight URIs per year, while children who attend day care have significantly more URIs. As many as 5–10% of URIs may result in acute rhinosinusitis. Thus, URI may be considered the most common etiologic factor for rhinosinusitis. As previously described, inflammation leads to stasis of secretions and obstruction of the sinus ostia. Viral infection may also have a direct affect on ciliary function, as well as increased bacterial growth during infection.

Wald et al. followed 214 children in home care, group care, or day care for 12 months after birth (42). The children in home care averaged 3.9, group care 5.1, and day care 6.3 respiratory illnesses per year. This significant difference in the incidence of URIs in children attending day care compared to children cared for in the home becomes insignificant by age 3 (43). With 5–10% of these URIs resulting in acute rhinosinusitis, it is clear that enrollment in day care plays a role in the chain of events leading to infection, especially early in life.

Anatomic/Structural Abnormalities

Structural abnormalities of the sinuses or nasal cavity are relatively rare causes of rhinosinusitis. The findings of septal deviation or lateral nasal wall abnormalities (concha bullosa, Haller cells, paradoxical middle turbinates) may cause rhinosinusitis if there is resultant obstruction of the OMC. Other developmental abnormalities such as choanal atresia or maxillary sinus hypoplasia have been found to be associated with rhinosinusitis (44). Structural abnormalities that do not directly obstruct the OMC should be considered instead to be structural variations. There appears to be no increased incidence of rhinosinusitis in patients with structural variations (45,46).

Although not an anatomic abnormality, the presence of a foreign body must also be considered in children, especially in cases of recalcitrant unilateral disease with a suggestive history, or excoriation of the ipsilateral nasal ala or vestibule.

Adenoid Vegetations/Adenotonsillar Hypertrophy

Adenoid hypertrophy can cause moderate to severe nasal obstruction. The adenoid bed has also been purported to be a bacterial reservoir for infections of the sinuses and middle ear. Takahashi et al. investigated the effect of adenoidectomy on rhinosinusitis in 78 children aged 5–7 (47). They found improvement in rhinosinusitis symptoms as well as clinical endoscopic examination after six months in 56% of children following an adenoidectomy, versus 24% in children who did not undergo adenoidectomy.

Vandenberg and Heatley evaluated the effect of adenoidectomy on symptoms of rhinorrhea, nasal congestion, mouth breathing, and frequent antibiotic use in children aged 1 to 12 years (48). Complete or near-complete resolution of symptoms was reported in 58% of the children, some improvement in 21%, and minimal or no improvement in 21%. Other studies support the role of adenoidectomy as beneficial in the treatment of rhinosinusitis in the pediatric population (49–52).

Environmental Factors

Environmental factors, including pollutants, irritants, toxicants, and passive cigarette smoke, may cause local irritation or inflammation. Resultant cellular damage may initiate an inflammatory cascade including the release of mediators, attraction of inflammatory cells to the area, and local edema. This could lead to mucosal swelling, decreased airflow, and possible OMC obstruction with subsequent development of rhinosinusitis. Preexisting conditions such as allergic or vasomotor rhinitis may exacerbate the effects of environmental factors.

Environmental factors may also lead to ciliary dysfunction. Aguis et al. found that after in vitro exposure of nasal ciliated cells from nonsmokers to cotinine, a major metabolite of nicotine, there was a significant drop in ciliary beat frequency compared with non-exposed ciliated cells (53). They concluded that cotinine has a marked effect on ciliary function in vitro. Secondhand smoke exposure may thus lead to diminished mucociliary clearance in children and subsequently to rhinosinusitis.

Dubin et al. examined the effect of passive tobacco smoke exposure on eustachian tube function in rats (54). There was a significant alteration in ciliary function and mucociliary clearance time within the eustachian tube. Bascom et al. reported similar results (55). In summary, environmental factors have been shown to affect ciliary function and mucociliary clearance and are likely to be etiologically important in pediatric rhinosinusitis.

CONCLUSION

The management of pediatric rhinosinusitis relies on a clear understanding of the pathophysiology and etiology of the underlying disease process. Any condition that affects the patency of the ostia, the mucociliary clearance mechanism, or the consistency and makeup of the secretions predisposes to rhinosinusitis. Our understanding of the role of comorbidities such as allergic disease, immune deficiencies, and GERD in contributing to pediatric rhinosinusitis continues to increase. Finally, the role of environmental pollutants and particularly of secondhand smoke exposure is increasingly recognized as a cause of rhinosinusitis in children.

REFERENCES

1. Lusk RP, Stankiewicz JA. Pediatric rhinosinusitis. Otolaryngol Head Neck Surg 1997; 3(2):S53–S57.
2. Hopp R, Cooperstock M. Medical management of sinusitis in pediatric patients. Curr Probl Pediatr 1997; 25(7):178–186.
3. Wald ER. Sinusitis in infants and children. Ann Otol Rhinol Laryngol 1992; 101(1):37–42.
4. Kaliner MA, Osguthorpe JD, Fireman P, Anon J, Georgitis J, Davis ML, Naclerio R, Kennedy D. Sinusitis: bench to bedside: current findings, future directions. Otolaryngol Head Neck Surg 1997; 116(6):S1–S20.
5. Gungor A, Corey JP. Pediatric sinusitis: a literature review with emphasis on the role of allergy. Otolaryngol Head Neck Surg 1997; 116(1):4–15.
6. Ott NL, O'Connell EJ, Hoffmans AD, Beatty CW, Sachs MI. Childhood sinusitis. Mayo Clinic Proc 1991; 66:1239–1247.
7. Braverman I, Wright ED, Wang CG, Eidelman D, Frenkiel S. Human ciliary beat-frequency in normal and chronic sinusitis subjects. J Otolaryngol 1998; 27(3):145–152.
8. Subauste MC, Jacoby DB, Richards SM, Proud D. Infection of a human respiratory epithelial cell line with rhinovirus: induction of cytokine release and modulation of susceptibility to infection by cytokine exposure. J Clin Invest 1995; 96:549–557.
9. Noah TL, Becker S. Respiratory syncytial virus-induced cytokine production by a human bronchial epithelial cell line. Am J Physiol 1993; 265(5 Pt 1):L472–L478.
10. Elias JA, Zheng T, Einarsson O, Landry M, Trow T, Rebert N, Panuska J. Epithelial interleukin-11: regulation by cytokines, respiratory syncytial virus, and retinoic acid. J Biol Chem 1994; 269:22261–22268.
11. Lundberg JO, Farkas-Szallasi T, Weitzberg E, Rinder J, Lidholm J, Anggaard A, Hokfelt T, Lundberg JM, Alving K. High nitric oxide in human paranasal sinuses. Nat Med 1995; 1:370–373.
12. Jain B, Rubenstein I, Robbins RA, Leishe KL, Sisson JH. Modulation of airway epithelial cell ciliary beat frequency by nitric oxide. Biochem Biophys Res Commun 1993; 191:83–88.
13. Shapiro GG, Rachelevsky GS. Introduction and definition of sinusitis. J All Clin Immunol 1992; 90:417–418.
14. Pelikan Z, Pelikan-Filipek M. Role of nasal allergy in chronic sinusitis maxillaries-diagnostic value of nasal challenge with allergen (NPT). J All Clin Immunol 1990; 86:484–491.
15. Shapiro GG, Virant FS, Furukawa CT, Pierson WE, Bierman CW. Immunologic defects in patient with refractory sinusitis. Pediatrics 1991; 87:311–316.
16. Lazar RL, Younis RT, Gross CW. Pediatric functional endonasal sinus surgery: review of 210 cases. Head Neck 1992; 14(2):92–98.
17. Hisamatsu K, Ganbo T, Nakazawa T, Murakami Y, Gleich GJ, Makiyama K, Koyama H. Cytotoxicity of human eosinophil granule major basic protein to human nasal sinus mucosa in vitro. J All Clin Immunol 1990; 86:52–63.
18. Nguyen KL, Corbett ML, Garcia DP, Eberly SM, Massey EN, Le HT, Shearer LT, Karibo JM, Pence HL. Chronic sinusitis among pediatric patients with chronic respiratory complaints. J All Clin Immunol 1993; 92(6):824–830.

19. Manning SC, Wasserman RL, Silver R, Phillips DL. Results of endoscopic sinus surgery in pediatric patients with chronic sinusitis and asthma. Arch Otolaryngol Head Neck Surg 1994; 120(10):1142–1145.
20. Palmer JN, Conley DB, Dong RG, Ditto AM, Yarnold PR, Kern RC. Efficacy of endoscopic sinus surgery in the management of patients with asthma and chronic sinusitis. Am J Rhinol 2001; 15(1):49–53.
21. Rosenstein BJ, Cuting GR. The diagnosis of cystic fibrosis. J Pediatr 1998; 132:689–695.
22. Nishioka GJ, Cook PJ. Paranasal sinus disease in patients with cystic fibrosis. Otolaryngol Clin North Am 1996; 29(1):193–205.
23. Cuyler JP, Monaghan AJ. Cystic fibrosis and sinusitis. J Otolaryngol 1989; 18(4):173–175.
24. Gentile VG, Isaacson G. Patterns of sinusitis in cystic fibrosis. Larygnoscope 1996; 106:1005–1009.
25. Jones JW, Parsons DS, Cuyler JP. The results of functional endoscopic sinus surgery on the symptoms of patients with cystic fibrosis. Int J Pediatr Otorhinolaryngol 1993; 28:25–32.
26. Triglia J-M, Nicollas R. Nasal and sinus polyposis in children. Laryngoscope 1997; 107(7):963–966.
27. Jaffe BF, Strome M, Khaw KT, Shwachman H. Nasal polypectomy and sinus surgery for cystic fibrosis—a 10 years review. Oto Clin North Am 1977; 10: 81–90.
28. Crockett DM, McGill TJ, Healy GB, Friedman EM, Salkeld LJ. Nasal and paranasal sinus surgery in children with cystic fibrosis. Ann Otol Rhinol Laryngol 1987; 96(4):367–372.
29. Cepero R, Smith RJ, Catlin FI, Bressler KL, Furuta GT, Shandera KC. Cystic fibrosis: an otolaryngologic perspective. Otolaryngol Head Neck Surg 1987; 97(4):356–360.
30. Polmar SH. The role of the immunologist in sinus disease. J All Clin Immunol 1992; 90(3 Pt 2):511–515.
31. Shapiro GG, Virant FS, Furukawa CT, Pierson WE, Bierman CW. Immunologic defects in patients with refractory sinusitis. Pediatrics 1991; 87(3): 311–316.
32. Umetsu DT, Ambrosino DM, Quinti I, Siber GR, Geha RS. Recurrent sinopulmonary intection and impaired antibody response to bacterial capsular polysaccharide antigen in children with selective IgG-subclass deficiency. N Eng J Med 1985; 313(20):1247–1251.
33. Ambrosino DM, Umetsu DT, Siber GR, Howie G, Goularte TA, Michaels R, Martin P, Schur PH, Noyes J, Schiffman G. Selective defect in the antibody response to *H. influenzae* type b in children with recurrent infections and normal serum IgG subclass levels. J All Clin Immunol 1988; 81(6):1175–1179.
34. Teknos TN, Metson R, Chasse T, Balercia G, Dickersin GR. New developments in the diagnosis of Kartagener's syndrome. Otolaryngol Head Neck Surg 1997; 116(1):68–74.
35. Chapelin C, Coste A, Reinert P, Boucherat M, Millepied MC, Poron F, Escudier E. Incidence of primary ciliary dyskinesia in children with recurrent respiratory diseases. Ann Otol Rhinol Laryngol 1997; 106(10 Pt 1):854–858.

36. Phipps CD, Wood E, Gibson WS, Cochran WJ. Gastroesophageal reflux contributing to chronic sinus disease in children. Arch Otolaryngol Head Neck Surg 2000; 126(7):831–836.
37. Contencin P, Narcy P. Nasopharyngeal monitoring in infants and children with chronic rhinopharyngitis. Int J Pediatr Otorhinolaryngol 1991; 22:249–256.
38. Burton DM, Pransky SM, Katz RM, Kearns DB, Seid AB. Pediatric airway manifestations of gastroesophageal reflux. Ann Otol Rhinol Laryngol 1992; 101:742–749.
39. Contencin P, Maurage C, Ployet MJ, Seid AB, Sinaasappel M. Gastroesophageal reflux and ENT disorders in childhood. Int J Pediatr Otorhinolaryngol 1995; 32(Suppl):S135–S144.
40. Beste DJ, Conley SF, Brown CW. Gastroesophageal relux complicating choanal atresia repair. Int J Pediatr Otorhinolaryngol 1994; 29:51–58.
41. Bothwell MR, Parsons DS, Talbot A, Barbero G, Wilder B. Outcome of reflux therapy on pediatric chronic sinusitis. Otolaryngol Head Neck Surg 1999; 121:255–262.
42. Wald ER, Dashefsky B, Byers C, Guerra N, Taylor F. Frequency and severity of infections in day care. J Pediatrics 1988; 112(4):540–546.
43. Wald ER, Guerra N, Byers C. Frequency and severity of infections in day care: three-year follow-up. J Pediatr 1991; 118(4):509–514.
44. Goldsmith AJ, Rosenfeld RM. Treatment of pediatric sinusitis. Pediatr Clin North Am 2003; 50(2):413–426.
45. Jones NS, Strobl A, Holland I. CT findings in 100 patients with rhinosinusitis and 100 controls. Clin Otolaryngol 1997; 22:47–51.
46. Wilner A, Choi SS, Vezina LG, Lazar RH. Intranasal anatomic variations in pediatric sinusitis. Am J Rhinol 1997; 11(5):355–360.
47. Takahashi H, Honjo I, Fujita A, Kurata K. Effects of adenoidectomy on sinusitis. Acta Oto-Rhino-Laryngol Belgica 1997; 51(2):85–87.
48. Vandenberg SJ, Heatley DG. Efficacy of adenoidectomy in relieving symptoms of chronic sinusitis in children. Arch Otolaryngol Head Neck Surg 1997; 123: 675–678.
49. Lusk RP. Surgical modalities other than ethmoidectomy. J All Clin Immunol 1992; 90:538–542.
50. Fujita A, Takahashi H, Honjo I. Etiological role of adenoids upon otitis media with effusion. Acta Otolaryngol Suppl 1988; 454:210–213.
51. Paul D. Sinus infection and adenotonsillitis in pediatric patients. Laryngoscope 1981; 91(6):997–1000.
52. Merck W. Relationship between adenoidal enlargement and maxillary sinusitis. HNO 1974; 6:198–199.
53. Aguis AM, Wake M, Pahor AL, Smallman A. The effects of in vitro cotitine on nasal ciliary beat frequency. Clin Otolaryngol All Sci 1995; 20(5):465–469.
54. Dubin MG, Pollock HW, Ebert CS, Berg E, Buenting JE, Prazma JP. Eustachian tube dysfunction after tobacco smoke exposure. Otolaryngol Head Neck Surg 2002; 126(1):14–19.
55. Bascom R, Kesavanathan J, Fitzgerald TK, Cheng KH, Swift DL. Sidestream tobacco smoke exposure acutely alters human nasal mucociliary clearance. Environ Health Perspectives 1995; 103(11):1026–1030.

3

Diagnostic Workup for Pediatric Rhinosinusitis

Edward Hepworth

Division of Otolaryngology–Head and Neck Surgery, University of New Mexico, Albuquerque, New Mexico, U.S.A.

Ron B. Mitchell

Department of Otolaryngology, Virginia Commonwealth University, Richmond, Virginia, U.S.A.

INTRODUCTION

The workup and treatment of rhinosinusitis in children is usually multidisciplinary. Recent advances in endoscopy and imaging techniques and in pharmacotherapy continue to improve the overall well-being of children with sinus disease. Research to date has focused mostly on antimicrobial therapy, criteria for disease classification, and improved techniques in operative management in adults. Sinus disease in children differs significantly from that seen in adults. Children with sinus disease have multiple factors that influence the presentation and the progression of the disease and these factors may be congenital, immunologic, or environmental. In addition, the initial symptoms, clinical findings, and radiological manifestations are quite different in children than in adults.

Epidemiology as it Relates to Disease Workup

The true prevalence of rhinosinusitis in children is unknown, but it has been estimated to be approximately 7% (1). Rhinosinusitis is the fifth most common diagnosis resulting in an antibiotic prescription. The direct medical cost to treat rhinosinusitis in children exceeds $2.4 billion annually in the United States (2).

Definitions

Acute bacterial rhinosinusitis has been defined as an infection of the sinuses lasting not more than 30 days and concluding in complete resolution (3). Subacute disease persists for 30 to 90 days with complete resolution. Recurrent acute disease consists of multiple acute episodes separated by symptom-free intervals of at least 10 days, or alternatively three acute episodes in six months or four acute episodes in one year. Chronic bacterial rhinosinusitis persists for more than 90 days. Acute rhinosinusitis superimposed on chronic disease occurs when patients with chronic rhinosinusitis acquire new symptoms that resolve within 30 days of treatment. The underlying residual symptoms attributed to chronic rhinosinusitis persist in these patients.

DEVELOPMENTAL ANATOMY AS RELEVANT TO DISEASE WORKUP

The embryologic development of the sinuses is summarized in Table 1. Certain key points regarding sinus cavity growth are germane to clinical, radiologic, and laboratory workup. The clinician must identify the child's status along the continuum of sinus development in order to adequately assess and treat the disease. The ostiomeatal complex (OMC) is present in nearly full

Table 1 Paranasal Sinus Development

Age	Development milestone
Birth	Maxillary sinus cavity present and partially aerated Ethmoidal cells present Sphenoidal and frontal sinus cavities absent
4 months	Frontal evaginations from anterior ethmoid cells visible microscopically
5 months	Maxillary sinus cavity visible radiographically
6 months	Ethmoidal cell septae visible radiographically
1 year	Frontal evagination evident in cadaveric dissection
3 years	Appreciable aeration of the frontal sinus in cadaveric specimens
6 years	Frontal aeration evident radiographically
7 years	Pneumatization of the sphenoid as far posteriorly as the sella turcica
10 years	Frontal disease becomes clinically significant
20 years	Complete pansinus aeration

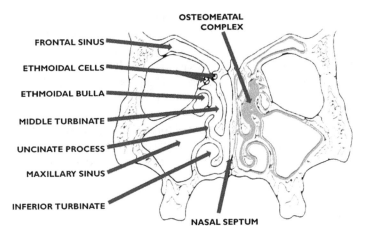

Figure 1 OMC in an infant.

complexity in the infant, although it continues to grow in size and change its orientation and topography throughout adolescence (Fig. 1). An image of the OMC in a one-year-old child is shown in Figure 2.

The assumption that immature or pathologically undersized sinus cavities are impervious to disease is, however, questionable. Suzuki et al. (4) demonstrated that patients with cleft lip and palate have significantly smaller sinus cavities than normal and are more prone to chronic sinus disease. Several authors have also described frontal mucocele development following pediatric trauma at a young age where frontal sinus development had been minimal (5,6).

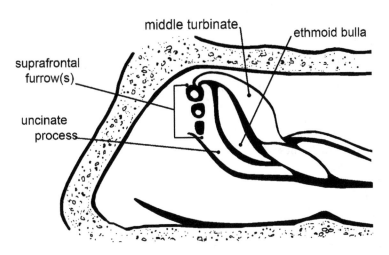

Figure 2 An image of OMC in a one-year-old child.

Several other factors related to the development of the sinuses are relevant to disease workup. These include the status of the foramen cecum; the status of the palate, lip, and alveolus; and the completion of closure of the nasal roof. Defects in any of these areas may result in conditions masquerading as, or contributing to, sinus disease. The presence of any of these defects should initiate a multidisciplinary workup rather than symptomatic management of sinonasal complaints. Evaluation of the intactness of the anterior skull base is best performed with computed tomography (CT) scan. Many of the midline nasal masses contribute to obstruction, inflammation, and chronic sinonasal complaints. These are often best evaluated by magnetic resonance imaging (MRI).

DISEASE HISTORY

A comprehensive medical history is essential for the diagnosis of sinus disease in children. This medical history serves a number of purposes. First, a diagnosis is obtained. Second, a reference point for monitoring treatment progress is established. Finally, a document is created that summarizes all relevant data for fellow healthcare providers in a standardized format. Children are often unable to articulate the symptoms of rhinosinusitis. Caregivers must provide information about congenital, genetic, and environmental factors that may influence treatment and outcome.

In fact, family circumstances may assume more importance than many aspects of disease pathology. For instance, time off from work, eligibility for day care while ill, and frequency of physician visits may prompt treatment decisions more than a change in symptoms. Ideally, treatment should address quality of life for all family members. Many providers rely on standardized questionnaires to avoid overlooking important details in this regard (7).

Chief Complaint

The chief presenting complaint of a child or caregiver may include:

- frequent anterior or posterior nasal drainage
- daytime cough
- nasal congestion
- low-grade fever
- ear pain or fullness
- irritability
- headache
- halitosis
- behavior problems
- learning problems
- poor growth or failure to thrive
- snoring

- frequent snorting
- cyclic vomiting (8)
- anorexia nervosa (9)
- chronic fatigue (10)

More severe cases of sinus disease may present as purulent rhinorrhea, a high fever, or periorbital edema. Nighttime cough is more prevalent in chronic than acute rhinosinusitis. A systematic approach to the documentation of presenting complaints will help to guide treatment, but more importantly, to provide a means for monitoring treatment and maintaining patient/caregiver rapport. This should include the following:

1. age at onset
2. severity
3. associated symptoms
4. alleviating factors
5. aggravating factors
6. any variation in the degree of severity or pattern of the complaint
7. a description of the nature of the complaint, for instance, burning, sharp or dull pain

History of Illness, Past Medical History, and Risk Factor Assessment

The past medical history should focus on those factors that are treatable or may require otolaryngologic intervention. Occult genetic disorders, correctable lifestyle factors, systemic disease, and risk prevention are all requisite elements of the workup.

Important elements of the past medical history address patient quality of life. Quality of life factors such as time lost from school due to illness, sleep disturbance, interference with daily activity, lack of attention at school or home, and medication side effects are important elements to include in the evaluation of sinus disease. Equally important to document are the previous treatment regimens and response to treatment, including:

1. antihistamines, noting which were effective and any side effects
2. decongestants and route of delivery
3. other nasal sprays—saline, corticosteroids, or anticholinergics
4. asthma medications—oral or inhaled
5. antibiotics, type including length and number of courses
6. previous emergency room/hospital treatment

Inquiry into ear infections is important. About 50% of children with otitis media will ultimately be diagnosed with allergic or infectious sinonasal disease (11). Food sensitivities, drug hypersensitivity, insect sting allergy, eczema, asthma, urticaria or angioedema, and contact sensitivity or dermatitis are all conditions that indicate systemic atopy and tendency toward sinonasal disease (12). Sinonasal disease is often familial, manifesting in one or both parents, or a sibling. This is particularly true with chronic rhinosinusitis (13). More importantly, high-density occurrence of sinus disease in a family may be the initial indicator of a more serious inherited disorder, as discussed below.

Inhalant allergies are becoming better understood as a major contributor to pediatric rhinosinusitis (14). Atopic conditions are perhaps the most common cause of mucosal edema in the sinonasal spaces and are largely influenced by the child's family and social environment. About 80% of children undergoing sinus surgery have a positive skin test response to inhalant allergens (12). Many children will not have classic allergy symptoms but may have enough disease manifestation to alter normal nasal function (15). Investigation into an allergic environment should include:

1. type of family dwelling: single or multiple, apartment or home
2. type of heating system: forced air, baseboard, or wood stove
3. type of cooling system: air conditioning, evaporative cooling
4. bedroom: frequency of cleaning, bedding changes, other issues related to hygiene, presence of stuffed animals or dolls (a child spends up to 12 hours daily there)
5. flooring: linoleum, carpeting, or hard wood
6. bedding: conventional mattress or waterbed, hollow-fiber-filled or feather pillow
7. pets: outdoor or indoor and access into bedroom areas
8. other: presence of molds or dampness; use of a humidifier, electrostatic or HEPA filters; and exposure to secondhand smoking

Related Disorder Assessment

Several disease conditions are relevant to both the history and the subsequent laboratory investigation of pediatric rhinosinusitis patients. These are discussed individually.

Cystic Fibrosis and Genetic Disorders

Cystic fibrosis is a disorder in which a transmembrane conductance regulator is defective. Related symptoms and disease states include congenital bilateral absence of the vas deferens, allergic bronchopulmonary aspergillosis, chronic pulmonary infection, and isolated chronic pancreatitis (16). Most patients with cystic fibrosis present to the otolaryngologist for focused workup and treatment often to include surgery for nasal polyposis. Chronic rhinosinusitis in the very young, especially when associated with multiple infections of the ear, nose, and throat, should prompt concern about undiagnosed cystic fibrosis (16).

In addition to cystic fibrosis, several genetic disorders contribute to rhinosinusitis risk. These include sporadic and inherited conditions such as the 22q11.2 deletion syndrome or DiGeorge syndrome (17), X-linked agammaglobulinemia (18), and α-1-antitrypsin deficiency.

Asthma

The role of rhinosinusitis in exacerbation of asthma symptoms has been well described (19). The diagnosis of asthma may be confounded by symptoms of cough caused by rhinosinusitis and resulting in posterior nasal drainage. A common immunochemical and cellular relationship between asthma and certain types of chronic sinonasal diseases have been established (20). The historic Samter's triad of nasal polyposis, aspirin sensitivity, and asthma may initially manifest with sinonasal symptoms. The workup of pediatric rhinosinusitis should include a history of asthma.

Ciliary Dyskinesia/Kartagener Disease

The posterior two-thirds of the nasal cavity and the paranasal sinuses are covered by a pseudostratified ciliated columnar epithelium. The cilia beat normally at a frequency of approximately 1000 cycles per minute to propel mucus to the ostia. Any dysfunction of the cilia will lead to an increased risk of rhinosinusitis. Tobacco smoke, viral infection, medications, and certain syndromes may cause ciliary dysfunction. Immotile cilia syndrome, also known as primary ciliary dysfunction (PCD), and Kartagener syndrome (KS) are two entities that affect the function of the respiratory epithelium. In both, respiratory infections occur as a result of ciliary defects that impair the drainage of inhaled particles and microbes to the oropharynx. Both PCD and KS manifest in the respiratory tract as nasal polyposis and bronchiectasis. In KS, these symptoms are part of a triad and are the long-term result of recurrent upper and lower respiratory tract infections that start early in life. The other two triad manifestations are cardiac defects and sperm dysmotility. Cardiac manifestations most often include dextrocardia or complete situs inversus. PCD differs from KS in the absence of situs inversus. Both disorders are associated with abnormalities of ciliary structure, including missing or abnormal dynein arms, abnormal radial spokes, and missing central microtubules. The diagnosis is based on these findings on a nasal or tracheal biopsy. Screening for these disorders is best accomplished through a complete family history.

Congenital Cyanotic Heart Disease

There is a high prevalence of intracranial infection and chronic rhinosinusitis in children with congenital heart disease (21). The causal relationship between congenital cardiac disease and infections in the brain and sinuses has not been adequately determined. It appears that the association between intracranial infection and heart disease is stronger in groups of cyanotic patients where bacterial vegetations are more commonly seen and cause changes in hematological flow (22). Sinus disease is also associated with sub-acute bacterial endocarditis (23). The proliferation and distension of the venous channels and marrow spaces in patients with congenital cyanotic heart disease may alter the bacteriology of the nasal cavity and paranasal sinuses and facilitate the spread of disease (24).

Cleft Palate

Children with a cleft palate are at a higher risk of rhinosinusitis. In a study of 47 patients with cleft lip and alveolus, with and without cleft palate, coexisting rhinosinusitis was observed in 15 patients (32%), a much higher percentage than that seen in the general population. The paranasal sinus cavities are known to be significantly smaller in patients with cleft palate. Whether this contributes to the higher prevalence of rhinosinusitis is unknown.

Gastroesophageal Reflux Disease

Gastroesophageal reflux disease is increasingly recognized as a factor in many otolaryngologic disorders. Several studies have shown a correlation between frequency and severity of rhinosinusitis and the degree of reflux (25–27).

Disorders of Inflammation and of the Immune System

Immunoglobulin deficiency: A history of recurrent upper respiratory tract infection (URI) should prompt suspicion of an underlying immune disorder. Children in developed countries normally experience six to eight viral upper respiratory infections each year. About 10% of these URIs are complicated by a secondary bacterial rhinosinusitis. An increase in the frequency of URIs above the normal threshold should prompt further investigation (28).

Chronic sinus conditions are now more appropriately characterized as derangements of the local or systemic immune system rather than unremitting bacterial colonization. Close associations between asthma, allergy, and sinus disease are now clear, largely due to identifiable and treatable humoral and cellular immune dysfunction. Immunoglobulin deficiency or dysfunction may be the most common cause of pediatric rhinosinusitis and may involve any of the four typical families of immunoglobulins. Consideration of immune defects in the patient history is important for several reasons. Prophylactic antibiotic therapy can reduce or resolve symptoms in patients with mild immune deficits, and intravenous immunoglobulin therapy (IVIG) can be added in more refractory disease with beneficial results (29). Realistic expectations regarding surgery efficacy can be established. Finally, patients and family members may express relief to have a treatable and understandable diagnosis.

Immunodeficiency, T-cell dysfunction, and HIV: T-cell dysfunction may be the most common immune disorder contributing to chronic rhinosinusitis. DiGeorge syndrome, discussed previously, is the most common identifiable T-cell disorder. Unlike the conditions of immunoglobulin deficiency, systemic T-cell dysfunction usually manifests early with severe systemic illness that may overshadow sinonasal complaints.

The population of pediatric patients with HIV continues to grow (30). Generally, a diagnosis has been established prior to subspecialty referral. Often, sinonasal complaints will involve atypical pathogens such as fungus, or neoplastic disorders. An increased incidence of atopic disease has also been found in HIV patients (31). The otolaryngologist should maintain a high suspicion for these disorders, as routine sinonasal pathologies will present in an even greater frequency in these patients.

Tuberculosis and mycobacterium infection: The prevalence of tuberculosis in children in the United States may be rising (32), and the problem of drug resistance has made treatment of this disease difficult. The possibility of tuberculosis infection should be considered when chronic rhinosinusitis is diagnosed in a child with a family member with tuberculosis or with recent travel to places where tuberculosis is endemic.

Mucormycosis: This condition is almost always seen in diabetic children. Unfortunately, children commonly present without antecedent URI complaints and with a rapidly progressing sinonasal complaint. Predisposing factors in addition to diabetes include acquired or induced immunodeficiency of a genetic, infectious, or chemotherapeutic nature. A history of type-I diabetes or systemic immune disease with rapidly progressive sinus symptoms, including proptosis, diminishing vision, headaches, or mental status changes, should prompt suspicion of this condition.

Additional Behavioral and Social Assessment

There is a higher prevalence of rhinosinusitis in females than males (33,34). Breast-feeding provides protection against rhinosinusitis in young patients. Inner city living (35), low income (36), tobacco use (37), day care (38), and swimming impart increased risk.

REVIEW OF SYSTEMS

Recent health problems merit specific inquiry. These include:

- URIs
- ocular complaints
- pharyngitis

- otitis media
- asthma
- GERD

PHYSICAL EXAMINATION

The components of a thorough physical exam include:

- vital signs
- general appearance
- scalp and skin examination
- cranial nerve exam including ocular motility and gross visual acuity
- otologic examination, including pneumotoscopy
- nasal cavity examination—symmetry of nares, drainage, and mucosal appearance
- endoscopic examination of the nasal cavities with or without cultures
- oral cavity and oropharyngeal examination
- palpation of the face
- neck examination
- chest, cardiovascular, and abdominal examination

Fever and other vital signs are of value in identifying the child at risk for sepsis or intracranial complications. A tachycardic or hypotensive child may be dehydrated. General appearance and systemic evaluation may elicit syndromic conditions predisposing to sinus disease. The physical exam can provide information concerning sinus-related conditions such as atopy. A lethargic or disoriented child, particularly with cranial nerve deficits, should prompt investigation for intracranial complications. Reproducible unilateral pain, present on percussion or direct pressure over the body of the frontal and maxillary sinuses, may indicate a diagnosis of acute bacterial sinusitis (39).

Otologic examination may reveal a coincident otitis media. An endoscopic culture of the middle meatus is considered by many to be the gold standard for the diagnosis of rhinosinusitis (40). The intranasal examination may demonstrate several features that may predispose to rhinosinusitis including a septal deformity, a concha bullosa, or abnormalities of the uncinate process (41). Allergic mucosa may be seen in the nasal cavity, manifesting as boggy, bluish changes with clear drainage. The general facial examination may identify several features of atopy including allergic shiner (periorbital edema), a supratip "allergic" nasal crease (chronic upward rubbing of the nasal tip), and Denny's lines (small lower eyelid creases from chronic mild edema of this region).

The oral cavity and pharynx should be assessed for adenotonsillar hypertrophy, palatal clefting, and asymmetry. The neck should be assessed for lymphadenopathy suggestive of systemic disease. Pulmonary examination may reveal generalized wheezing indicative of asthma. The remainder of the examination may elucidate occult systemic conditions with rare sinonasal manifestations, as discussed above.

OTHER CLINICAL AND LABORATORY INVESTIGATIONS

Laboratory investigations that are relevant to pediatric rhinosinusitis may include:

- nasal aspirate
- chloride sweat testing
- exhaled nitrate testing
- mucosal biopsy
- complete blood count (CBC) with differential
- immunoglobulin assays
- erythrocyte sedimentation rate (ESR)

Sweat testing is employed for identification of cystic fibrosis. Exhaled nitrate testing has been proposed both for the identification of KS as well as a general screening tool for rhinosinusitis (42). Nitrate levels are well below normal in children with KS and in children with infection (43). Mucosal biopsy may also be helpful in identifying primary ciliary disorders.

Three other techniques have been employed for the measurement of in vivo ciliary clearance. These include the saccharin test, the methylene blue dye test, and the radioisotope test. Each involves placing a droplet of test substance into the front of the nose and assessing time to detection by patient sensation, by visual detection in the oropharynx, or by radioisotope scanner.

A raised white cell count suggests acute infection. More detailed hematology and serology workup may be necessary in a suspected case of HIV. Immune dysfunction can be screened using immunoglobulin assays. Generally, all subclasses are assayed, with particular attention to IgA and IgG. The diagnosis of IgA deficiency cannot be made before the age of two years. Patients with IgA deficiency associated with selective IgG subclass deficiency appear to be more susceptible to respiratory tract infections than those who do not have IgG deficiency (44). ESR may be of benefit in screening for chronic disorders that contribute to rhinosinusitis.

RADIOGRAPHIC EVALUATION

Radiographic imaging is generally reserved for children with refractory rhinosinusitis who are candidates for operative management. Less frequently, it is used to exclude complications of rhinosinusitis or in looking for suspected neoplastic or fungal disease. Concern persists regarding unnecessary radiation exposure. A typical plain film of the pediatric skull exposes a child's orbit to

0.85 cGy of radiation, as compared with 7.4 cGy for a full biplanar CT and 2.8 cGy for a limited scan (45). The typical risk threshold for cataract injury has been established at 2.0 cGy for an isolated exposure (46).

Plain Radiographs

Until the mid-1990s, plain films were used as the primary means of radiographic evaluation. Six-foot-Caldwell views, for instance, assisted in frontal sinus preoperative planning. They were used to demonstrate the degree of pneumatization of the frontal bone as well as the other paranasal sinuses. None of the plain radiographic views allows adequate visualization of the ethmoidal air cells. Since ethmoidal and middle meatus disease is most often the area of clinical interest and disease focus, CT scans have gained preference.

The Waters' view is used for routine screening of rhinosinusitis. It may be adequate for confirming a diagnosis of acute rhinosinusitis (47) and has improved penetration of the anterior skull base when compared with standard occipitofrontal views. The lateral neck film is employed to measure adenoidal obstruction of the nasopharynx that may lead to chronic nasal and sinus complaints and may prompt operative intervention (48). A clinical endoscopic or mirror examination of the nasopharynx generally yields the same information without the cost and radiation exposure of this study.

Computed Tomography

Computed tomography (CT) scans are the radiological gold standard for the diagnosis of rhinosinusitis (49). CT scanning is of unparalleled value in preoperative planning and in intraoperative decision-making. Coronal CT images allow optimal visualization of soft tissue thickening in the area of the OMC that cannot be appreciated by endoscopy. Sphenoid disease is also easily identified on coronal CT, while it is usually not evident in plain films.

CT scans are superior to plain radiographs in identifying minimal disease (50), but they should not be relied upon for primary diagnosis of rhinosinusitis. CT scans will demonstrate sinus opacification in many pediatric patients who have a self-limited nasal discharge but would meet criteria for acute rhinosinusitis. CT scans may overestimate sinus disease. About 50% of children undergoing CT for extranasal complaints have evidence of sinus mucosa thickening (51). Likewise, 25% of children with sinus opacification and clinical symptoms are culture negative (52). Finally, 70% of patients with a viral URI will demonstrate mucosal inflammation of the maxillary and ethmoid sinuses for up to eight weeks after resolution of symptoms (53).

Magnetic Resonance Imaging

Magnetic resonance imaging (MRI) may be used to distinguish fluid from neoplastic soft tissue and from normal sinonasal mucosa. MRI is superior to CT in assessing the status of the anterior skull base and orbit in neoplastic disease. Contrast-enhanced MRI may be used to distinguish inflamed meninges from tumor invasion and is invaluable in preoperative planning for a potentially disfiguring and debilitating operation. MRI also has a role in the diagnosis and surgical planning for fungal rhinosinusitis.

Ultrasound

In Europe, ultrasound has been used to screen for rhinosinusitis and to monitor treatment progress, but it has not been used widely in the United States (54,55).

OTHER TESTS

These may include allergy workup, investigations for GERD, workup for ciliary dysfunction, and genetic testing and counseling.

OTHER DIAGNOSTIC CONSIDERATIONS

Pediatric sinusitis is often more a disease of a family rather than a child. The health status of the child will often impact the whole family, particularly parental ability to work. Several quality of life instruments have been developed and validated to quantify the impact of the disease on the child and family (56,57). Monitoring diagnosis and treatment as it impacts the family is an important part of the clinical management of rhinosinusitis.

NATURAL HISTORY OF DISEASE

Uncomplicated rhinosinusitis spontaneously resolves in 40% of patients. A placebo study of 188 randomized patients in a group of community-based clinics demonstrated no outcome difference between comparable groups of children treated with amoxicillin, amoxicillin-clavulanate, or placebo (58).

SUMMARY

The current management of pediatric rhinosinusitis stresses prevention, evidence-based treatment, and continuing quality of life assessment. The risk to the individual from incomplete or improper workup and treatment may be low in most cases, but the cost to society and the inconvenience to the child's family and other social infrastructures are substantial. As a rule, medical treatment should be exhausted before surgery is considered as therapy for pediatric rhinosinusitis (59).

REFERENCES

1. Aitken M, Taylor JA. Prevalence of clinical sinusitis in young children followed up by primary care pediatricians. Arch Pediatric Adolesc Med 1998; 152: 244–248.
2. McCaig LF, Hughes JM. Trends in antibiotic prescribing among office based physicians in the United States. JAMA 1995; 273:214–219.
3. Wald ER. Clinical practice guideline: management of sinusitis. Pediatrics 2001; 108(3):798–808.
4. Suzuki H, Yamaguchi T, Furukawa M. Maxillary sinus development and sinusitis in patients with cleft lip and palate. Auris Nasus Larynx 2000; 27(3):253–256.
5. Smoot EC, Bowen DG, Lappert P, Ruiz J. Delayed development of an ectopic frontal sinus mucocele after pediatric cranial trauma. J Craniofac Surg 1995; 6(4):327–331.
6. Hore I, Mitchell RB, Radcliffe G, De Casso Moxo C. Pott's puffy tumour: a rare cause of forehead swelling in a child. Int J Clin Pract 2000; 54(4):267–268.
7. Cunningham JM, Chiu EJ, Landgraf JM, Gliklich RE. The health impact of chronic recurrent rhinosinusitis in children. Arch Otolaryngol Head Neck Surg 2000; 126(11):1363–1368.
8. Murray RD, Heitlinger LA, Robbins JL, Hayes JR. Heterogeneity of diagnoses presenting as cyclic vomiting. Pediatrics 1998; 102(3):583–587.
9. Sokol MS. Infection-triggered anorexia nervosa in children: clinical description of four cases. J Child Adolesc Psychopharmacol 2000; 10(2):133–145.
10. Feder HM Jr, Dworkin PH, Orkin C. Outcome of 48 pediatric patients with chronic fatigue. A clinical experience. Arch Fam Med 1994; 3(12):1049–1055.
11. Dowell SF, Schwartz B, Phillips WR. Appropriate use of antibiotics for URIs in children: Part I. Otitis media and acute sinusitis. The Pediatric URI Consensus Team. Am Fam Physician 1998; 58(5):1113–1118, 1123.
12. Lombardi E, Stein RT, Wright AL, Morgan WJ, Martinez FD. The relation between physician-diagnosed sinusitis, asthma, and skin test reactivity to allergens in 8-year-old children. Pediatr Pulmonol 1996; 22(3):141–146.
13. Fakhri S, Frenkiel S, Hamid QA. Current views on the molecular biology of chronic sinusitis. J Otolaryngol 2002; 31(suppl 1):S2–S9.
14. Gungor A, Corey JP. Pediatric sinusitis: a literature review with emphasis on the role of allergy. Otolaryngol Head Neck Surg 1997; 116(1):4–15.
15. Parsons DS, Phillips SE. Functional endoscopic surgery in children: a retrospective analysis of results. Laryngoscope 1993; 103(8):899–903.
16. Raman V, Clary R, Siegrist KL, Zehnbauer B, Chatila TA. Increased prevalence of mutations in the cystic fibrosis transmembrane conductance regulator in children with chronic rhinosinusitis. Pediatrics 2002; 109(1):E13.
17. Dyce O, McDonald-McGinn D, Kirschner RE, Zackai E, Young K, Jacobs IN. Otolaryngologic manifestations of the 22q11.2 deletion syndrome. Arch Otolaryngol Head Neck Surg 2002; 128(12):1408–1412.
18. Quartier P, Debre M, De Blic J, de Sauverzac R, Sayegh N, Jabado N, Haddad E, Blanche S, Casanova JL, Smith CI, Le Deist F, de Saint Basile G, Fischer A. Early and prolonged intravenous immunoglobulin replacement therapy in childhood agammaglobulinemia: a retrospective survey of 31 patients. J Pediatr 1999; 134(5):589–596.

19. Fox RW, Lockey RF. The impact of rhinosinusitis on asthma. Curr Allergy Asthma Rep 2003; 3(6):513–518.
20. Steinke JW, Bradley D, Arango P, Crouse CD, Frierson H, Kountakis SE, Kraft M, Borish L. Cysteinyl leukotriene expression in chronic hyperplastic sinusitis-nasal polyposis: importance to eosinophilia and asthma. J Allergy Clin Immunol 2003; 111(2):342–349.
21. Malik S, Joshi SM, Kandoth PW, Vengsarkar US. Experience with brain abscesses. Indian Pediatr 1994; 31(6):661–666.
22. Basit AS, Ravi B, Banerji AK, Tandon PN. Multiple pyogenic brain abscesses: an analysis of 21 patients. J Neurol Neurosurg Psychiatry 1989; 52(5):591–594.
23. Saiman L, Prince A, Gersony WM. Pediatric infective endocarditis in the modern era. J Pediatr 1993; 122(6):847–853.
24. Rosenthal A, Fellows KE. Acute infectious sinusitis in cyanotic congenital heart disease. Pediatrics 1973; 52(5):692–696.
25. Phipps CD, Wood E, Gibson WS, Cochran WJ. Gastroesophageal reflux contributing to chronic sinus disease in children. Arch Otolaryngol Head Neck Surg 2000; 126:831–836.
26. Ulualp SO, Toohill RJ, Hoffmann R, Shaker R. Possible relationship of gastro-esophagopharyngeal acid reflux with pathogenesis of chronic sinusitis. Am J Rhinol 1999; 13(3):197–202.
27. Gilger MA. Pediatric otolaryngologic manifestations of gastroesophageal reflux disease. Curr Gastroenterol Rep 2003; 5(3):247–252.
28. Ueda D, Yoto Y. The ten-day mark as a practical diagnostic approach for acute paranasal sinusitis in children. Pediatr Infect Dis J 1996; 15:576–579.
29. Ramesh S, Brodsky L, Afshani E, Pizzuto M, Ishman M, Helm J, Ballow M. Open trial of intravenous immune globulin for chronic sinusitis in children. Ann Allergy Asthma Immunol 1997; 79:119–124.
30. Madhi SA, Petersen K, Madhi A, Khoosal M, Klugman KP. Increased disease burden and antibiotic resistance of bacteria causing severe community-acquired lower respiratory tract infections in human immunodeficiency virus type 1-infected children. Clin Infect Dis 2000; 31(1):170–176.
31. Rudikoff D. The relationship between HIV infection and atopic dermatitis. Curr Allergy Asthma Rep 2002; 2(4):275–281.
32. Starke JR, Jacob RF, Jereb J. Resurgence of tuberculosis in children. J Pediatr 1992; 120:839–855.
33. Collins JG. Prevalence of selected chronic conditions: United States, 1990–1992. Vital Health Stat 10 1997; 194:1–89.
34. Adams PF, Hendershot GE, Marano MA. Centers for Disease Control and Prevention/National Center for Health Statistics. Current estimates from the National Health Interview Survey, 1996. Vital Health Stat 10 1999; 200:1–203.
35. Wolf C. Urban air pollution and health: an ecological study of chronic rhino-sinusitis in Cologne, Germany. Health Place 2002; 8(2):129–139.
36. Chen Y, Dales R, Lin M. The epidemiology of chronic rhinosinusitis in Canadians. Laryngoscope 2003; 113(7):1199–1205.
37. Siahpush M. Socioeconomic status and tobacco expenditure among Australian households: results from the 1998–1999 household expenditure survey. J Epidemiol Community Health 2003; 57(10):798–801.

38. Bishai WR. Issues in the management of bacterial sinusitis. Otolaryngol Head Neck Surg 2002; 127(suppl 6):S3–S9.
39. Williams JW, Simel DL. Does this patient have sinusitis? Diagnosing acute sinusitis by history and physical examination. JAMA 1993; 270:1242–1246.
40. Wald ER. Microbiology of acute and chronic sinusitis in children. J Allerg Clin Immunol 1992; 90:452–456.
41. Sivasli E, Zirikçi A, Bayazýt YA, Gumusburun E, Erbagci H, Bayram M, Kanlykama M. Anatomic variations of the paranasal sinus area in pediatric patients with chronic sinusitis. Surg Radiol Anat 2003; 24(6):400–405.
42. Lundberg JON, Weitzberg E, Nordvall SL, Kuylenstierna R, Lundberg JM, Alving K. Primarily nasal origin of exhaled nitric oxide and absence in Kartageners syndrome. Eur Respir J 1994; 8:1501–1504.
43. Lindberg S, Cervin A, Runer T. Nitric oxide (NO) production in the upper airways is decreased in chronic sinusitis. Acta Otolaryngol 1997; 117:113–117.
44. Ali MS, Wilson JA, Pearson JP. Mixed nasal mucus as a model for sinus mucin gene expression studies. Laryngoscope 2002; 112(2):326–331.
45. Sillers MJ, Kuhn FA, Vickery CL. Radiation exposure in paranasal sinus imaging. Otolaryngol Head Neck Surg 1995; 112(2):248–251.
46. Hall EJ. Radiobiology for the Radiologist. 2nd ed. Philadelphia: Harper and Row, 1978:350–356.
47. Ros SP, Herman BE, Azar-Kia B. Acute sinusitis in children: is the Water's view sufficient? Pediatr Radiol 1995; 25(4):306–307.
48. Mahboubi S, Marsh RR, Potsic WP, Pasquariello PS. The lateral neck radiograph in adenotonsillar hyperplasia. Int J Pediatr Otorhinolaryngol 1985; 10(1):67–73.
49. Lazar RH, Younis RT, Parvey LS. Comparison of plain radiographs, coronal CT and intraoperative findings in children with chronic sinusitis. Otolaryngol Head Neck Surg 1992; 107:29–34.
50. Garcia DP, Corbett ML, Eberly SM, Joyce MR, Le HT, Karibo JM, Pence HL, Nguyen KL. Radiographic imaging studies in pediatric chronic sinusitis. J Allergy Clin Immunol 1994; 94(3 Pt 1):523–530.
51. Manning SC, Biavati MJ, Phillips DL. Correlation of clinical sinusitis signs and symptoms to imaging findings in pediatric patients. Int J Pediatr Otorhinolaryngol 1996; 37(1):65–74.
52. Wald ER, Reilly JS, Casselbrant M, Ledesma-Medina J, Milmoe GJ, Bluestone CD, Chiponis D. Treatment of acute maxillary sinusitis in childhood: a comparative study of amoxicillin and cefaclor. J Pediatr 1984; 104(2):297–302.
53. Gwaltney JM Jr, Phillips CD, Miller DR, Riker DK. Computed tomographic study of the common cold. NEJM 1994; 330(1):25–30.
54. Tiedjen KU, Becker E, Heimann KD, Knorz S, Hildmann H. Value of B-image ultrasound in diagnosis of paranasal sinus diseases in comparison with computerized tomography. German Laryngo-Rhino-Otologie 1998; 77(10):541–546.
55. Varonen H, Kunnamo I, Savolainen S, Makela M, Revonta M, Ruotsalainen J, Malmberg H. Treatment of acute rhinosinusitis diagnosed by clinical criteria or ultrasound in primary care. A placebo-controlled randomised trial. Scand J Prim Health Care 2003; 21(2):121–126.

56. Garbutt JM, Gellman EF, Littenberg B. The development and validation of an instrument to assess acute sinus disease in children. Qual Life Res 1999; 8(3):225–233.
57. Kay DJ, Rosenfeld RM. Quality of life for children with persistent sinonasal symptoms. Otolaryngol Head Neck Surg 2003; 128(1):17–26.
58. Garbutt JM, Goldstein M, Gellman E, Shannon W, Littenberg B. A randomized, placebo-controlled trial of antimicrobial treatment for children with clinically diagnosed acute sinusitis. Pediatrics 2001; 107(4):619–625.
59. Anand VK, Panje WR. Practical Endoscopic Sinus Surgery. New York: McGraw-Hill, 1993.

4

Adult Versus Pediatric Sinusitis

Raphael Chan

Bossier City, Louisiana, U.S.A.

Frank C. Astor

Departments of ENT and Otolaryngology, University of Miami, Miami, Florida, U.S.A.

Ramzi T. Younis

Department of Pediatrics, University of Miami, Miami, Florida, U.S.A.

INTRODUCTION

Rhinosinusitis implies inflammation of the mucosa of the nose and paranasal sinuses including infectious and noninfectious processes. Even though this definition is true for children and adults, there are enough age-related variances relevant to its diagnosis and treatment to require specialized expertise.

Differing predisposing factors in the pathogenesis of sinusitis in children and adults contribute to their differences in presentation, clinical course, and management. It is the intention of this chapter to highlight important clinical aspects that physicians will encounter between both groups. Knowledge of sinusitis, with its multifactorial etiologies, continues to evolve as a disease with manifestly age-related characteristics.

ANATOMY

In childhood, the sinuses undergo progressive and continuous growth and development. At birth, only the maxillary and ethmoid sinuses are present to be clinically significant. The maxillary sinuses show two growth spurts, initially within the first three years, and subsequently from 7 to 18 years. Before age nine, the sinus floor sits higher than the nasal floor; thereafter, the sinus floor is lower than the nasal floor. This is a consideration in the planning of intranasal approaches to the maxillary sinuses in children, and in the diagnosis of odontogenic sinusitis in adults. The ethmoid sinuses are not significant in size at birth but are determinable radiologically by age one, reaching adult size by 12 years of age. The frontal sinuses develop slowly and at one year they are just perceptible. By six they can be radiologically demonstrated and grow rapidly from 12 years to reach adult size in the late teens. The frontal sinuses do not generally give rise to infections until after puberty. The sphenoid sinus is small at birth, but progressively invades into the sphenoid bone and, has reached the sella turcica by age seven. Growth of the sphenoid sinus continues into adulthood to wrap adjacent structures that form indentations in the wall of the fully developed sinus.

PATHOPHYSIOLOGY

Sinus pathophysiology is largely based on the impaired drainage through the ostia. Normal physiology depends on the integrity and patency of the sinus ostia, the ciliary function, and the quality of the secretions. Pathology involving any of these factors, either singly or in combination, will create an obstruction of the drainage pathways, resulting in the entrapment of secretions (Fig. 1). This pooling of secretions with subsequent inflammatory changes, acidosis and anaerobiosis, forms the environment ideal for microbiological growth.

Upper respiratory infection (URI) and allergy are the most common predisposing factors to sinusitis in children, commencing with edema and mucosal swelling and concurrent narrowing at the ostio meatal regions. By comparison, because the ostia are smaller in children as compared to adults, these factors play a more significant role in children (2).

Gastroesophageal reflux disease (GERD) is an apparently important condition associated sinusitis, especially in children more than two years old (3). Many uncontrolled studies have supported this link as the vigorous treatment of GERD in these patients has resulted in the reduction of symptoms. However, the authors are cognizant of the need for prospective double-blind control studies to conclude that GERD contributes to sinus disease.

Adenoids probably play a role in rhinosinusitis in children (Table 1). By virtue of their size, they can obstruct the normal drainage from the sinuses into the nasopharynx, causing backflow and pooling. However, their significance is called into question when functional endoscopic sinus surgery (FESS) and adenoidectomy have been compared in studies showing the superiority of the former (5). In the adult, adenoids are expected to involute and are not as important. Evidence of lymphoid hyperplasia in the adult nasopharynx should raise suspicion of malignancy.

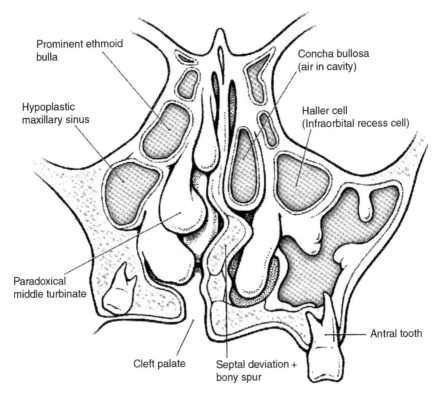

Figure 1 Anatomical factors contributing to sinus disease. *Source*: From Ref. 1.

Nasal polyps are another major contributing factor in chronic sinusitis by obstructing the ostia. However, they are rare in children and their presence in this age group calls for further investigation for cystic fibrosis, allergic fungal sinusitis, or allergy. The adolescent male that presents with a hemorrhagic polyp should be evaluated for juvenile nasopharyngeal angiofibroma. Patients with cystic fibrosis may initially present with sinusitis since more than 10% develop nasal polyps by three years of age. Children with intractable or chronic sinusitis should also be investigated for immune deficiency states and for ciliary motility dysfunction (6). Presence of nasal polyps in the adult may raise suspicion of neoplasia under special circumstances and require biopsy, particularly if unilateral or with associated invasion or erosion.

MICROBIOLOGY

Community-acquired acute sinusitis studies consistently show the presence of *S. pneumoniae*, *Moraxella catarrhalis*, and *H. influenzae* as the most important pathogens in adults and children. *Staphylococcus aureus* and

Table 1 Extrinsic and Intrinsic Causes of Chronic Rhinosinusitis

---

Extrinsic causes of CRS can broadly be broken down into:
Infectious (viral, bacterial, fungal, and parasitic)
Non-infectious/inflammation
   Allergic-IgE-mediated
   Non-IgE mediated hypersensitivities
   Pharmacologic
   Irritants
Disruption of normal ventilation or mucociliary drainage
   Surgery
   Infection
   Trauma

Intrinsic causes contributing to CRS:
Genetic
   Mucociliary abnormality
      Cystic fibrosis
      Primary ciliary dysmotility
   Structural
   Immunodeficiency
Acquired
   Aspirin hypersensitivity associated with asthma and nasal polyps
   Autonomic dysregulation
   Hormonal
      Rhinitis of pregnancy
      Hypothyroidism
Structural
   Neoplasms
   Osteoneogenesis and outflow obstruction
   Retention cysts and antral choanal polyps
Autoimmune or idiopathic
   Granulomatous disorders
      Sarcoid
      Wegener's granulomatosis
   Vasculitis
      Systemic lupus erythematosus
      Churg-Straus syndrome
   Pemphigoid
Immunodeficiency

Abbreviations: CRS, chronic rhinosinusitis. *Source*: From Ref. 4.

anaerobic flora are more common in chronic adult sinusitis than in children (7). *Pseudomonas aeruginosa* play an important role in cystic fibrosis and in the immunocompromised adult or in nosocomial or intensive care unit (ICU) acquired sinusitis. Nevertheless, although it is worth mentioning the role of opportunistic fungal infections in HIV and diabetic patients, it is beyond the scope of this chapter to further the discussion, except to state that they are seen in all age groups.

THE CLINICAL DIAGNOSIS OF SINUSITIS

The categorization of sinusitis in children and adults is similar and arbitrarily based on the duration of symptoms rather than on severity. Clinical diagnosis of acute sinusitis has been defined by major and minor criteria for symptoms that exist for longer than seven days (Table 2). The presence of any two major criteria or one major and two or more minor criteria are highly suggestive of acute or sub-acute sinus disease (8). Acute sinusitis is

Table 2   Clinical Diagnosis of Rhinosinusitis

Signs and symptoms

Major criteria
  Purulent nasal discharge
  Purulent pharyngeal drainage
  Cough
Minor criteria
  Periorbital edema[a]
  Headache[b]
  Facial pain[b]
  Tooth pain[b]
  Earache
  Sore throat
  Foul breath
  Increased wheeze
  Fever

Diagnostic tests

  Major criteria
    Waters' radiograph with opacification, air fluid level, or thickened mucosa
      ≥50% of antrum
    Coronal CT scan with thickening of mucosa or opacification of sinus
  Minor criteria
    Nasal cytologic study (smear) with neutrophils and bacteremia
    Ultrasound studies
  Probable sinusitis
    Signs and symptoms: 2 major criteria or 1 major and ≥ minor criteria
    Diagnostic tests: 1 major = confirmatory, 1 minor = supportive

[a]More common in children.
[b]More common in adults.
Source: From Ref. 8.

characterized by symptoms persisting more than seven days, by resolution of disease between bouts, and occurring less than four times per year. Sub-acute sinusitis has been defined as disease with symptoms and signs lasting four weeks to three months. It is generally agreed that chronic sinusitis refers to disease lasting more than three months, associated with irreversible disease such as osteal obstruction or polyposis.

Children

The most common presentations of sinus disease in children are cough and rhinorrhea. The cough is typically worse at night, the rhinorrhea purulent and associated with nasal obstruction. Other complaints may include fever, halitosis, irritability, pallor, wheezing, or periorbital edema. The child harboring a "cold" that seems more severe than normal with high fever, purulence, and discharge could signify a sinus infection complicating a viral URI. In children with allergy, sinusitis should be considered when not responding to historically effective treatment or if resolution is rapidly followed by recurrence (9).

Older children, who are able to vocalize, may complain of headache, sore throat, or earache. Since these are uncommon complaints under the age of eight, their presence denotes the ominous possibility of sinus complications (10). In contrast with adults, the initial presentation of sinusitis in children is the complication of the sinusitis. Up to 60% of children with chronic sinusitis present with associated middle ear disease (11). Other presentations in chronic disease include laryngitis, bronchitis, and periorbital cellulitis.

Adults

Adult symptoms are more frequently localized to the specific sinus involved. Sinus pain and tenderness are significant complaints. There is accompanying nasal congestion and mucopurulence. Severe infections correlate with more prominent symptoms and signs such as headaches, pyrexia, and even delirium.

In acute sinusitis, the pain is often sharp and stabbing. Even though often localized, sinus pain will radiate to other regions of the head and neck. Bending, straining, and coughing aggravate its intensity. Maxillary pain initiates from the inner canthus of the eye or cheeks and may radiate to the molars or the ears. Ethmoid sinus pain is localized over the bridge of the nose and behind the eye. Eye movements intensify it. Frontal sinus pain clinically occurs over the forehead and may radiate to the temples or the occiput. Isolated sphenoid sinusitis is rare and often late in being recognized, presenting as ill-defined headache often associated with neurological deficits of adjacent cranial nerves.

DIAGNOSTIC AIDS

Transillumination

The increased thickness of the soft tissue and bony vault in children under 10 years of age limits the clinical usefulness of transillumination in children. The use of transillumination in adults will give information as to the state of the maxillary and frontal sinuses, but will not be effective in evaluating the ethmoid and sphenoid sinuses. In adults, transillumination had a sensitivity of 73% and a specificity of 54% when compared with a positive sinus radiograph (12).

Ultrasonography

The use of A-mode ultrasound is popular in Europe with numerous studies showing high correlation between mucosal thickening on plain sinus films, ultrasound, and antral puncture. Ultrasonography (US) was met with initial enthusiasm in the United States but later studies did not support its usefulness. US may have a role in the diagnosis of acute sinusitis during pregnancy given all its inherent limitations, obviating the need for radiation exposure (13).

Radiology

Radiological studies may not be helpful in children under six years of age. Furthermore, CT scans may over diagnose rhinosinusitis by documenting an overwhelming presence of abnormal CT scan findings in children and infants who had a preceding URI of two weeks (14). For adults, the incidental changes on CT are not dissimilar (15). Although rarely ordered by the specialist, plain films may be indicated in the primary setting in adults (16). Indications for magnetic resonance imaging (MRI) in children and adults remain similar and MRIs are used mostly to exclude intracranial disease or to distinguish inflammatory and neoplastic margins.

Endoscopy

In the adult, office endoscopy allows for the complete examination of the nasal cavity and the nasopharynx, enabling the detection of anatomical abnormalities or findings that may contribute to the development of rhinosinusitis. Indeed, 9% of patients with normal sinus CT scans had abnormal endoscopic findings in one study (17). A most accurate diagnosis of sinusitis, endoscopy relies on the visualization of mucous draining from the middle meatus (18). Purulent crusting may be seen with the effects of drying and dehydration. Swelling over the affected sinuses, polypoid degeneration, or frank polyposis may also be observed. However, endoscopy is not an easy task in children, who may resist any attempts at inspection. Endoscopy requires full cooperation from the patient and hence it is not generally suitable in the ambulatory setting in very young children.

COMPLICATIONS

Odontogenic Sinusitis

The normal adult size of the maxillary sinus is not reached until approximately 20 years of age. In the fully developed maxillary sinus, the two upper premolars and the upper molars may be separated from the antral cavity by just the periosteum. Sinusitis of dental origin is hence more common after the second decade (19).

Acute odontogenic sinusitis is always unilateral with exquisite tenderness on palpation or percussion of the diseased molar or premolar tooth. Odontogenic sinusitis accounts for 5 to 10% of acute sinusitis. Anaerobes are found in 50% of all these patients and accounts for the feculent odor that accompanies these infections. The presence of zinc in aspergillosis maxillary sinusitis is related to the overfilling of dental paste. Zinc has been found to stimulate the growth of *Aspergillus fumigatus*. In one series, a radiopaque foreign body was seen in 94% of the cases (20). Root canal therapy can provoke periapical inflammation adjacent to the floor of the maxillary sinus. Instrumentation can introduce bacteria into the sinus and cases of sinusitis have followed endosseeous implant into the posterior maxilla.

Orbital Complications

The ethmoid sinuses are present since birth, and infections of the ethmoid sinuses can arise at any age. Approximately 80% of all orbital complications from ethmoid sinusitis are in children (21). The paper-thin bony plates that separate the ethmoid and maxillary sinuses from the orbit are easy conduits for infections to spread in this age group (22). Chandlers' classification describes the progressive orbital infection from sinusitis.

Intracranial Complications

The intracranial spread of frontal, ethmoid, and sphenoid sinuses can lead to the development of meningitis, brain abscess, and peridural abscesses. Brain abscess is one of the most common intracranial complications of sinusitis exceeded only by orbital complications. In younger children, the ethmoid and maxillary sinuses are present at birth and are the most common sources of intracranial complications in this age group. The frontal and sphenoid sinuses are rarely implicated due to their later development in life. Whereas intraorbital complications are more frequent in younger children, intracranial sequelae are most common in older children and adults (Table 3). Brain abscesses are most likely to occur in the frontal lobe, either due to direct extension of the infection or through venous transmission.

The maxillary sinuses are rarely involved in direct intracranial spread because of the distance from the cranium (23). Isolated sphenoid sinusitis has been associated with ipsilateral involvement of the ophthalmic or

Table 3 The Diagnosis of Chronic Rhinosinusitis in Adults

Duration of disease is qualified by continuous symptoms for >12 consecutive weeks or >12 weeks of physical findings[a]

One of these signs of inflammation must be present and identified in association with ongoing symptoms consistent with CRS:
  Discolored nasal drainage arising from nasal passages, nasal polyps, or polypoid swellings as identified on physical examination with anterior rhinoscopy or nasal endoscopy with anterior rhinoscopy performed in the decongested state
  Edema or erythema of the middle meatus or ethmoid bulla as identified by nasal endoscopy
  Generalized or localized erythema, edema, or granulation tissue. If it does not involve the middle meatus or ethmoid bulla, radiologic imaging is required to confirm the diagnosis[b]
Imaging modalities for confirming the diagnosis
  CT scan—demonstrating isolated or diffuse mucosal thickening, bone changes, and air-fluid level
  Plain sinus radiograph—Waters' view revealing mucous membrane thickening of > than 5 mm or complete opacification of one or more sinuses. An air-fluid level is more predictive of acute rhinosinusitis but may also be seen in chronic rhinosinusitis[c]
  MRI is not recommended as an alternative to CT because of its excessively high sensitivity and lack of specificity

[a]Signs consistent with CRS will support the symptom time duration.
[b]Other chronic rhinologic conditions such as allergic rhinitis can have such findings and therefore they may not be associated with rhinosinusitis. It is recommended that a diagnosis of rhinosinusitis require radiologic confirmation under these circumstances.
[c]A plain sinus X-ray without the equivocal signs listed in a, b, or c is not considered diagnostic. Aside from an air-fluid level, plain sinus radiographs have low sensitivity and specificity.
Abbreviations: CRS, chronic rhinosinusitis.
Source: From Ref. 24.

maxillary division of the trigeminal nerve; however, sphenoiditis is most commonly implicated with meningitis. In some series, it is the most common complication of cavernous sinus thrombosis (24).

Infection of the frontal sinus carries the highest risk of intracranial complications. An infection in the frontal sinus spreads by way of the valveless diploic veins through the bone causing osteomyelitis of the frontal bone. A subperiosteal abscess of the frontal bone presenting as a localized swelling of the forehead overlying the frontal sinus is called Pott's puffy tumor, described in all ages but most common in adolescence (25). These patients are at highest risk of intracranial complications (26).

Sinus Mucocele

Mucoceles of the sinuses usually occur due to either obstruction of the osteum or mucosal entrapment following a sinus fracture. These are more commonly found in the ethmoid, frontal, and sphenoid sinuses of adults. Ethmoid muco-celes may invade the orbit, causing proptosis of the globe. Sphenoid mucocele can produce cranial nerve deficits or visual field disorders. A frontal mucocele presents localized pain and has the potential to erode and invade intracranial and orbital structures. Mucocoeles are uncommon in children and their distri-bution depends on the stage of development of the paranasal sinuses (27).

TREATMENT

Medical

Antibiotics remain the treatment of choice in bacterial sinusitis (28). The choice of antimicrobials in otherwise healthy children and adults generally does not differ except for tetracyclines and quinolones that are not recom-mended in childhood and in pregnancy. High-dose ampicillin or amoxicillin remain first line therapy in uncomplicated cases. Augmented penicillin is effective against β-lactamase resistant bacteria and anaerobes. Fluoroquino-lones have been shown to have excellent penetration of the sinuses, and should be reserved for those patients with penicillin allergy, those not responsive to first line therapy, or those with moderate or severe infections. Fluoroquinolones have been used in special pediatric conditions, particu-larly in cystic fibrosis. Combination antibiotic therapy with clindamycin or metronidazole is recommended in anaerobic infections. Amphoteri-cin-B is used to treat pediatric and adult invasive fungal sinusitis.

In both adults and children, chronic sinusitis and recurrent acute sinusitis may require a combination of agents and prolonged administration (29). Decongestants, intranasal steroids, and systemic steroids have potential roles. The predominance of Th2 cytokines in chronic inflammation has been found in sinus tissues, especially in coexistent morbidities such as allergic rhinitis and asthma (30) (Figs. 2, 3). Concerns with linear growth suppression in young children on long-term usage of intranasal beclomethasone (31) were alleviated with reports of other nasal preparations without this effect (32,33).

Leukotriene modifiers have improved nasal congestion and restored the sense of smell in patients with chronic hyperplastic sinusitis/nasal polyposis (34).

Functional Endoscopic Sinus Surgery

Modern sinus surgery is geared at establishing drainage and preserving healthy mucosal layer. Attention is paid to the osteomeatal unit anterior eth-moid cells. Surgery is planned and tailored around patients' symptoms and endoscopic and CT scan findings. FESS involves minimal normal tissue damage with precise and subtle removal of disease (Figs. 4, 5). This treatment philosophy is ideally represented by endoscopic techniques that maintain the physiology and integrity of the ostia of the maxillary and frontal sinuses. Endoscopic techniques are described to treat pediatric and adult sinusitis.

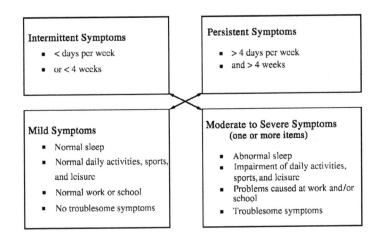

Figure 2 Classification of rhinitis according to allergic rhinitis and its impact on asthma (ARIA). *Source*: From Ref. 35.

Medical therapy remains the overwhelming treatment of choice in children with sinusitis. Surgery may be indicated in three groups of patients: those with true chronic disease, those with serious underlying disease, and those with complications of sinusitis (36). Extensive sphenoethmoidectomy is usually not justified in children except in specific circumstances including complications, polyposis, cystic fibrosis, fungal sinusitis, and others. Surgery usually entails performing limited anterior ethmoidectomy and possibly enlargement of the maxillary ostium. Several authors adamantly believe there is no place for surgery in uncomplicated childhood sinusitis. One study reports an 80% success rate in FESS in children as not favorable when compared to those without surgical treatment (37). The development of prognostic systems to compare outcomes allows a more objective determination of treatment. In one pediatric study, FESS results were based on the preoperative categorization of sinus disease into four stages of progressive severity (38). Results suggested that FESS had no apparent advantage in stages 1 and 4, but 2 and 3 had "much improved" rates of 79% and 68% for FESS, respectively, compared to 54% and 42% for medical treatment. The authors concluded that FESS may be particularly effective for patients with intermediate prognostic stages.

In adults, the reported success rate of FESS is over 80%; however, these reports may lack standardization in the staging systems and may have poor correlation between objective findings on endoscopy and/or CT scans with symptoms. Comprehensive outcome studies are currently being done on FESS to measure its efficacy compared to other treatments. There are a number of staging systems used to classify adult sinusitis. One of the easiest to implement was created by Lund and Mackay (39) based on subjective (visual

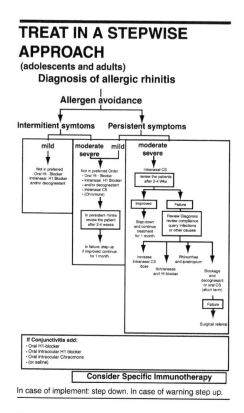

TREAT IN A STEPWISE APPROACH
(adolescents and adults)
Diagnosis of allergic rhinitis

Figure 3 Basic treatment plan for rhinitis according to ARIA guidelines. *Source*: From Ref. 35.

analogue scale) and objective (CT scan and endoscopy) findings. Kennedy et al. (40) proposed a staging system based on the extent of the disease as diagnosed by CT scan and endoscopic findings, while Schaitkin's et al. (41) is based on the subjective report of patients' symptoms improvement. Zein-reich has reviewed the staging of rhinosinusitis based on CT imaging (42).

Open Operations for Paranasal Sinuses

In spite of the prominence and success of endoscopic sinus surgery in the treatment of paranasal sinuses infections, open operations remain important in acute sinusitis with orbital or intracranial complications or when endoscopic sinus surgery has failed to cure or to remove disease from the sinus. These operations retain a vital role in adults but to a much lesser degree in children.

Maxillary Sinus

Antral lavage is widely practiced in Europe in adults. Irrigation of the maxillary sinus removes the occluding mucous plug, which prevents the

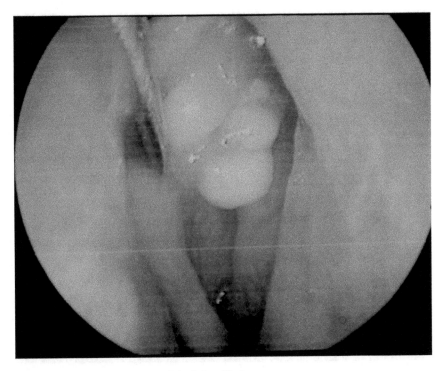

Figure 4 Nasal polyp in the right infundibulum.

egress of secretions from the sinus and clearing the retained products of infection. Specimens may be obtained for culture in resistant infections and in the immunocompromised patients. This procedure can be performed in the ambulatory setting in adults under local anesthesia. Antral lavage is not generally considered a viable option in children as it addresses the maxillary sinus and not the ethmoid sinus. Cannulation of the maxillary ostium is considered too traumatic for the pediatric sinus (43).

The infrequently utilized Caldwell–Luc procedure can be indicated in patients following unsuccessful FESS, in fungal sinusitis where inspissated fungal masses cannot be removed through an intranasal antrostomy, for excision of tumors through a Denker's approach, or in patients with cystic fibrosis (44). The Caldwell–Luc procedure is rarely indicated in children due to the potential risk of damage to the roots of developing permanent teeth. If this procedure is to be considered in children, the opening into the maxillary sinus must be made high and lateral to the roots of the canine teeth. The inferior antrostomy should not be made too far anterior so as not to cause injury to the front incisors (45). Maxillary sinusitis from dental origin or fungal infection may be treated with a less traumatizing procedure through a combined FESS and fenestration of the canine fossa with a miniwindow (46).

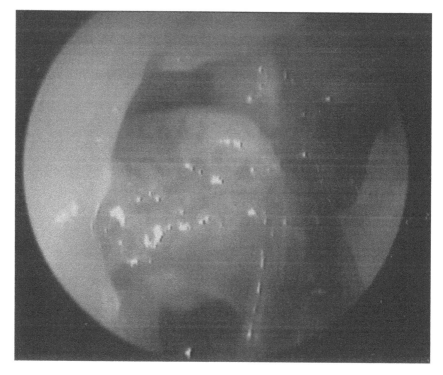

Figure 5 Fungal ball with fungal mucin in the maxillary sinus.

Ethmoid Sinus

Sinusitis with orbital infection is the strongest indication for the external approach to the ethmoid sinus. Postseptal infection mandates surgery. The endoscopic technique has been advocated for the treatment of orbital cellulitis and subperiosteal abscess with the removal of the lamina papyracea and is used in adults and children. The external approach remains safe and reliable in the emergency situation in children or in combination with an orbital abscess approach.

Frontal Sinus

The frontal sinus is not developed until age 12 and generally does not give rise to disease until the late teens and adulthood. Hence, frontal sinus surgery is not performed in children.

Trephination is usually indicated for acute sinusitis that is not responding to antibiotics or in the presence of an empyema, intracranial, or orbital complication. Trephination is easy to perform and free of surgical complications, although less utilized by experienced rhinologists skilled in frontal recess surgery.

With the availability of endoscopic techniques, frontoethmoid and osteoplastic flap procedures are not used as often today in chronic sinusitis (47). Osteoplastic flap with obliteration may be the best option for achieving long-term control of persistent allergic fungal sinusitis. The series by Hardy and Montgomery showed resurgery for complications was 10% and occurred up to 20 years later (48).

CONCLUSION

Multiple factors seem to play a direct or contributing role in the pathogenesis of rhinosinusitis. Management planning differs between adult and pediatric rhinosinusitis because of differences in the clinical characteristics. However, the study of rhinosinusitis continues to evolve as more information becomes available. While much debate remains regarding potential etiologies, associated conditions, and common mediators, newer forms of technology in diagnosis and treatment are emerging. This separation of rhinosinusitis into adult and pediatric forms may be better understood or even truncated with future advances.

REFERENCES

1. Kennedy DW, Bloger WE, Zinreich SJ. Diseases of the Sinuses. Diagnosis and Managerment. Hamilton, London: B.C. Decker Inc, 2001.
2. Furukawa CT. The role of allergy in sinusitis in children. J Allergy Clin Immunol 1992; 90(3 Pt 2):515–517.
3. Rudolph CD. Supraesophageal complications of gastroesophageal reflux in children: challenges and treatment. Am J Med 2003; 1153(suppl 1):150–156.
4. Benninger MS. Adult chronic rhinosinusitis: definitions, diagnosis, epidemiology and patholophysiology. Otolaryngol Head Neck Surg 2003; 129S:S1–S32.
5. Ramadan HH. Adenoidectomy vs. Endoscopic sinus surgery for the treatment of pediatric sinusitis. Arch Otol Head Neck Surg 1999; 125(11):1208–1211.
6. Coste A, Girodon E, Louis S, Pruliere-Escabasse V, Goossens M, Peynegre R, Escundier E. Atypical sinusitis in adults must lead to looking for cystic fibrosis and primary ciliary dyskinesia. Laryngoscope 2004; 114(5):839–843.
7. Gwaltney JM. Management update of bacterial rhinosinusitis and the use of cefdinir. Otolaryngol Head Neck Surg 2002; 127(suppl 6):S24–S29.
8. Shapiro GG, Rachelefsky GS. Introduction and definition of sinusitis. J Allergy Clin Immunol 1992; 90(3):417–418.
9. Rachelefsky GS, Goldberg M, Katz RM, Boris G, Gyepes MT, Shapiro MJ, Mickey MR, Finegold SM, Siegal SC. Sinus disease in children with respiratory allergy. J Allergy Clin Immunol 1978; 61(5):310–314.
10. Clement PA, Bluestone CD, Gordts F, Lusk RP, Otten FW, Goossens H, Scadding GK, Takahashi H, van Buchem FL, van Cauwenberge P, Wald ER. Management of rhinosinusitis in children. Int J Pediatr Otorhinolaryngol 1999; 49(suppl 1):S95–S100.

11. Rachelesfky GS. Chronis sinusitis. The disease of all ages (editorial). Am J Dis 1989; 143(8):886–888.
12. William JW Jr, Simel DC, Roberts L, Samsa GP. Clinical evaluation for sinusitis: making the diagnosis by history and physical examination. Ann Intern Med 1992; 117(9):705–710.
13. Puhakka T, Alanen A, Kallio T, Koroff L, Suonpaa J, Ruuskanen O. Makela HJ. Validity of ultrasonography in the diagnosis of acute sinusitis. Arch Otolaryngol Head Neck Surg 2000; 126(12):1482–1486.
14. Conrad DA, Jenson HB. Management of acute bacterial rhinosinusitis. Curr Opin Pediatr 2002; 74(1):86–90.
15. Jones NS. CT of the paranasal sinuses: a review of the correlation with clinical, surgical and histopathological findings. Clin Otolaryngol 2002; 27(1): 11–17.
16. Desrosier M, Frenkiel S, Hamid QA, Low D, Small P, Carr S Hawke M, Kirpatrick D, Lavigne F, Mandell L, Stevens HE, Weiss K, Witterrick IJ, Wright ED, Davidson R. Acute bacterial sinusitis in adults: management in the primary setting. J Otolaryngol 2002; 31(suppl 2):2S 2–14.
17. Vining EM, Yanagisawa K, Yanagisawa F. The importance of preoperative nasal endoscopy in patients with sinonasal disease. Laryngoscope 1993; 103(5): 512–519.
18. Kuhn FA. Role of endoscopy in the management of chronic rhinosinusitis. Ann Otol Rhinol Laryngol 2004; 193(suppl):19–23.
19. Kretzschmar DP, Kretzschmar CJ, Rhinosinusitis. Review from a dental perspective. Oral Surg Med Pathol Oral Radio Endod 2003; 96(2):128–135.
20. Legent F, Billet J, Beauvillain C, Bonnet J, Megeville M. Role of dental canal fillings in the development of *Aspergillus sinusitis*. A report of 85 cases. Arch Otolaryngol 1989; 246(5):318–320.
21. Moloney JR, Badlan NJ, McRae A. The acute orbit. Preseptal (periorbital) cellulitis, subperiosteal abscess and orbital cellulitis due to sinusitis. J Laryngol Otol 1987; 12(suppl):1–18.
22. McCarty MC, Wilson MW, Fleming JC, Thompson JW, Sandlund JT, Flynn PM, Knapp KM, Hail BG, Ribeiro RC. Manifestations of fungal sinusitis of the orbit in children with neuropenia and fever. Ophthal Plast Reconstr Surg 2004; 20(3):217–223.
23. Raghava N, Evans K, Basu S. Infratemporal fossa abscess: complication of maxillary sinusitis. J Laryngol Otol 2004; 118(5):377–378.
24. Otol Bakar AS. Role of anaerobic bacteria in sinusitis and its complications. Ann RhinoLaryngol 1991; (suppl 154):17–22.
25. Blackshaw G, Thomson N. Potts Puffy Tumor reviewed. J Laryngol Otol 1990; 104(7):574–577.
26. Gupta M, El-Hakim H, Burgava R, Mehta V. Pott's puffy tumor in a preadolescent child: the youngest reported in the post-antibiotic era. Int J Pediatr Otorhinolaryngol 2004; 68(3):373–378.
27. Timon CL, O' Dwyer TP. Ethmoidal mucocoeles in children. J Laryngol Otol 1989; 103(3):284–286.

28. William JW Jr, Aguilar C, Cornell J, Chiquette ED, Makela M, Holleman DR, Simel DL. Antibiotics for acute maxillary sinusitis. Ann Emerg Med 2003; 42(5):705–708.
29. Mucha SM, Baroody FM. Sinusitis update. Curr Opin Allergy Clin Immunol 2003; 3(1):33–38.
30. Calderon E, O'Neal ML, Fox RW, Calderon-Moncloa J. Chronic sinusitis in children. J Investig Allergol Clin Immunol 1996; 6(1):5–13.
31. Skoner DP, Rachelefsky GS, Meltzer EO, Chervinsky P, Morris RM, Seltzer JM, Storms WW, Wood RA. Detection of growth suppression in children during treatment with intranasal beclomethasone dipropionate. Pediatrics 2000; 105(2):E23.
32. Schenkel E, Skoner DP, Bronsky E, Miller SD, Pearlman DS, Rooklin A, Rosen JP, Ruff ME, Vandewalker ML, Wanderer A, Damaraju CV, Nolop KB, Mesarina-Wicki B. Absence of growth retardation in children with perennial allergic rhinitis following 1 year treatment with mometarsone furoate acqueous nasal spray. Pediatrics 2000; 105(2):E22.
33. Grossman J, Banov C, Bronsky EA, Nathan RA, Pearlman D, Winder JA, Rather PH, Mendelson L, Findlay SR, Kral KM, et al. Fluticasone propionate acqueous nasal spray is safe and effective for children with seasonal allergic rhinitis. Pediatrics 1993; 92(4):594–599.
34. Borish L. The role of leukotrienes in upper and lower airway inflammation and the implications for treatment. Ann Allergy Asthma Immunol 2002; 88(4 suppl 1): 16–22.
35. Scadding GK. Recent advances in the treatment of rhinitis and rhinosinusitis. Int J Pediatr Otorhinolaryngol 2003; 67S1:S201–S204.
36. Manning SC. Surgical intervention for sinusitis in children. Curr Allergy Asthma Rep 2001; 1(3):289–296.
37. Jones NS. Current concepts in the management of pediatric rhinosinusitis. J Laryngol Otol 1999; 113(1):1–9.
38. Lieu JE, Piccirillo JF, Lusk RP. Prognostic staging system and therapeutic effectiveness for recurrent or chronic sinusitis in children. Otolaryngol Head Neck Surg 2003; 129(3):222–233.
39. Lund VJ, Mackay IS. Staging in rhinosinusitis. Radiology 1993; 31(4):183–184.
40. Kennedy DW, Wright ED, Goldberg AN. Objective and subjective outcomes in surgery for chronic sinusitis. Laryngoscope 2000; 110(3 Pt 3):29–31.
41. Schaitkin B, May M, Shapiro A, Fucci M, Mester SJ. Endoscopic sinus surgery: 4 year fellow-up on the first 100 patients. Laryngoscope 1993; 103:1117–1120.
42. Zinreich SJ. Imaging for staging of rhinosinusitis. Ann Otol Rhinol Laryngol 2004; 193(suppl):19–23.
43. Lusk RP, Stankiewicz JA. Pediatric rhinosinusitis. Otolaryngol Head Neck Surg 1997; 117:S53–S57.
44. Biltzer A, Lawson W. The Caldwell–Luc procedure in 1991. Otolaryngol Head Neck Surg 1991; 105(5):717–722.
45. Paavolainen M, Paavolainen R, Tarkkanen J. Influence of Caldwell–Luc operation on developing permanent teeth. Laryngoscope 1977; 87:613–620.
46. el-Hennaw DM. Combined functional endoscopic sinus surgery (FESS): a revisited approach. Rhinology 1998; 36(4):196–201.

47. Scott NA, Wormald P, Close D, Gallagher R, Anthony A, Maddern GJ. Endoscopic modified Lothrop procedure for the treatment of chronic frontal sinusitis. A systematic review. Otol Head Neck Surg 2003; 129(4):427–438.
48. Hardy JM, Montgomery WW. Osteoplastic frontal sinusotomy. An analysis of 250 operations. Ann Otol 1976; 85:523–532.

5

Complications of Pediatric Sinusitis

Kevin D. Pereira

Medical Center of Otolaryngology Department, University of Texas, Houston, Texas, U.S.A.

Tina P. Elkins

University of Texas, Cypress, Texas, U.S.A.

Ramzi T. Younis

Department of Pediatrics, University of Miami, Miami, Florida, U.S.A.

INTRODUCTION

Children suffer from six to eight viral upper respiratory infections a year. Of these, approximately 5 to 13% will transform into a bacterial sinus infection, with a majority of these bacterial superinfections responding to appropriate antibiotic treatment while others progress and have potentially devastating outcomes. Recognizing the clinical signs and symptoms that are associated with the complication of pediatric sinusitis is of the utmost importance since the key to treating them involves prompt medical and occasionally surgical management.

The medical community has seen a decrease in the number of complications associated with pediatric sinusitis since the development of antibiotics and immunizations. In the pre-antibiotic era, there was a mortality rate of approximately 17% in patients with orbital cellulites, and those who survived had a 20% chance of being blind in the affected eye (1).

The advent of the *Haemophilus influenzae* type B (Hib) vaccine reduced the incidence of Hib-related periorbital cellulites from 11.7% to 3.5% and the total number of annual cases by 59% (1,2). However, the risk of blindness (10%) due to sinusitis-related orbital disease still exists along with developing intracranial extension of disease (3–11%) (3). Despite the use of antibiotics and surgical therapy, the risk of death from intracranial complications remains, ranging from 12.8% to 40% (4,5).

In order to fully understand how the complications of sinusitis evolve, the anatomy and its relationships must be fully understood. Complications of sinusitis occur because of either loss of anatomical barriers or hematological spread. The maxillary, ethmoid, and frontal sinuses share a common wall, lamina papyracae, with the orbit. Within this wall, there are small dehiscences that are often too small to be seen radiographically, but do allow for spread of the bacteria into the adjacent orbits. These are referred to as the dehiscences of Zuckerkandhl and are a result of the anterior and ethmoidal neurovascular bundles.

Hematological spread occurs because of the extensive valveless system that connects the facial venous system to the cavernous sinus via the ophthalmic veins. Specifically, the superior ophthalmic vein crosses over the optic nerve and enters the cavernous sinus via the superior orbital fissure. It has a valveless connection with the angular, supraorbital, and supratrochlear veins. The inferior ophthalmic vein crosses under the optic nerve, entering the cavernous sinus via the inferior orbital fissure. It has a valveless connection with the pterygoid plexus and the ethmoidal veins. Once the bacteria enters the cavernous sinus, it has the potential to cause a intracranial infection. The diploic blood flow of the cranial bones also contributes to the hematological spread of disease resulting in intracranial infection. The diploic veins of Breschet are valveless and can result in an extracranial infections spreading inward.

In general, radiographic studies are performed on patients when their clinical examination shows the potential need for surgery. Some authors state that the guidelines for taking a patient to the operating room for surgical drainage are the same used for having a CT scan or MRI (6). The CT scans are recommended when abscesses are suspected and there is no change in symptoms despite appropriate IV antibiotic therapy. If an intracranial complication is suspected, then MRI is superior to CT in detecting small abnormalities. However, CT has a role in the planning of the surgical management (6).

The complications that result from pediatric sinusitis are can be broken down into extracranial and intracranial.

Extracranial

1. mucoceles
2. osteomyelitis
3. orbital infections
4. cavernous sinus thrombosis

Intracranial

1. meningitis
2. epidural abscess

3. subdural abscess
4. brain abscess

MUCOCELES

A mucocele is a mucous-containing sac that is lined with epithelial cells and results from chronic sinusitis due to inflammation and scarring of the sinus ostia. As the sac slowly enlarges, it results in bony changes, mainly bony expansion. The mucocele can either be primary, i.e., mucous retention cyst, or secondary, due to ostial obstruction (7). The frontal sinus is most commonly involved, along with the ethmoid sinuses. Rarely does one find isolated ethmoid or sphenoid involvement.

The patients' symptoms are often related to the bony expansion. As the mucocele compresses the adjacent orbit, it can cause visual changes, such as diploplia, epiphora, or proptosis. Within the nasal cavity, it can result in nasal obstruction and headaches or be associated with facial swelling (8). Due to the slow nature of these lesions, they are a rare finding in young children. Therefore, their presence warrants an evaluation for cystic fibrosis, as this can be a presenting symptom of the disease (9,10).

Radiographically, a plain film of the sinuses will show an opacified sinus with thinning and expansion of the surrounding bone. The mucocele will appear as a homogeneous swelling arising from the sinuses on CT scan. Bony expansion will be seen and the size of the mucocele can be determined on CT, thus assisting with surgical management. It is this detail that the CT offers over MRI that makes it the test of choice. In complex cases, 3D reconstruction can be beneficial in aiding the surgeon in relating the mucocele to the surrounding anatomy (11).

Treatment of the mucocele is surgical. Historically, external drainage of the sinus was performed. Traditionally, the frontoethmoidal mucocele would be treated with masrupialization and formation of a new drainage pathway. This would be created via an external frontoethmoidectomy by frontal sinus obliteration or cranialization (11). However, with the current use of endoscopes, this has proven to be an effective choice. In a retrospective study of seven pediatric patients by Hartley et al. with mucoceles that underwent endoscopic drainage, no complications or recurrences after one year were identified. The anterior ethmoid (5), posterior ethmoid (1), and the sphenoid sinus (1) were involved in this group of patents (8).

OSTEOMYELITIS

Frontal sinusitis can progress to an osteomyelitis, eventually eroding the cortex and causing a pericranial, periorbital, or epidural abscess. This was first described in the late 1700s by Sir Percival Pott as an indolent, puffy, circumscribed tumor of the forehead due to inflammation of the cranial bones.

The fluctuation felt above the patient's frontal sinus is due to a subperiosteal collection of pus and is eponymously named Pott's puffy tumor (12).

The ideal choice for evaluation is CT scan, as this will allow for visualization of the bony changes. However, the bony changes are a late finding; therefore, scintigraphy is used in order to check for early changes of osteomyelitis (13). Initial treatment is with about six to eight weeks of IV antibiotics, including antistaphylococcal penicillins, chloramphenicol, and third generation cephaloporins. The broad spectrum antibiotics are tailored to the offending organism which is predominantly non-enterococcal streptococci, *Staphylococcus aureus*, and oral anaerobes (fusobacterium, bacteriodes, and anaerobic streptococci) (12). Surgical drainage is initially performed and followed by debridement and sometimes a frontal sinusectomy (7). Reconstruction is held until complete eradication of the diseased bone.

ORBITAL CELLULITIS

The most common complication of bacterial sinusitis is involvement of the orbit, which can lead to morbid complications for the pediatric patient. The severity of the disease varies and is dependent on the structures involved and whether it is preseptal, postseptal, extraconal, or intraconal.

PRESEPTAL CELLULITIS

This is the most common complication seen in children with bacterial sinusitis, usually involving the ethmoid sinuses. The infection at this stage is still confined to the paranasal sinuses, with passive venous congestion resulting in inflammation of the soft tissues of the eyelids anterior to the orbital septum. Chemosis is sometimes seen (14). Preseptal cellulitis is not associated with changes or loss of vision. However, the patient must be thoroughly evaluated to rule out any involvement of the postseptal structures, which can lead to serious morbidity. A complete ocular exam is of utmost importance; therefore, the globe must be evaluated, even in the most difficult-to-examine child. The eyelids should be gently retracted and the globe examined for proptosis, limitation of ocular movement, papillary reactions, and possibly for acuity. If the complete ocular exam cannot be performed, then a radiographic evaluation must be performed (15).

The CT scan is the study preferred in evaluation of the orbital structures and for localizing the disease (16) (Fig. 1). The accuracy of diagnosis of orbital complications on CT ranges from 87 to 91% compared to 70–81% for clinical diagnosis alone (6). Treatment involves prompt diagnosis and prompt use of antibiotics. When the eyelid is 50% or less swollen, then the patient may be sent home on oral antibiotics. Close follow-up is required over the next 24 to 48 hours, and if there is not significant improvement, then the patient should be admitted for IV antibiotic therapy. If admitted,

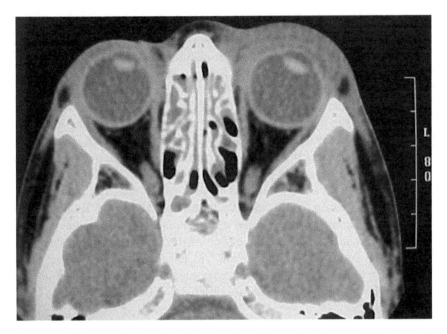

Figure 1 CT scan of the orbits showing ethmoid opacifications and left preseptal cellulitis.

it is recommended that the patient start on ceftriaxone (100 mg/kg/day in two divided doses) or ampicillin-sulbactam (60 mg/kg/day in four divided doses). Vancomycin (60 mg/kg/day in four divided doses) is recommended if there is a concern then there is a resistant *Streptococcus pneumoniae* (17). Surgical treatment is not indicated in this case.

POSTSEPTAL INFLAMMATION

Postseptal infections, either extraconal or intraconal, are more serious and prompt recognition and treatment are necessary. They are usually due to acute sinusitis, in contrast to preseptal infection which can be due to trauma, bacteremia, or sinusitis (18). Postseptal infection is a result of bacteria or fungus passing through the bony dehisences within the lamina papyracae or along the neurovascular bundle. While a majority of the infections are unilateral, bilateral spread has been reported and requires more aggressive treatment (16). Patients will present with periorbital edema, chemosis, proptosis, and decreased extraocular movement. Vision changes will vary and are more extreme in patients with intraconal disease. The visual changes are a result of increased intraorbital pressure, optic neuritis, traction on the optic nerve, or retinal artery thrombosis. In all cases, CT scan is recommended in order to fully evaluate the disease process and for management planning. An abscess is suggested by the findings of a low-density mass effect with/without enhancement, air-fluid mass, lateral displacement of the medial rectus, or displacement of the periostium away from the lamina papyracae (6).

Extraconal spread of disease from the ethmoids through the lamina papyracae can allow for purulence to collect in the subperiosteal potential space between the periorbita and the bony orbital wall, resulting in a subperiosteal abscess (SPA) (Fig. 2). The developing SPA will result in an infero-lateral displacement of the globe leading to diplopia. This physical finding is accompanied by chemosis, proptosis, diminished ocular mobility, and mild to moderate visual loss. Evaluation is best achieved through a CT scan, since physical examination is difficult due to periorbital edema. Radiographic findings include an enhancing convex lesion adjacent to the lamina papyracae. Other findings might include edema of the lateral rectus and displacement of the periostium of the lamina. An ultrasound of the orbit is also beneficial when distinguishing between a medial extraconal inflammatory mass and an abscess, as a CT cannot differentiate this difference.

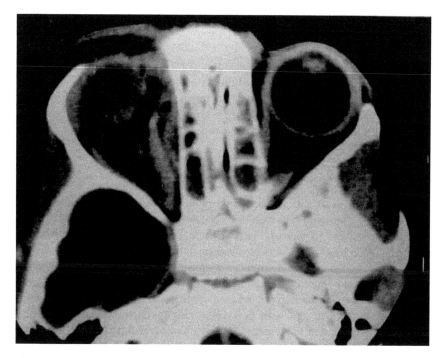

Figure 2   CT scan of the orbits showing ethmoid opacification and right subperiosteal abscess.

Treatment includes hospitalization with close observation for any changes in vision. This entails vision checks for acuity and color perception every two hours. The patient will need to be placed on IV antibiotics that cover for resistant organisms and allow for cerebral spinal fluid penetration. The timing and type of surgical intervention is debated, whereas most physicians will perform the drainage by either an external (traditional) or internal (endoscopic) approach. In either method, drainage of the SPA along with an anterior ethmoidectomy can be performed.

Intraconal involvement is often due to an untreated infection of the extraconal space spreading into the intraconal area through the fascia between the rectus muscle posteriorly, as this is quite thin. The nerves, blood vessels, and muscles located in this region, along with the globe, may become infected, resulting in proptosis, opthalmoplegia, and visual loss along with preseptal edema and chemosis. Examination of the funcus will allow the physician to check for optic disk edema due to venous congestion. Progression to ophthalmoplegia suggests a high likelihood of a intraconal abscess, although this can be mimicked by pressure effects of an extraconal abscess (3).

CAVERNOUS SINUS THROMBOSIS

Cavernous sinus thrombosis is due to extension of the septic phlebitis beyond the orbit and is a serious complication carrying a high morbidity rate of 10 to 15%. The patient will have bilateral axial proptosis along with cranial 3, 4, and 6 palsies. Other signs include meningismus and dilation of episcleral veins. Work-up should include high-resolution CT scan and IV antibiotics started immediately. The antibiotics should cover suspected organisms, mainly *Staphylococcus aureus*, and be able to cross the blood–brain barrier as intracranial progression can occur. The IV antibiotics should continue until the inflammation has resolved and then replaced by oral antibiotics for another four to six weeks. After antibiotic treatment and drainage have taken place, the patient can be started on high-dose systemic steroids, in order to reduce the edema around the optic nerve. It is felt that the temporary immunosuppression risk is outweighed by the benefit of reducing the swelling of the optic nerve and helping to preserve vision of the affected eye.

INTRACRANIAL COMPLICATIONS

Approximately 0.5 to 24% of all patients admitted for rhinosinusitis develop intracranial complications. There are several routes of spread into the intracranial compartment. It can be spread directly, through osteomyelitis, perineural spaces of the olfactory nerves, congenital, or traumatic dehiscences in the walls of the sinuses or through a septic phlebitis (19). These complications include subdural empyema, intracerebral abscess, epidural abscess, meningitis, and cavernous or superior sagittal sinus thrombosis (13). These complications occur mainly in adolescents and in males (20–22). Despite the advances with antibiotic therapy, there is still a 5 to 21% mortality and 40% morbidity rate. The radiographic modality of choice in diagnosing a patient with a suspected intracranial complication is MRI, as CT can be normal on 50% of patients early (23). T1 and T2 non-enhanced images along with T1-gadolinium-enhanced images are obtained. The T1-weighted images will often show mass effect and effacement. If there is a formed abscess, T1 will be hypointense and T2 will be hyperintense. The T1 with gadolinium images will show enhancement. CT, however, is often obtained in order to help with surgical planning (6).

SUBDURAL EMPYEMA

Subdural empyema is a rare intracranial complication of sinusitis, accounting for less than 10% of the cases (24). It usually arises from the frontal sinus, either by direct extension from the epidural space or from septic thrombi in the venous channels draining the subdural space (25). In children, this sinus begins to become pneumatized during the first few years of life, with a true sinus defined at the age of two. It reaches adult size by age 12 or 13. Patients will present with rapidly declining neurological deterioration. They will also have headache, nausea and vomiting, lethargy, and possibly seizures. The work-up consists of imaging with an MRI and a CT for operative planning (Fig. 3). The patient should undergo IV antibiotics and urgent drainage of the abscess. Despite appropriate therapy, there is still a 25 to 35% mortality rate (4,26). Of those who survive, about 30% will be neurologically impaired (27).

INTRACEREBRAL ABSCESS

This is an uncommon complication of pediatric sinusitis resulting from sinusitis involving the frontal, ethmoid, and sphenoid sinus which, despite appropriate therapy, carries a 20 to 30% mortality rate (7). The primary sites involved are the frontal and the frontoparietal regions. Patients will usually present with fever, headaches, vomiting, lethargy, or just subtle mood changes (28). Poor prognostic symptoms include seizures and neurological deficits (29).

CT and MRI are the studies of choice in diagnosing this condition and are highly sensitive. A lumbar puncture should not be performed, as this can be life-threatening to a patient with a cerebral abscess. Treatment should be aggressive and involve IV antibiotics plus surgical aspiration or debridement. It is important in the treatment of the abscesses to leave the abscess wall intact (29). The affected sinus should also be drained at the time of abscess drainage. The antibiotics should cover both aerobes (staphylococcus, hemolytic, and streptococcus) and anaerobic species (anaerobic streptococci, fusobacterium, and bacteroides).

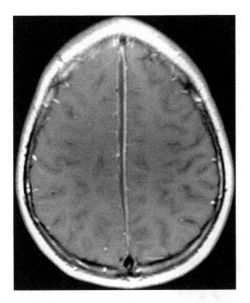

Figure 3 14-year-old boy presented with neurological deficits and found to have a subdural abscess along the falx cerebri. The source was the right frontal sinus.

EPIDURAL ABSCESS

Subperiosteal suppuration of the calvarium can result in an epidural abscess, most often due to frontal sinus disease. The infection in this space occurs almost exclusively due to frontal sinusitis with secondary osteomyelitis. This is probably due to the venous communication and loosely adherent dura. The patient can present with symptoms such as purulent nasal discharge, fever, headache, scalp swelling, and, rarely, signs or symptoms of increased intracranial pressure or localized neurological findings (30). Radiographically, an epidural abscess will remain localized within the extradural space but can progress and become subdural (Fig. 4).

Management of the abscess has evolved over the years. Patients who present without focal neurological symptoms, with normal intracranial pressure, and with no intradural spread of infection can be treated with endoscopic sinus drainage and a six-week course of antibiotics, covering *Staphylococcus aureus* and *Streptococcus*. A repeat CT scan should be performed at the conclusion of the IV therapy to ensure a complete response. If a conservative approach is elected, as previously described, and there is no improvement after 48 hours, then further evaluation is warranted. The patient can either undergo drainage of the epidural abscess by the otolaryngology and neurosurgical service or continue under observation. Drainage of the sinuses can either be done externally or endoscopically. It is expected that there will

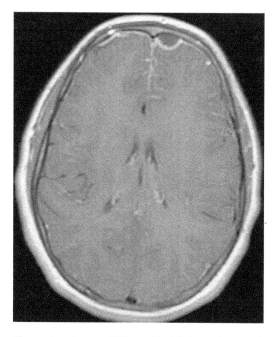

Figure 4   15-year-old boy with left frontal sinus disease with left epidural extension.

be improvement seen by 2 weeks and if this is not occurring then repeat, CT scan should be obtained (28). As with any intracranial infection, if there is any change in mental status or worsening of symptoms, then more aggressive treatment should be initiated.

MENINGITIS

Disease from the ethmoid and sphenoid sinuses is the main sinus involved in patients with meningitis. This is regarded by most as being the most common intracranial complication due to sinonasal disease (31). This is due to the immature arachnoid membrane found in children that allows transmission of bacteria, while the adult arachnoid is relatively resistant. Patients will usually present with headache, neck stiffness, and high fever plus symptoms of sinus infection. Examination will reveal a toxic-appearing patient who is febrile with two-thirds having nuchal rigidity. It is uncommon to see neurological deficits except for the occasional cranial nerve palsy resulting in abnormal extraocular movement. The work-up of the patient should include a CT scan of the sinus and brain. As in most cases where intracranial involvement is suspected, this should be done prior to performing a lumbar puncture. Treatment includes IV antibiotics with close observation.

If improvement is not seen, then surgical drainage of the sinuses is indicated. It is important to note that it is common to see neurological sequelae, mainly sensorineural hearing loss, and mental deficits, after meningitis.

REFERENCES

1. Gamble RC. Acute inflammation of the orbit in children. Arch Ophthalmol 1933; 10:483–497.
2. Ambati BK, Ambati J, Stratton L, Schmidt EV. Periorbital and orbital cellulites before and after the advent of Haemophilus influenza type B vaccination. Ophthalmology 2000; 107(8):1450–1453.
3. Patt BS, Manning SC. Blindness resulting from orbital complications of sinusitis. Otolaryngol Head Neck Surg 1991; 104(6):789–795.
4. Kraus M, Tovi F. Central nervous system complications secondary to otorhinological infections. An analysis of pediatric cases. Int J Pediatric Otorhinolaryngol 1992; 24(3):217–226.
5. Pattisapu JV, Parent AD. Subdural empyemas in children. Pediatr Neurosci 1987; 13(5):251–254.
6. Younis RT, Anand VK, Davidson B. The role of computed tomography and magnetic resonance imaging in patients with sinusitis with complications. Laryngoscope 2002; 112:224–322.
7. Stankiewicz JA, Newell DJ, Park AH. Complications of inflammatory diseases of the sinuses. Otolaryngol Clin North Am 1993; 26:639–655.
8. Hartley BE, Lund VJ. Endoscopic drainage of pediatric sinus mucoceles. Int J Pediatr Otorhinolaryngol 1999; 50(2):109–111.
9. Alvarez RJ, Liu NJ, and Isaacson G. Pediatric ethmoid mucoceles in cystic fibrosis: long term follow-up of reported cases. Ear nose throat J 1997; 76(8): 538–539, 543–546. (Review).
10. Guttenplan MD, Wetmore RF. Paranasal sinus mucocele in cystic fibrosis. Clin Pediatr (Phila) 1989; 28(9):429–430.
11. Kennedy DW, Josephson JS, Zinreich SJ, Mattox DE, Goldsmith MM. Endoscopic sinus surgery for mucoceles. A viable alternative. Laryngoscope 1989; 99(9):885–895.
12. Cohen AR, Gupta N. Mass in the forehead of a three-year-old girl. Pediatr Neurocurg 2002; 37(1):38–47.
13. Wells RG, Sty JR, Landers AD. Radiological evaluation of Pott Puff tumor. JAMA 1986; 255(10):1331–1333.
14. American Academy of Pediatrics. Subcommittee on Management of Sinusitis and Committee on Quality Improvement. Clinical practice guideline: management of sinusitis. Pediatrics 2001; 108(3):798–808.
15. Osguthorpe JD, Hochman M. Inflammatory sinus diseases affecting the orbit. Otolaryngol Clin North Am 1993; 26:657–671.
16. Mitchell R. Bilateral orbital complications of pediatric rhinosinusitis. Arch Otolaryngol Head Neck Surg 2002; 128(8):971–974.
17. American Academy of Pediatrics. Subcommittee on Management of Sinusitis and Committee on Quality Improvement. Clinical practice guideline: management of sinusitis. Pediatrics 2002; 109(5):40.

18. Gutowski WM, Mulbury PE, Hengerer AS, Kido DK. The role of CT scans in managing the orbital complications of ethmoiditis. Int J Pediatr Otorhinolaryngol 1988; 15(2):117–128.
19. Jones NS, Walker JL, Bassi S, Jones T, Punt J. The intracranial complications of rhinosinusitis: can they be prevented? Laryngoscope 2002; 112(1):59–63.
20. Wald ER, Reilly JS, Casselbrant M, Ledesma-Medina J, Milmoe GT, Bluestone CD. Treatment of acute maxillary sinusitis in childhood. A comparative study of amoxicillin and cefaclor. J Pediatr 1984; 104(2):297–302.
21. Skelton R, Maixner W, Isaacs D. Sinusitis induced subdural empyema. Arch Disease Childhood 1992; 67(12):1478–1480.
22. Kaufman DM, Litman N, Miller MH. Sinusitis induced subdural empyema. Neurology 1983; 33(2):123–132.
23. Ong YK, Tan HK. Suppurative intracranial complications of sinusitis in children. Int J of Pediatric Otol 2002; 66:49–54.
24. Lang EE, Curran AJ, Patil N, Walsh RM, Rawluk D. Intracranial complications of acute frontal sinusitis. Clin Otolaryngol 2001; 26:452–457.
25. Bambakidis NC, Cohen AR. Intracranial complications of frontal sinusitis in children: pott's puffy tumor revisited. Pediatric Neurosurgery 2001; 35:82–89.
26. Hoyt DJ, Fisher SR. Otolaryngologic management of patients with subdural empyema. Laryngoscope 1991; 101:20–24.
27. Dolan RW, Chowdhury K. Diagnosis and treatment of intracranial complications. J Oral Maxillofacial Surg 1995; 53(9):1080–1087.
28. Giannoni C, Sulek M, Friedman EM. Intracranial complications of sinusitis: a pediatric series. Am J Rhinol 1998; 12(3):173–178.
29. Clayman GL, Adams GL, Paugh DR, Koopmann CF Jr. Intracranial complications of paranasal sinusitis. A combined institutional review. Laryngoscope 1991; 101(3):234–239.
30. Heran NS, Steinbok P, Cochrane DD. Conservative neurosurgical management of intracranial epidural abscesses in children. Neurosurgery 2003; Vol 53(4m): 893–898.
31. Kraus M, Tovi F. Central nervous system complications secondary to otorhinologic infections. An analysis of 39 pediatric cases. Int J Pediatr Otorhinolaryngol 1992; 24(3):217–226.

6

Pediatric Sinusitis and Comorbidities

Maria T. Peña and George H. Zalzal
*Department of Otolaryngology,
Children's Research Institute, Children's National Medical Center,
Washington, D.C., U.S.A.*

INTRODUCTION

Several pathological conditions are closely associated with pediatric sinusitis. These comorbid conditions frequently exacerbate and may indeed precipitate pediatric sinusitis. Seven of the most common diseases associated with children who present with rhinosinusitis are discussed in detail in this chapter. A common pathophysiological outcome in many of these diseases is obstruction at the ostiomeatal complex (OMC). Edema and inflammation of the OMC, which can be seen with allergic rhinitis, asthma (especially allergic asthma), and extraesophageal reflux disease, can seal off sinus cavities, leading to stagnation of mucous and subsequent bacterial overgrowth. In patients with an immune dysfunction, this situation is exacerbated because of their inability to clear infections effectively. Edema and obstruction worsen as a result of the release of inflammatory mediators by mast cells and eosinophils to combat infection. With long-standing OMC obstruction, an anaerobic mileu develops in the sinus cavities, and chronic exposure to this environment damages the sinus mucosa and cilia, leading to ineffective mucociliary clearance. Patients with ciliary transport defects such as primary ciliary dyskinesia (PCD) and thick mucous secretions such as the ones seen in cystic fibrosis (CF) are further compromised because of their inherent defects in the clearance of the mucous blanket.

ALLERGIC RHINITIS

Pathophysiology

Allergic rhinitis is defined as immunoglobin E-(IgE) mediated inflammation of the sinonasal mucosa, conjunctivae, lacrimal glands, and eustachian tubes (ET). Allergic diathesis is a result of selective activation of a subset of T-helper lymphocytes (TH); TH2 cells, which produce TH2 cytokines (IL-4, IL-5, IL-9, and IL-13) that activate tissue mast cells; IgE producing B cells; and eosinophils (1,2). These cells act in concert with released allergic mediators, resulting in both an early and a late phase allergic response. The binding of an allergen to allergen-specific IgE bound to high affinity Fcε receptors expressed on the surface of tissue mast cells triggers the release of histamine, cyclooxygenase and 5-lipooxygenase products, platelet-activating factor, and cytokines (Fig. 1), which produce the symptoms associated with the early phase of the allergic response (3). These mediators have significant effects on tissues and can result in sneezing, rhinorrhea, pruritus, and edema (4). In the late phase response, there is an influx and activation of eosinophils, neutrophils, platelets, basophils, and macrophages resulting in epithelial shedding, basement membrane thickening, and subepithelial fibrosis (2). The allergic late phase response is associated with hyperresponsiveness to inhaled allergens and lowers the antigen threshold necessary to trigger mast cell degranulation (3).

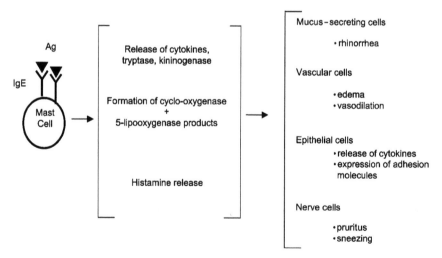

Figure 1 Summary of IgE-mediated allergic inflammation and mast cell mediator release. The release of cytokines, tryptase, kiniogenase, and histamine along with the formation of cyclooxygenase and 5-lipooxygenase products acts on mucus secreting cells, vascular cells, epithelial, and nerve cells to produce symptoms associated with allergy. *Source*: From Ref. 4.

Correlation with Sinusitis

The literature contains many reports regarding association of allergic rhinitis with sinusitis. Furukawa (5) reviewed several of these studies (6–8), noting the minimum concordance of allergy and sinusitis to be 25%, and the maximum concordance to be 70%. These concordance levels are well above the 10 to 15% reported incidence of allergic rhinitis in the pediatric population (9). Although some of the studies reviewed lacked a control group or were biased because of preselection of the patients studied, the high levels of concordance suggest that allergic rhinitis is an important factor predisposing children to sinus disease. Gungor and Corey (10) discuss several mechanisms that could account for this relationship. These include: (i) antigen–antibody reaction causing the release of allergic mediators from inflammatory cells producing allergic symptoms and radiographic evidence of sinonasal inflammation, (ii) the release of major basic protein from eosinophils producing toxic effects on the sinonasal mucosa and cilia, (iii) nasal priming secondary to repeated exposure to the offending allergen lowering the threshold for allergic clinical manifestations, and (iv) reflex-mediated neurogenic reactions caused by neuropeptides that lead to vasodilation and edema of the sinonasal mucosa (10). In addition, viral infections can contribute to the pathophysiology of rhinosinusitis.

Clinical Presentation and Management

Perhaps the most important factor in evaluating a child with allergic rhinitis is a complete medical history of both the family and the patient, as allergy has a strong familial tendency. In fact, if one parent has difficulties with atopy, each of his/her children has a 20 to 40% chance of having allergy. If both parents have allergic problems, the likelihood of any offspring having allergy during their lifetime increases to 50 to 70% (1). Other relevant information includes a history of rhinorrhea, frequent upper respiratory tract infections (URIs), sinusitis, cough, wheezing, behavioral problems including attention deficit hyperactivity disorder (11), otitis media (OM), and eczema. In the infant, a history of colic, formula changes, irritability, nausea, vomiting, diarrhea (especially associated with certain foods), or restless sleeping is pertinent. It is important to remember that the pattern of allergy evolution in children coincides with both their development and their interactions with the environment. Therefore, food hypersensitivity is often seen during infancy and early childhood. As children begin to explore their home environment, inhalant allergens become more problematic, especially sensitivity to house dust mites, molds, and animal danders. Sensitivity to pollens manifests later during school age (1).

Physical examination of pediatric patients with allergic diathesis reveals prominent signs. The eyelids, especially the lower eyelids, demonstrate a puffy, bluish discoloration, which is a consequence of blood being diverted from the inflamed and congested nasal mucosa. When this congestion becomes chronic, it can cause spasms in the muscles of Müller, giving rise to Dennie–Morgan lines, which are creases in the lower eyelid radiating from the area around the medial canthus. The nose can develop a supratip horizontal crease externally. Anterior rhinoscopy frequently demonstrates thin mucoid rhinorrhea, pale boggy mucosa with a bluish appearance, and enlarged inferior turbinates. In children with perennial allergy, the nasal mucosa may appear red and inflamed with thick white mucoid secretions. The lips may be cracked and chapped from chronic mouth breathing secondary to nasal obstruction. The posterior pharynx demonstrates a cobblestone appearance because of lymphoid hyperplasia. The skin around the mouth, chin, and cheeks often has a rash similar to eczema.

Diagnostic testing can be useful in establishing the diagnosis of atopy. The two modalities available are either in vivo skin endpoint titration or in vitro testing. With in vitro testing, the child's serum is incubated with allergens of interest that are linked to a carrier. If reactive, the patient's serum IgE will form IgE-allergen-carrier-complexes that can be either radiolabelled or linked to an enzyme reaction. The former are known as radioactive allergosorbent test (RAST) and the latter are called enzyme-linked immunosorbent assays (ELISAs). In vitro tests are generally considered less sensitive than skin testing and are more expensive. In vivo testing takes advantage of the reactivity of sensitized mast cells to a specific IgE. Extracts of common aeroallergens are applied to the dermis, either by prick, puncture, scratch, or sometimes intradermal injection, bringing the sensitized mast cells and allergens into contact. A positive result is indicated by a wheal and flare. Both positive and negative controls should be employed. Serial dilutions are used to determine end points for immunotherapy. In vivo testing is highly specific and sensitive, providing the most accurate reflection of a patient's allergic status.

Therapeutic management of allergic rhinitis consists of several strategies. Once the antigen(s) of interest are known, a systematic approach can be employed to either eliminate the allergen(s) from the patient's environment altogether, or to take measures to significantly reduce allergen exposure. Second, pharmacologic therapy can be administered, including antihistamines, decongestants, cromolyn, and corticosteroids. If these first two modalities do not offer significant improvement, or if the patient is seriously compromised, then immunotherapy can be considered. The goal of immunotherapy is to switch the immune system from pro-allergic to anti-allergic. The principles of immunotherapy are described in detail by Cook (12). In brief, allergen-specific IgG antibodies are slowly generated while allergen-specific IgE is decreased. Candidates for immunotherapy must have test evidence, preferably in vivo, of IgE antibody to specific allergens. Patients then receive a series of appropriate increasing doses of the specific allergen(s) of interest in a controlled environment until maximum benefits are obtained, usually between three and five years.

ASTHMA

Asthma is an inflammatory disease characterized by reversible airway obstruction that can objectively be measured by pulmonary function tests and hyperreactivity to environmental stimuli. The pulmonary inflammation seen in asthma typically demonstrates infiltration of lung mucosa by eosinophils, activated T cells, and degranulated mast cells. These inflammatory cells and the release of their cellular mediators produce increased glandular secretions, desquamation of epithelial patches, and interstitial edema, closely resembling the pathophysiology of allergic rhinitis. In fact, allergic rhinitis is frequently associated with asthma (13). Many aeroallergens and irritants are known to cause asthma. Aspiration of inflammatory mediators produced by allergy can aggravate the pulmonary inflammation and bronchial hyperresponsiveness seen in asthma (14,15).

Correlation with Sinusitis

Clinical Manifestations and Therapy

Galen first observed that sinusitis could precipitate asthma almost 2000 years ago (16). He postulated that sinonasal secretions dripped from the skull directly into the lungs and recommended nasal irrigation to combat this problem. This was common practice until anatomists could not identify the proposed conduit between the skull and lungs (16). It was not until the twentieth century that the association between the sinuses and lungs was re-explored. Recent investigations have reviewed sinonasal radiographic data that have resulted in both medical and surgical management algorithms for pediatric sinusitis and their impact on asthma. In independent studies, Rachelefsky et al. (17) and Zimmerman et al. (18) noted that 21 to 31% of asthmatic children demonstrated significant sinonasal abnormalities on the basis of air-fluid levels, mucosal thickening greater than 5 mm, and opacification of one or more sinuses on plain films as defined by Schwartz et al. (19). Moreover, Friedman et al. (20) and Goldenhersch et al. (21) found that 60% and 75%, respectively, of asthmatic children with opacification, air-fluid levels, or mucosal thickening (>5 mm) on sinus radiographs had positive bacterial cultures from maxillary sinus aspirates.

Several investigators have researched the effect of aggressive medical therapy on infected paranasal sinuses of asthmatic children. Busco et al. (22) reported 83% of pediatric asthmatic patients improved with medical therapy. However, this group did not include any objective measures of outcomes. In 1983, Cummings et al. (23) conducted a placebo-controlled, double-blind investigation of sinusitis medical therapy (antibiotics, nasal steroids, and decongestants) on asthma. He documented fewer asthmatic symptoms, as demonstrated by decreased use of inhaled bronchodilators and oral steroid therapy in children. However, bronchial reactivity and pulmonary function tests were not improved in these patients. Friedman et al. (20) reported a two-fold improvement in forced expiratory volume 1 (FEV1) following bronchodilator therapy in eight asthmatic children after two to four weeks of antibiotic therapy. Baseline pulmonary function tests were not improved in any of these eight patients. Oliveira et al. (24) and Tsao et al. (25) demonstrated in separate studies that bronchial hyperresponsiveness in asthmatic children with sinusitis dramatically improved with medical therapy for their sinusitis. In contrast to other studies, Rachelefsky et al. (26) observed 20 of 30 children normalized their pulmonary function tests after a two-to-four week course of antibiotics with and without antral lavage. The patients in this study were followed for only three months, and no data is available on long-term results.

Pathophysiological Mechanisms

Several paradigms have been proposed to explain the relationship between asthma and sinusitis. They include: (i) aspiration of mucopurulent secretions from the sinuses into the lower airways, (ii) failure of the obstructed nasal mucosa to filter, heat, and humidify inspired air, therefore providing a greater antigen and irritant burden to the lower respiratory tract, (iii) enhanced vagal stimulation in the infected sinuses causing direct bronchospasm (rhino-sinobronchial reflex), (iv) generation of bacterial toxins that can induce partial beta (β) blockade of effector cells, and (v) aspiration of mediators released from activated inflammatory cells in infected sinuses into the distal airways (14,15).

Both activated $CD4^+$ T lymphocytes and eosinophils have been isolated in asthmatic lung tissue and diseased sinus mucosa (27,28). Messenger RNA for granulocyte-macrophage colony-stimulating factor (GM–CSF) and IL-5, both capable of activating eosinophils, have been found in sinus mucosa of patients with sinusitis (27). These observations suggest that sinusitis can induce asthma by stimulating eosinophil production and activation (14).

Clinical Presentation and Management

Children with asthma and sinusitis present with a history of nasal congestion, rhinorrhea, postnasal drip, and headache. They may wheeze or cough. Coughing without wheezing can also be a sign of bronchial hyperresponsiveness. Many pediatric patients have a waxing and waning course. They do well on antibiotics and steroids, but once medications are decreased or terminated, their clinical status deteriorates. Other patients have an indolent course with very subtle symptoms and signs. Nasal cytology and computed tomography (CT) imaging are useful in assessing the status of sinuses in pediatric asthmatic patients. Most pediatric patients over five years of age with asthma have allergy; these children need a thorough evaluation for allergic rhinitis as well as other manifestations of atopy.

Table 1 Medical Management of Sinusitis in Pediatric Asthmatics

---

Antibiotics
  3–6 weeks
  If no improvement, alternative β lactamase resistant antibiotic
Topical nasal steroid sprays
Prednisone
  If no improvement with nasal steroid sprays
Nasal saline irrigations
Mucolytic agents
Humidifier

Source: From Ref. 29.

Medical therapy for chronic sinusitis in children with asthma is summarized in Table 1. It includes three to six weeks of an appropriate antibiotic(s) (remember β lactase resistance) and topical nasal steroid sprays. Patients also irrigate their nose at least twice daily with saline solution. A short course of oral steroids can be added (29). Pediatric pulmonologists, and in some cases infectious disease specialists, should also be involved in the care of these patients. If these measures provide no relief from the sinonasal symptoms and asthma, and the patient has no other confounding medical problem, e.g., uncontrolled allergy, reflux disease, CF, PCD, or immunodeficient state, then surgical intervention can be considered.

Worth observed that surgical procedures, including antral lavage and adenoidectomy (30), resulted in significant improvement in patient symptoms in moderate to severe asthmatic children. Parsons and Phillips (31) noted that asthmatic children with sinusitis had fewer asthmatic exacerbations and emergency room visits per year after endoscopic sinus surgery. Manning et al. (32) demonstrated significant improvement in asthma (29) and sinusitis symptom scores of 11 and 13 patients, respectively, in a group of 14 children with severe asthma and sinusitis. Both glucocorticoid requirements and hospitalization were also reduced in this group. No significant differences in pulmonary function tests were observed for any patient. Although many patients improved after surgery, a favorable outcome was not uniform. More controlled studies are needed to further elucidate this inconsistent response.

CYSTIC FIBROSIS

Pathophysiology

Cystic fibrosis (CF) is an inherited exocrinopathy characterized by progressive pulmonary obstruction, sinonasal pathology, and pancreatic insufficiency. It is an autosomal recessive disease associated with mutations in the CF transmembrane conductance regulator (CFTR) gene on chromosome 7 (33). The CFTR gene normally encodes for a chloride channel regulated by cyclic adenosine monophosphate (c-AMP) (34,35). In CF, CFTR mutations result in abnormal or non-functional c-AMP-regulated chloride channels causing aberrations in ion transport across epithelial cellular membranes. Specifically in respiratory epithelium, the failure to secrete the chloride ion is thought to result in excessive sodium ion absorption. As more sodium is absorbed into the cells, water will flow out of the airway lumen into the cells. Consequently, mucus viscosity may increase, which in turn could impair mucociliary clearance in both the lower and upper respiratory tracts (36), thus predisposing CF patients to chronic sinus infections. These chronic infections sustain recruitment of inflammatory cells and release of inflammatory mediators, which can further compromise the OMC with edema. Dead inflammatory cells (neutrophils) have also been associated with increases in mucous viscosity (37), further exacerbating this cycle.

Correlation with Sinusitis

Nearly 100% of children with CF will have radiographic evidence of sinusitis by age one. The incidence of nasal polyps in children and adults with CF ranges from 6.7% to 48% (38–41). Recent studies cite a higher prevalence of nasal polyposis; this may reflect the increasing availability of endoscopy, which allows for superior sinonasal examination. However, as discussed by Slavit and Kasperbauer (42), it is unclear if the sinonasal manifestations are directly related to CF or are a consequence of chronic infections.

Several studies have observed that nasal polyps occur more frequently in older CF patients (40,41). These observations support the conclusion that CF patients with nasal polyps constitute a subgroup within this exocrinopathy. Kingdom et al. (43) performed cross sectional analysis of the National CF Patient Registry of the CF Foundation (Bethesda, MD, U.S.A.), and found that two separate genotypes—ΔF508 homozygous and F508/G55ID compound heterozygous—were more prevalent in CF patients with nasal polyps who underwent sinonasal surgery. This subset of patients had a greater percent-predicted forced capacity on pulmonary function tests, less staphylococcal colonization, greater birth weight, and fewer gastrointestinal symptoms as infants (42), all factors which favorably impacted survival.

Clinical Presentation and Management

Although the true incidence of nasal polyposis and chronic sinusitis is unknown, a large proportion of the CF population manifests sinonasal symptoms between the ages of 5 and 14 years (44). Common complaints from families and children include nasal obstruction, mucopurulent rhinorrhea, headache, orbital pain, postnasal drip with cough, severe halitosis, and constant throat clearing. Rhinological examination often demonstrates rhinorrhea and nasal polyps.

Endoscopic examination, if tolerated by the child, should be performed as nasal polyps can be missed on anterior rhinoscopy. Any child with nasal polyps on nasal examination should be evaluated for CF by sweat test and/or genetic analysis. CT imaging of the sinuses can be helpful as CT scans have shown a characteristic appearance of the sinuses in children with CF. Typically, there is a demineralization of the uncinate process and bilateral medial displacement of the lateral nasal wall with a mucocele-like appearance of the maxillary sinuses (45), as shown in Figure 2. CF patients frequently demonstrate frontal sinus hypoplasia or agenesis.

Pediatric CF patients with significant sinonasal symptoms, e.g., nasal obstruction, mucopurulent rhinorrhea, and pain, are candidates for surgical intervention (46). It is important to remember that CF patients are vulnerable to increased bleeding due to vitamin K malabsorption (45) and exacerbation of their obstructive lung pathology from retained secretions during prolonged intubations. Duplechain et al. (47) noted 24% more blood loss in pediatric CF patients undergoing endoscopic sinus surgery. One patient in a series of CF children undergoing sinus surgery reported by Rowe-Jones and MacKay (36) had to be transfused. Pediatric pulmonologists, infectious disease specialists, and nutritionists should evaluate and optimize all pediatric surgical candidates prior to surgery.

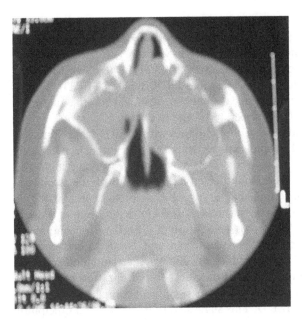

Figure 2 Axial computerized tomography of a 3-year-old patient with cystic fibrosis. Note the mucocele-like appearance of the maxillary sinuses and medial bowing of the lateral nasal walls.

Historically, surgical intervention for children with CF was usually limited to nasal polypectomy. The recidivism rate of the nasal polyps was approximately 60% (47). By adding an ethmoidectomy, recurrence rates for nasal polyposis decreased to 10% (47). However, Rowe-Jones and MacKay (36), in a study population of pediatric CF patients, demonstrated a 50% chance of symptoms returning within two years or sooner. Prior studies either did not define rigorous parameters for follow up intervals or did not report follow up intervals at all. The CF patients most likely to improve or remain symptom-free for an extended period of time were those with mucopurulent rhinorrhea or pain (35). Rowe-Jones and MacKay (36), as well as Madonna et al. (48), noted that sinus surgery did not improve pulmonary function tests. Given the high rate of recidivism of polyposis with nasal obstruction and added surgical risks of CF itself, management techniques that can reduce the need for surgical intervention have been explored. Moss and King (49) have added serial antimicrobial lavage after endoscopic sinus surgery in CF patients and demonstrated reduced recurrences of sinonasal disease, and therefore greater intervals between surgical procedures.

GASTROESOPHAGEAL REFLUX DISEASE

Pathophysiology

Gastroesophageal reflux (GER) is very common in infants and young children. Typically, it resolves over the first year of life (50). GER is physiological in this age group, but when patients manifest symptoms of emesis, choking, failure to thrive, and/or evidence of inflammation of the aerodigestive tract, GER becomes pathological and is known as GER disease (GERD). Transient relaxation of the lower esophageal sphincter permits stomach contents to reflux into the esophagus and upper aero-digestive tract.

During sleep, infants and young children with GERD have decreased rates of swallowing and esophageal peristalsis, which impacts negatively on clearance of gastric reflux (50). Delayed gastric emptying may also predispose or exacerbate GERD in affected individuals. Both the esophago-laryngeal adductor reflex and the laryngeal chemoreflex, implicated in pulmonary and laryngeal manifestations of GERD, have been well documented in the literature (51,52). An association of GERD with nasopharyngitis has also been noted. In 1991, Contencin and Narcy (53) studied 31 children with GERD, 13 of whom had chronic or recurrent rhinitis, or rhinopharyngitis. They found that both the number and duration of episodes of nasopharyngeal acidity below pH 6 was significant compared to the control group that also had GERD. This suggested that, GER could precipitate an inflammatory reaction in the nasopharynx similar to that in the larynx and the distal airways. Acid and pepsin, known to cause injury to the laryngeal epithelium (54), can be extrapolated to also cause nasopharyngeal mucosal injury. However, no direct correlation could be established. Beste et al. (55) also documented acid reflux as high as the choana with radionucleotide scanning and/or double lumen pH probe studies.

Clinical Presentation and Management

Pediatric patients with sinusitis and GER typically present with symptoms outside of the gastrointestinal tract. Sinonasal symptoms frequently encountered in this population include nasal obstruction, mucopurulent rhinorrhea, halitosis, cough, postnasal drip, headache (or behavior suggesting pain, e.g., head-banging, and face-rubbing), and behavior changes (56). Many of these children have been on prolonged courses of antibiotics and topical nasal steroids, and some have even undergone sinonasal surgery without any improvement.

Several options are available to assess these patients for GERD. Upper gastrointestinal series, technetium scintigraphy, esophageal endoscopy with and without biopsy, direct laryngobronchoscopy, bronchoalveolar lavage for lipid-laden macrophages, and continuous extended pH probe have all been used. Continuous pH probe studies are considered the gold standard. This test consists of a probe being placed just below the cricopharyngeus muscle (proximal probe) and another probe placed in the upper esophagus (distal probe) to evaluate the intraluminal acidity over time. Probe placements should be confirmed radiographically. Parameters measured by the probes are: (i) the number of reflux episodes, (ii) duration of the longest reflux episode, (iii) number of reflux episodes longer than 5 minutes, and (iv) the percentage of time with a pH less than 4 (57). Positive results are indicated when the esophageal probe indicates the percent of the study time below pH 4 (known as the reflux index) is 5% or more, there is a reflux episode longer than 5 minutes, and there are two or more episodes of reflux per hour of study time (57,58). No indices have been established for the proximal probe, but in 1999 Halstead (58) demonstrated that more than 10 episodes of reflux into the pharynx in a 24-hour period were associated with GERD. Current criteria at the University of Iowa are one proximal reflux event or more than 1% of the study period with a pH < 4 (59).

Bothwell et al. (60) performed a retrospective review of 28 children treated for reflux disease with sinonasal symptoms. They noted that 89% of these patients improved significantly with reflux therapy, ultimately avoiding an endoscopic sinus procedure. Halstead (58) studied the role of GER in 11 pediatric patients with rhinitis/sinusitis. About 55% of the children who responded to antireflux medication were under two years of age and had a positive pH probe result. The outcomes of these investigations underscore the importance of evaluating and treating "gastronasal" (60) reflux in children with chronic sinusitis, especially patients less than two years of age and in which surgical intervention is being considered.

Table 2 Pharmacologic Therapy in GERD

Prokinetic agents	Metoclopramide	0.1 mg/kg qid
		30 min before meals and qhs
H$_2$ blockers	Cimetidine	Neonate: 5 mg/kg q 6 hr
		Child: 10 mg/kg BID
	Ranitidine	2 mg/kg q 6 hr
	Famotidine	0.5 mg/kg BID
Proton pump inhibitors	Omeprazole	1–2 mg/kg/day
	Lansoprazole	2–3 mg/kg/day

Source: From Refs. 59, 61.

Management of GERD is comprised of conservative measures, pharmacologic agents, and surgical intervention. Conservative management consists of positional therapy, reduced feeding volumes, and thickening of food. Older children should have caffeine products removed from their diets and have no food for at least two hours before bedtime. Pharmacologic therapy consists of prokinetic agents, H$_2$ receptor antagonists, and proton pump inhibitors, which are summarized in Table 2 (59,61). In cases with severe and unresponsive GERD, a Nissen fundopolication might be warranted.

IMMUNE DYSFUNCTION

Pathophysiology

Immune dysfunction manifests as many separate pathological states, but in general, T-cell (cellular immunity) defects are seen with viral, fungal, or protozoal infections and B-cell (humoral immunity) abnormalities are associated with recurrent bacterial infections. Polysaccharides encapsulated organisms such as *Hemophilus influenzae* type B, meningococci, and pneumococci, are particularly virulent in these patients. Combined immunodeficiencies involve both the humoral and cellular arms of the immune system, frequently are inherited in an X-linked or autosomal recessive manner (62), and present with severe infections that are often fatal early in life.

Recurrent and chronic sinopulmonary infections have been associated with humoral immunity defects, especially immunoglobin G (IgG) subclass deficiencies (63–65). IgG subclass immunodeficiency is defined as a serum level of that subclass that is less than two standard deviations of predicted values in a normal age-matched population in a patient with recurrent infections (66). Since IgG$_2$, IgG$_3$, and IgG$_4$ do not reach adult levels until late adolescence and they do so at different rates, the age of the patient as well as the range of particular IgG subclass must be known for meaningful comparison. Furthermore, the patient must be symptomatic. The lack of each IgG subclass has been identified in a healthy, infection-free portion of the population (67).

Clinical Presentation and Management

Children afflicted with IgG subclass deficiencies have a history of recurrent aggressive infections from early on, usually beginning when maternal IgG reaches its nadir at three to six months of age (67). OM, sinusitis, pharyngitis, bronchitis, pneumonia, and other pyogenic infections caused by normal pathogens but not opportunistic organisms is the norm for these patients. Chronic OM usually predates sinusitis and improves with time. Sinusitis, however, is a recurring problem. Meningitis, sepsis, and bronchiectasis are also seen in this population. These patients either do not respond well to appropriate antibiotic therapy or have repeated recurrences of infection shortly after completing adequate medical therapy. Clinical suspicion and laboratory analysis are paramount in making the diagnosis.

Laboratory analyses should include quantitative immunoglobulin levels, IgG subclass levels, a complete blood cell count with differential, and antibody responses to both protein and polysaccharide antigen immunization (68,69). Diphtheria and tetanus antibodies are measured before and 30 days after antigen challenge to assess bacterial protein antibody responses. Selected pneumococcal serotypes (typically 3, 7, 9, and 14) (70) as well as *H. influenzae* type B are measured before and 30 days after administration with polyvalent pneumococcal vaccine and unconjugated *H. influenzae* type B vaccine, respectively (68,69). An appropriate response is considered a greater than two-fold increase in the corresponding antibody titers. IgG and IgG subclass levels that are normal or low normal in a patient with recurrent infections suggests immune dysfunction. These patients should also be evaluated for CF or allergy if clinically indicated.

Shapiro et al. (70) observed 34 out of 61 children with chronic sinusitis to have some combination of immunoglobulin class and subclass deficiencies and immunization hyporesponsiveness. It is one of few studies (70,71) that suggest prevalence of IgG class deficiency in symptomatic pediatric patients. The importance of using antibody response to selected antigens is underscored. The diagnosed would have been missed in 17 of these patients.

Management of these patients consists of prophylactic antibiotics and appropriate immunizations. Even though the children cannot mount an adequate antibody response, a low response may confer enough immunity to prevent serious complications from aggressive infections. Repeated immunizations may also increase antibody response over time. Intravenous immunoglobulin is reserved for patients with severely immunodeficient patients and those with significant obstructive pulmonary disease refractory to aggressive antibiotic management (66).

Endoscopic sinus surgery in immunodeficient pediatric patients with chronic sinusitis despite maximal medical management had an approximately 50% success rate (72), similar to that of adults (68). Most patients were subjectively improved.

PRIMARY CILIARY DYSKINESIA

Pathophysiology

Primary ciliary dyskinesia (PCD) is an autosomal recessive disorder of genetically inherited ciliary motility defects. Kartagner's syndrome (KS), described by Kartagener in 1933 (73), is a subset of PCD and was originally described in four patients with situs inversus, bronchiectasis, sinusitis, and male infertility. Approximately half of patients with PCD have situs inversus and, therefore, KS (74,75). Electron microscopic examination of cilia from tissues obtained from at least two separate anatomical sites in these patients (76) is necessary to make the diagnosis. Electron microscopic examination of ciliated mucosa demonstrates ultrastructural defects of the cilia. The defects reported in the literature include absent or reduced number of inner and outer dynein arms, abnormal cilia length, absent radial spokes, and translocation of microtubule doublet (77–81), although absence of normal dynein arms has been the most reported finding in KS. Because every component of ciliary ultrastructure has been implicated as a cause of PCD, Teknos et al. (82) adapted objective criteria to diagnose congenital ciliary defects from Lurie et al. (77) in an effort to more rigorously define and diagnose PCD. These criteria include dextrocardia, ciliary beat frequency less than 10 Hz, and a mean dynein arm count (inner, outer, or both) of less than two per ciliary cross section counting a minimum of 50 cross sections. Patients who meet at least one of these criteria are diagnosed with PCD and, if dextrocardia is present, KS is diagnosed. When applying these criteria to patients with corroborating clinical evidence of PCD or KS, Teknos et al. (82) reversed diagnoses of normal to PCD or KS in an approximately 35% of the patients studied.

Clinical Presentation and Management

The incidence of PCD ranges from one in 15,000 to one in 30,000 births (83). Generally, patients present during early childhood with a history of multiple recurrent upper and lower airway infections. Sturgess and Turner (84) observed the following clinical manifestations in decreasing frequency: productive cough, sinusitis, OM, situs inversus, bronchiectasis, nasal polyps, and digital clubbing. It is important to suspect PCD/KS in children with the above manifestations. The copious and retained airway secretions and recurrent pneumonitis ultimately result in bronchiectasis which, if not managed aggressively, can lead to irreversible pulmonary fibrosis (82). Both CF and immunodeficient states must also be excluded in these patients.

Chest roentgenogram in these children is abnormal but in a nonspecific manner. Common findings include dextrocardia as seen in Figure 3, hyperinflation of the lung, and/or segmental collapse (85). Segmental collapse is usually seen in the middle and lower lobes as well as the lingula. CT scan of the chest is of benefit to delineate the extent of bronchiectasis. Bronchiectasis, the chronic dilation of bronchi or bronchioles, due to obstruction and chronic inflammation can be seen in the chest CT of a child with KS in Figure 4. Pulmonary function tests in these patients are normal at a young age, but many times progress to a restrictive pattern by the third decade of life (86). Patients with PCD/KS should be aggressively managed with vigorous pulmonary toilet, appropriate antibiotic therapy, intravenous gammaglobulin, and prophylactic measures including vaccination against common virulent organisms. Parsons and Greene (87) reported on endoscopic sinus surgery in three children with PCD. All three patients had significant improvement of their symptoms for at least 30 months. Although demonstrating favorable results, only three patients were studied and follow up was less than three years.

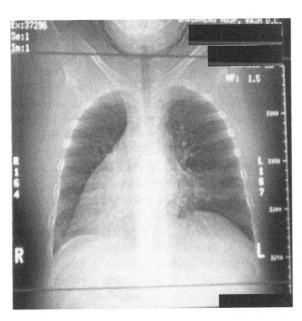

Figure 3 Chest roentgenogram of a child with Kartagener's syndrome demonstrating dextrocardia.

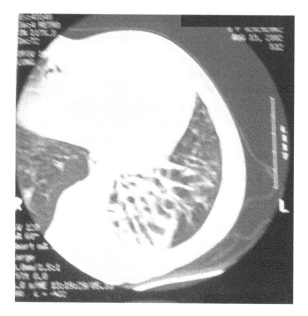

Figure 4 Chest computerized tomogram of a pediatric patient with bronchiectasis and Kartagener's syndrome.

OTITIS MEDIA

Correlations with Sinusitis

Pathophysiology

Otitis media (OM) and sinusitis have very similar pathophysiology. In OM, the three main functions of the ET—ventilation, drainage, and protection (88)—become compromised. When the ET are impaired, negative pressure increases in the middle ear cleft as a result of oxygen absorption from the middle ear space by the vascular respiratory epithelial lining. The secretions produced by the goblet cells and submucosal glands in the middle ear mucosa collect and stagnate, and along with the negative pressure in the middle ear cleft, frequently result in otalgia. The increased negative middle ear pressure creates a suction of the already dysfunctional ET. The net result is a reversal of normal mucociliary flow from the nasopharynx into the middle ear (88). The mucus covering the adenoids and nasopharynx, including the bacterial flora of the nasopharynx, is "sucked" into the middle ear cleft. The mucus within the middle ear space provides growth medium to the nasopharyngeal bacteria. The organisms release toxins, which further compromise the ET, perpetuating this cycle.

In sinusitis, the sinus ostia and transition spaces become dysfunctionally obstructed as a result of inflammation and/or anatomical abnormalities of the nose and sinuses. The sinus mucosa absorbs the oxygen within the sinus cavity and creates a negative pressure environment. The respiratory epithelium lining the sinuses secretes mucus from the goblet cells and glands, which then stagnates in the functionally isolated sinus. The negative pressure within the sinus and obstructed transition space allows normal nasal bacterial flora to flow into the sinus cavity, where the mucus present serves as an excellent growth medium. Again released, bacterial toxins exacerbate the cycle (89). Parsons and Wald (90) discuss the similar pathophysiological processes described above in an elegant manner, drawing parallels between chronic OM and sinusitis.

Microbiology

Many of the pathogens associated with OM have also been recovered in patients with sinusitis. Parainfluenza virus and adenovirus have both been recovered from the nasopharynx of children with OM (91) and children and adults with acute sinusitis (92,93). Middle ear aspirates of acutely infected children include *Streptococcus pneumoniae* (30–40%), *Haemophilus influenzae* non-typable (20%), and *Moraxella catarrhalis* (12%) (94). In acute maxillary sinusitis, these pathogens have been isolated in 30%, 20%, and 20% of cases, respectively (94). Brooke et al. (95) prospectively demonstrated 69% concordance in microbiological findings between middle ear effusions and maxillary sinus aspirates in 32 children with chronic OM and sinusitis at surgery. These studies support a common bacterial/viral etiology for both otitis media and sinusitis.

Clinical Presentation and Management

Children with OM present with either specific symptoms such as otalgia, otorhea, hearing loss, and disturbances of balance and/or general symptoms including irritability, vomiting, and fever. Systemic symptoms are common in acute OM. On physical examination, the appearance of the eardrum will be bulging and erythematous with decreased mobility. In chronic OM with effusion, the tympanic membrane can appear thickened, opaque, and retracted and have impaired mobility. In acute infections, the management is antimicrobial therapy with rigorous follow-up. Restoration of ventilation may be appropriate for chronic processes. The reader is encouraged to review several excellent references in the literature for further detailed management of OM.

ACKNOWLEDGMENTS

The authors would like to acknowledge Mary C. Rose, Ph.D, for editing, and Pawandeep K. Aujla, for manuscript preparation.

REFERENCES

1. Cook PR, Nishioka GJ. Allergic rhinosinusitis in the pediatric population. Otolaryngol Clin North Am 1996; 29:39–56.
2. Bousquet J. Inflammatory mediators in the pathophysiology of rhinitis. Allergy Clin Immunol News Suppl 1994; 3:5–7.
3. Naclerio RM. Allergic rhinitis. N Eng J Med 1991; 325:860–869.
4. Baraniuk JN. Pathogenesis of allergic rhinitis. J Allergy Clin Immunol 1997; 99:763–772.
5. Furukawa CT. The role of allergy in sinusitis in children. J Allergy Clin Immunol 1992; 90:515–517.
6. Savolainen S. Allergy in patients with acute maxillary sinusitis. Allergy 1989; 44:116–122.
7. Rachelefsky GS, Siegel SC, Katz RM, Spector MD, Rohr AS. Chronic sinusitis in children [abstr]. J Allergy Clin Immunol 1991; 87:219.
8. Furukawa CT, Sharpe M, Bierman CW. Allergic patients have more frequent sinus infections than non-allergic patients [abstr]. J Allergy Clin Immunl 1992; 89:332.
9. Fireman P. Allergic rhinitis. In: Bluestone CD, Stool SE, eds. Pediatric Otolaryngology. 2d ed. Philadelphia: WB Saunders, 1990:793–804.
10. Gungor A, Corey JP. Pediatric sinusitis: a literature review with emphasis on the role of allergy. Otolaryngol Head Neck Surg 1997; 116:4–15.
11. Boris M, Mandel FS. Food and additives are common causes of ADHD in children. Ann Allergy 1994; 72:462–468.
12. Cook PR. In vitro testing and immunotherapy. Curr Opin Otolaryngol Head Neck Surg 1994; 2:118–127.
13. Smith JM. Epidemiology and natural history of asthma, allergic rhinitis, and atopic dermatitis (eczema). In: Middleton E Jr, Reed CE, Ellis E, Adkinson NF Jr, Yunginger JW, eds. Allergy Principles and Practic. Vol. 3. St Louis: Mosby, 1998:891–929.
14. Marney SR. Pathophysiology of reactive airway disease and sinusitis. Ann Otol Rhinol Laryngol 1996; 105:98–100.
15. Campanella SG, Asher MI. Current controversies: sinus disease and the lower airways. Pediatric Pulmonology 2001; 31:165–172.
16. Daremberg C. Oeurves Anatomiques, Physiologitues et Medicales de Galien. Vol 1. Paris: Baillere, 1854.
17. Rachelefsky GS, Goldberg M, Katz RM. Sinus disease in children with respiratory allergy. J Allergy Clin Immunol 1978; 61:310.
18. Zimmerman B, Stringer D, Feanny S. Prevalence of abnormalities found by sinus x-rays in childhood asthma: lack of relation to severity of asthma. J Allergy Clin Immunol 1987; 88:268.
19. Schwartz HJ, Thompson JS, Sher TH. Occult sinus abnormalities in the asthmatic patient. Arch Intern Med 1987; 147:2194.
20. Freidman R, Ackerman M, Wald E, Casselbrandt M, Friday G, Fireman P. Asthma and bacterial sinusitis in children. J Allergy Clin Immunol 1984; 74:185.
21. Goldenhersh MJ, Rachelefsky GS, Dudley J. The microbiology of chronic sinus disease in children in respiratory allergy. J Allergy Clin Immunol 1990; 85:1030.

22. Busco L, Fiore L, Frediani T. Clinical and therapeutic aspects of sinusitis in children with bronchial asthma. Int J Pediatr Otorhinolaryngol 1981; 3:287.
23. Cummings NP, Wood RW, Lere JL. Effect of treatment of rhinitis/sinusitis on asthma: results of a double-blind study. Pediatr Res 1983; 17:373.
24. Oliveira CA, Sole D, Naspitz CK, Rachelefsky GS. Improvement of bronchial hyperresponsiveness in asthmatic children treated for concomitant sinusitis. Ann Allergy Asthma Immunol 1997; 79:70–74.
25. Tsao CH, Chen LC, Yeh KW, Huang JL. Comcomitant chronic sinusitis treatment in children with mild asthma. Chest 2003; 123:757–764.
26. Rachelefsky GS, Kartz RM, Siegel SC. Chronic sinus disease with associated reactive airway disease in children. Pediatrics 1984; 73:525.
27. Hamilos DL, Leung DYM, Wood R. Chronic hyperplastic sinusitis: association of tissue eosinophilia with mRNA expression of granulocyte-macrophage colony-stimulating factor and interleukin-13. J Allergy Clin Immunol 1993; 92: 39–48.
28. Corrigan CJ, Kay AB. CD-4 T-lymphocyte activation in acute severe asthma: relationship to disease severity and atopic status. Am Rev Respir Dis 1990; 141:970–977.
29. Corren J, Rachelefsky GS. Interrelationship between sinusitis and asthma. Immunol Allergy Clin North Am 1994; 14:171–184.
30. Worth G. The role of sinusitis in severe asthma. Immunol Allergy Proc 1984; 7:45.
31. Parsons DS, Phillips SC. Functional endoscopic surgery in children: a retrospective analysis of results. Laryngoscope 1993; 103:899–903.
32. Manning SC, Wasserman RL, Silver R, Phillips DL. Results of endoscopic sinus surgery in pediatric patients with chronic sinusitis and asthma. Arch Otolaryngol Head Neck Surg 1994; 10:1142–1145.
33. Riordan JR, Rommens JM, Kerem B. Identification of the cystic fibrosis gene: cloning and characterization of complementary DNA. Science 1989; 245: 1066–1073.
34. Wilschanski M, Zielenski J, Markiewicz D. Correlation of sweat chloride concentration with classes of the cystic fibrosis transmembrane conductance regulator gene mutations. J Pediatr 1995; 127:705–710.
35. Kerem B, Rommens JM, Buchanan. Identification of the cystic fibrosis gene: genetic analysis. Science 1989; 245:1073–1080.
36. Rowe-Jones J, MacKay IS. Endoscopic sinus surgery in the treatment of cystic fibrosis with nasal polyposis. Laryngoscope 1996; 106:1540–1544.
37. Potter JL, Spector S, Matthews LW. Studies on pulmonary secretions, III: the nucleic acids in whole pulmonary secretions from patients with cystic fibrosis, bronchiectasis, and laryngectomy. Am Rev Respir Dis 1969; 99:909–916.
38. Stern RC, Boat TF, Wood RE. Treatment and prognosis or nasal polyps in cystic fibrosis. Pediatrics 1962; 30:389–401.
39. Kerrebijn JDF, Poublon RML, Overbeek SE. Nasal and paranasal disease in adult cystic fibrosis. Eur Resp J 1992; 5:1239–1242.
40. Brihaye P, Clement PAR, Dab I. Pathological changes of the lateral nasal wall in patients with cystic fibrosis. Int J Pediatr Otorhinolaryngol 1994; 28:141–147.

41. Coste A, Gilain L, Roger G. Endoscopic and CT-scan evaluation of rhinosinusitis in cystic fibrosis. Rhinology 1995; 33:152–153.
42. Slavit DH, Kasperbauer JL. Ciliary dysfunction syndrome and cystic fibrosis. In: McCaffrey TV, ed. Systemic Disease and the Nasal Airway. New York: Thieme, 1993:131–149.
43. Kingdom TT, Lee KC, Fitzsimmons SC, Cropp GJ. Clinical characteristics and genotype analysis of patients with cystic fibrosis and nasal polyposis requiring surgery. Arch Otolaryngol Head Neck Surg 1996; 122:1209–1213.
44. Mak GK, Henig NR. Sinus disease in cystic fibrosis. Clin Rev Allergy Immunol 2001; 21:51–63.
45. April MM, Zinreich J, Baroody FM, Naclerio R. Coronal CT scan abnormalities in children with chronic sinusitis. Laryngoscope 1993; 103:985–990.
46. Schulte DL, Kasperbauer JL. Safety of paranasal sinus surgery in patients with cystic fibrosis. Laryngoscope 1998; 108:1813–1815.
47. Duplechain JK, White JA, Miller RH. Pediatric sinusitis: the role of endoscopic sinus surgery in cystic fibrosis and other forms of sinonasal disease. Arch Otolaryngol Head Neck Surg 1991; 117:422–426.
48. Madonna D, Isaacson G, Rosenfield R, Panitch H. Effect of sinus surgery on pulmonary function in patients in cystic fibrosis. Laryngoscope 1997; 107:328–331.
49. Moss RB, King VV. Management of sinusitis in cystic fibrosis by endoscopic surgery and serial antimicrobial lavage. Arch Otolaryngol Head Neck Surg 1995; 121:566–572.
50. Vadenplas Y, Goyvaerts H, Helven R. Gastroesophageal reflux, as measured by 24 hour pH monitoring, in 509 healthy infants screened for risk of sudden infant death syndrome. Pediatrics 1991; 88:834–840.
51. Bauman NM, Sandler AD, Schmidt C. Reflex laryngospasm induced by stimulation of distal esophageal afferents. Laryngoscope 1994; 105:209–214.
52. Bauman NM, Sandler AD, Smith RJ. Respiratory manifestations of gastroesophageal reflux disease in pediatric patients. Ann Otol Rhinol Laryngol 1996; 105:23–32.
53. Contencin P, Narcy P. Nasopharyngeal pH monitoring in infants and children with chronic rhinopharyngitis. Int J Ped Otorhinolaryngol 1991; 22:249–256.
54. Koufman JA. The otolaryngologic manifestations of gastroesopheageal reflux disease (GERD): a clinical investigation of 225 patients using ambulatory 24-hour pH monitoring and an experimental investigation of the role of acid and pepsin in the development of laryngeal injury. Laryngoscope 1991; 101(suppl 53):50–55.
55. Beste DJ, Conley SF, Brown CW. Gastroesophageal reflux complicating choanal atresia repair. Int J Pediatr Otorhinolaryngol 1994; 29:51–58.
56. Parsons D, Phillips S. Functional endoscopic surgery in children: a retrospective analysis of results. Laryngoscope 1993; 103:899–903.
57. Little FB, Koufman JA, Kohut RI. Effect of gastric acid on the subglottic stenosis. Ann Otol Rhinol Laryngol 1985; 94:516–519.
58. Halstead LA. Role of gastroesophageal reflux in pediatric upper airway disorders. Otolaryngol Head Neck Surg 1999; 120:208–214.

59. Bauman N, Smith R. Extra esophageal reflux disease in pediatric patients. Proceedings of Academy of Otolaryngology Instruction Course, Orlando, FL, Sept 21–24, 2003.

60. Bothwell MA, Parsons D, Talbot A, Barbero GJ, Wilder B. Outcome of reflux therapy on pediatric chronic sinusitis. Otolaryngol Head Neck Surg 1999; 121:255–262.

61. Barbero GJ. Gastroesophageal reflux and upper airway disease: a commentary. Otolaryngol Clin North Am 1996; 29:27–37.

62. Sell S. Immunopathology and Immunity. 4th ed. New York: Elsevier, 1987.

63. Berger M. Immunoglobulin G subclass determination in diagnosis and management of antibody deficiency syndromes. J Pediatr 1987; 110:325–328.

64. Heiner DC. Recognition and management of IgG subclass deficiencies. Pediatr Infect Dis 1987; 6:235–238.

65. Smith DA, Nahm MH. IgG subclass deficiency and immunocompetence to carbohydrate antigens. Clin Immunol Newsletter 1987; 8:97–100.

66. Fadal RG. Chronic sinusitis, steroid-dependent asthma and IgG subclass and selective antibody deficiencies. Otolaryngol Head Neck Surg 1993; 109:606–610.

67. Shackelford PG. IgG subclasses: importance in pediatric practice. Pediatr Rev 1993; 14:291–296.

68. Sethi DS, Winkelstein JA, Lederman H, Loury M. Immunologic defects in patients with chronic recurrent sinusitis: diagnosis and management. Otolaryngol Head Neck Surg 1995; 112:242–247.

69. Smith TF. Chronic sinopulmonary infection: is Ig deficiency the cause? J Respir Dis 1989; 10:12–29.

70. Shapiro GG, Virant FS, Furukawa CT, Pierson WE, Bierman CW. Immunologic defects in patients with refractory sinusitis. Pediatrics 1991; 87:311–316.

71. Umetsu DT, Ambrosino DM, Quinti I, Siber GR, Geha RS. Recurrent sinopulmonary infection and impaired antibody response to bacterial capsular polysaccharide antigen in children with selective IgG-subclass deficiency. N Eng J Med 1985; 313:1247–1251.

72. Lusk RP, Polmar SH. Endoscopic ethmoidectomy and maxillary antrostomy in immunodeficient patients. Arch Otolaryngol Head Neck Surg 1991; 117:60–63.

73. Kartagener M. Zur pathologie der bronchietaktiasien: bronkiektasien bei situs viscerum invertus. Beitrage Zur Klinik Der Turberkulose Und Spezifischen 1933; 83:489–501.

74. Afzelius BA, Camner P, Mossenberg B. Acquired ciliary defects compared to those seen in the immotile cilia syndrome. Eur J Respir Dis 1983; 127(suppl):148–150.

75. Camner P, Afzelius BA, Eliasson R, Mossberg B. Relation between abnormalities of human sperm flagella and respiratory tract disease. Int J Androl 1979; 2:211–224.

76. Ehouman A, Pinchon MC, Escudier E. Ultrastructural abnormalities of respiratory cilia: description and quantitative study of respiratory mucosa in a series of 33 patients. Virchows Arch [Cell Pathol] 1985; 48:87–95.

77. Lurie M, Rennert G, Goldberg SL, Rivilin J, Greenberg E, Katz I. Ciliary ultrastructure in primary ciliary dyskinesia and other chronic respiratory conditions: the revelance of microtubular anomalies. Ultrastruct Pathol 1992; 16: 547–553.

78. Rutland J, Cox T, Dewar A, Rehaln M, Cole P. Relationship between dynein arms and ciliary motility in Kartagener's syndrome. Eur J Respir Dis 1983; 4(suppl 128):470–472.

79. Escalier D, Jouannet P, David G. Abnormalities of the ciliary axomenal complex in chidren: an ultrastructural and cinetic study in a series of 34 cases. Biol Cell 1982; 44:271–282.

80. Eavery RD, Nadol JB, Holmes LB. Karagener's syndrome. A blinded, controlled study of cilia ultrastructure. Arch Otolaryngol Head Neck Surg 1986; 112:646–650.

81. Neustein HB, Nickerson R, O'Neal M. Kartagener's syndrome with absence of inner dynein arms of respiratory cilia. Am Rev Respir Dis 1980; 122:979–981.

82. Teknos TN, Metson R, Chasse T, Balercia G, Dickersin GR. New developments in the diagnosis of Kartagener's syndrome. Otolaryngol Head Neck Surg 1997; 116:68–74.

83. Rott HD. Genetics of Kartagener's syndrome. Eur J Respir Dis 1983; 127 (suppl):1–4.

84. Sturgess JM, Turner JAP. Ultrastructural pathology of cilia in the immotile cilia syndrome. Perspect Pediatr Pathol 1984; 8:133–161.

85. Nadel HR, Stringer DA, Levinson H, Turner JAP, Sturgess JM. The immotile cilia syndrome: radiological manifestations. Radiology 1985; 154:651–655.

86. Rossman CM, Forest JB, Ruffin RE, Newhouse MT. Immotile cilia syndrome in individuals with and without Kartagener's syndrome. Am Rev Respir Dis 1980; 121:1011–1016.

87. Parsons DS, Greene, BA. A treatment for primary cilia dyskinesia: efficacy of functional endoscopic sinus surgery. Laryngoscope 1993; 110:12969–12972.

88. Bluestone CD, Klein JO. Otitis Media, atelectasis, and Eustachian tube dysfunction. Pediatr Otolaryngol 1990; 1:320–486.

89. Kennedy DW, Gwaltney JM, Jones JG. Medical management of sinusitis: educational goals and management guidelines. Ann Otol Rhinol Laryngol 1995; 104(suppl 167):22–30.

90. Parsons DS, Wald ER. Otitis media and sinusitis: similar diseases. Pediatric Sinusitis. Otolaryngol Clin North Am 1996; 29:11–25.

91. Klein BS, Folette FR, Yolken RH. The role of respiratory syncytical virus and other viral pathogens in acute otitis media. J Pediatr 1982; 101:16–20.

92. Evans RD, Sydnor JB, Moore WEC. Sinusitis of the maxillary autrum. N Engl J Med 1975; 293:735–739.

93. Wald ER, Reilly JS, Casselbrant MC. Treatment of acute maxillary sinusitis in childhood: a comparative study of amoxicillin and cefaclor. J Pediatr 1984; 104:297–302.

94. Paradise JL. Otitis media in infants and children. Pediatrics 1980; 65:917–943.

95. Brooke I, Yocum P, Shah K. Aerobic and anaerobic bacteriology of concurrent chronic otitis media with effusion and chronic sinusitis in children. Arch Otolaryngol Head Neck Surg 2000; 126:174–176.

7

Pediatric Allergy and Sinusitis

Samantha M. Mucha and Fuad M. Baroody

Section of Otolaryngology-Head and Neck Surgery, Pritzker School of Medicine, University of Chicago, Chicago, Illinois, U.S.A.

INTRODUCTION

Rhinosinusitis is a common disease in both adult and pediatric populations and is thought to affect approximately 14% of the U.S. population (1). Prevalence rates are more difficult to determine in children because of their frequent inability to describe symptoms and the need for parental observation to suspect the diagnosis. It has been estimated that 5 to 10% of all upper respiratory infections are complicated by sinusitis. Since the average child contracts six to eight upper respiratory infections each year, it is clear that the pediatric population is greatly impacted by this disease as well (2).

Allergic rhinitis is also a highly prevalent and burdensome disease. It is estimated that 20% of the population, or more than 40 million Americans, have allergic rhinitis (3). In children and adolescents, reported prevalence rates range from 9% to 42%, depending on whether the rates are self-reported symptoms or physician-diagnosed allergic rhinitis (4–6). The economic impact includes billions of dollars spent on medications, both prescription and over-the-counter, as well as lost days from school or work and decreased productivity (7).

Rhinosinusitis and allergic rhinitis have equally significant social and emotional effects on children as well. Based on child health questionnaires completed separately by children ages 4 to 18 and their parents, children with chronic recurrent rhinosinusitis had significantly more bodily pain and more physical limitations than children who had other chronic illnesses, including attention deficit hyperactivity disorder, psychiatric disorders, juvenile rheumatoid arthritis, epilepsy, and asthma (Fig. 1) (8). Allergic rhinitis has been shown to cause daytime fatigue and loss of sleep in children, which leads to impaired learning (9). Quality of life questionnaires exist for children and adolescents with allergic rhinitis. Specifically, the Pediatric Rhinoconjunctivitis Quality of Life Questionnaire (PRQLQ) and the Pediatric Allergic Disease Quality of Life Questionnaire (PADQLQ) are two validated quality of life measures developed for pediatric patients with seasonal allergic rhinitis (10,11). Allergic rhinitis has also been shown to have a significant impact on quality of life as well as cognitive function in the adult population (12,13). Although there are no published studies comparing quality of life in pediatric allergic and control patients, there has been one study looking at quality of life in Seattle teenagers (14). Of 2084 13- to 14-year olds enrolled, 320 (15%) reported a physician-diagnosis of allergic rhinitis, 176 (8%) reported rhinitis-like symptoms with no confirmation of the diagnosis, and 1588 (75%) were free of allergic symptoms. The teens with allergic rhinitis or rhinitis-like symptoms had significantly higher reports of asthma, limitations in activities, sleep loss, and overall low self-satisfaction. The

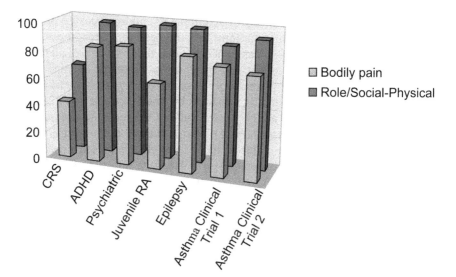

Figure 1 Comparison of chronic recurrent rhinosinusitis to other chronic illnesses using the Child Health Questionnaire-Parent Form 50. Patients with chronic rhinosinusitis had much lower mean scale scores ($p < 0.05$) for bodily pain and role social-physical domains. *Abbreviations*: ADHD, attention deficit hyperactivity disorder; RA, rheumatoid arthritis. *Source*: Adapted from Ref. 8.

investigators also point out that the teens with rhinitis-like symptoms were more likely to have impaired quality of life than either of the other groups. This is probably because those teens were not properly diagnosed and thus were not treated, whereas the already diagnosed group was receiving treatment for their allergies.

Patients with rhinosinusitis often suffer from allergic rhinitis, and the link between these two entities has been well established. This chapter will discuss the pathophysiology of both diseases, provide evidence for the link between them in the pediatric population, and explore how the treatment of allergic rhinitis may decrease the burden of rhinosinusitis.

PATHOPHYSIOLOGY

Allergic Rhinitis

The pathophysiology of allergic rhinitis is complex and describing it in full detail is beyond the scope of this chapter. In brief, it is an IgE-mediated process that involves an initial sensitization to a specific allergen followed by an inflammatory reaction triggered by subsequent exposure to the allergen. During the sensitization process, allergen deposited on the nasal mucosa is engulfed by antigen-presenting cells (macrophages, Langerhans and dendritic cells, and B lymphocytes) and is degraded within their phagolysosomes. Portions of the antigen are then exteriorized on the surfaces of antigen-presenting cells and are presented by class-II MHC molecules to T-helper cells. The IL-1-activated T-helper cells then secrete cytokines, which promote the growth and differentiation of other cells involved in the immune response. Cells of the TH2 subgroup of helper cells recognize the allergen and induce B cell isotype switching and allergen-specific IgE production by releasing cytokines, namely IL-4 (15). The allergen-specific IgE molecules are then attached to many different cells, with mast cells and basophils being the most important in this process (16).

When an individual is later exposed to the allergen to which an individual is sensitized, the IgE receptors on mast cells in the nasal mucosa become cross-linked by the allergen, leading to the release of inflammatory mediators such as histamine, prostaglandins, leukotrienes, and others (16,17). These mediators, in turn, act on the nasal end organs to produce the symptoms of allergic rhinitis, namely sneezing, itching, rhinorrhea, and nasal congestion. These events occur within minutes of exposure and are termed the early allergic response. After this almost immediate response, about 50% of patients develop a late allergic response (16). This response occurs 3 to 12 hours after allergen exposure despite the absence of repeat exposure. The late phase response is primarily characterized by nasal congestion, with a smaller occurrence of rhinorrhea and sneezing. Whereas cellular influx is not prominent during the early response, an influx of neutrophils, eosinophils, and basophils into nasal secretions and tissues characterizes the late allergic inflammatory response (18,19). Eosinophils increase significantly in nasal lavage fluids and the mucosa after nasal allergen challenge (20) and have been shown to peak in lavage fluids six to eight hours after challenge (21). Furthermore, multiple studies using lavage and biopsy to examine nasal secretions and the nasal mucosa, respectively, have shown an influx of eosinophils during the allergy season (15). Basophils have also been found in nasal lavages, and both basophils and mast cells have been demonstrated in epithelial scrapings or mucosal biopsies during seasonal exposure (22). Inflammatory cytokines are also involved in the inflammation associated with allergic rhinitis. The TH2 lymphocyte subset seems to predominate and these lymphocytes secrete IL-4, IL-5, and IL-13, among other cytokines, which promote the production of IgE and the survival of eosinophils in tissues. The presence of these cytokines in allergic patients has been demonstrated in nasal mucosal biopsies after allergen challenge or during natural allergen exposure through cells expressing either the specific proteins or their mRNA (23,24).

This inflammatory response, a hallmark of allergic rhinitis, leads to a heightened state of reactivity of the nasal mucosa such that during the season, allergic patients become more sensitive to further allergen exposure (priming) and to irritants such as environmental pollution, cigarette smoke, and strong odors (non-specific hyperresponsiveness). This has been demonstrated in the laboratory setting by progressively increasing nasal responsiveness to repetitive allergen exposure (25) and increasing responsiveness to nonspecific stimuli, such as histamine and methacholine, after previous allergen exposure (26).

Rhinosinusitis

Acute rhinosinusitis is usually a short-lasting disease and most commonly occurs as a sequalae of a viral upper respiratory tract infection with secondary bacterial infection of the paranasal sinus cavities. The most common organisms cultured in such cases in children and their respective prevalences are as follows: *Streptococcus pneumoniae* (35–42%), *Hemophilus influenzae* (21–28%), *Moraxella catarrhalis* (21–28%), anaerobes (3–7%), and *S. pyogenes* (3–7%).

The role of bacteria in chronic rhinosinusitis is less well established. A variety of organisms have been cultured from the paranasal sinuses in these situations and include α-hemolytic *Streptococcus*, *S. aureus*, *S. pneumoniae*, *H. influenzae*, *M. catarrhalis*, and anaerobes. The relationship between these organisms and clinical disease is not clearly established and is confounded by the fact that most of these organisms are cultured at the time of surgery after prolonged antibiotic treatment and that these might represent colonization of functionally impaired sinus cavities.

Investigations into the cellular constituents of the paranasal sinuses in chronic rhinosinusitis ± polyposis have begun to shed some light on the contribution of chronic inflammation to this entity. Eosinophils play a key role in this inflammatory process. Children with chronic rhinosinusitis were found to have significantly more eosinophils in their sinus mucosa than controls (27). This suggests that eosinophilic inflammation plays an important role in the pathophysiology of chronically inflamed sinus tissue. It is speculated that the proteins produced by eosinophils, such as major basic protein, are deleterious to the epithelial lining and promote chronic inflammation. T lymphocytes are also important in chronic rhinosinusitis. The TH2 lymphocyte cytokine profile predominates in the sinus mucosa of patients with this disease. An increased number of $CD4^+$ T lymphocytes were found in the sinus mucosa of children with chronic rhinosinusitis when compared to normal adult sphenoid sinus mucosa (28). Studies in adults also suggest that patients with chronic rhinosinusitis have higher numbers of inflammatory cytokines present in their tissues than control inferior turbinate mucosa (29). Adult patients with chronic rhinosinusitis and concomitant allergic rhinitis had a higher number of inactive and activated eosinophils in the sinus mucosa when compared to patients with chronic rhinosinusitis and no allergic rhinitis (30). When maxillary sinus biopsies from adults with chronic hyperplastic rhinosinusitis and a history of allergy were compared to those from patients with chronic rhinosinusitis and no allergy or to healthy controls, patients with chronic rhinosinusitis and allergy had a significantly higher number of cells expressing IL-4 and IL-5 (31).

The Pathophysiologic Link between Allergic Rhinitis and Rhinosinusitis

Several theories have been postulated to explain the link between these two diseases. The first theory is that the nasal edema that is caused by allergic rhinitis inhibits the natural drainage of the paranasal sinuses, possibly secondary to decreased mucociliary activity or direct obstruction of the natural ostia. The secretions that cannot be drained from the sinuses then become a nidus for bacterial infection. A study done by our group showed that 6 out of 10 ragweed-allergic adults had sinus mucosal thickening on CT scan during the ragweed season (32). All patients were treated with intranasal steroids and five of the six patients with mucosal abnormalities had repeat CT scans after the ragweed season. In all five patients, the mucosal abnormalities persisted despite significant improvement in both symptoms and quality of life scores. These data do not support this theory. However, a study by Crystal-Peters et al. evaluated conditions in more than 40,000 seasonal allergic rhinitis adult and pediatric patients in a retrospective cross-sectional analysis and compared in-season to out-of-season incidence of these conditions (33). Conditions evaluated included asthma, sinusitis, migraines, and otitis media, which were identified through medical claims. The group found that all of these conditions occurred more frequently during the outdoor allergy season than outside the season. These data support the edema theory, but the study only considered diagnoses made without addressing how the diagnoses were made or whether they were confirmed with objective testing.

A second theory is that allergen penetrates the paranasal sinuses as well as the nasal cavity, leading to a direct inflammatory response within the sinuses. There is evidence to both support and refute this theory. Gwaltney et al. demonstrated the accumulation of fluid in the paranasal sinuses after having subjects blow their noses strongly (34). Gentle nose blowing did not result in nasal fluids entering the sinuses. Thus, allergen that is contained within nasal secretions could theoretically be forced into the sinuses during vigorous nose-blowing. Against this hypothesis is the study by Adkins et al. who scanned subjects after they inhaled radiolabeled allergen (35). No radiolabeled allergen was seen within the sinuses. This makes sense given the narrow passageways between the nasal cavity and paranasal sinuses. Also, mucociliary transport moves mucus toward the sinus ostia and out of the sinuses (36). Therefore, any allergen that somehow migrated near the ostium of a paranasal sinus would be transported along with the mucus away from that sinus.

A third theory is that allergic rhinitis leads to a state of systemic allergic inflammation with possible migration of activated leukocytes from the circulation to other airway sites such as the sinuses and the lungs. Braunstahl et al. performed two experiments that support this idea of local allergen exposure causing distant inflammatory responses. The first study involved segmental bronchial provocation in allergic and non-allergic subjects (37). The group performed nasal and bronchial biopsies before and after segmental bronchial provocation and compared the inflammatory responses at the two sites. The allergic subjects had significantly increased numbers of eosinophils in the lamina propria of the nasal mucosa and increased IL-5 expression in the nasal epithelium along with the bronchial inflammation that was expected. The other study involved nasal allergen provocation in non-asthmatic subjects with and without allergy (38). As in the first study, nasal and bronchial biopsies were performed before and after nasal provocation. There were significantly increased levels of eosinophils and endothelial adhesion molecules in the nasal and bronchial mucosa in the allergic, but not the non-allergic, subjects. These studies provide supporting evidence for distant airway inflammation after a local allergen exposure and could partially account for the high rate of rhinosinusitis seen in allergic patients.

One final theory deserves to be mentioned. Neural reflexes could play a role in the inflammation that occurs in areas not directly exposed to allergen.

Specifically, an allergen that causes inflammation in the nasal cavity may trigger sensory afferent nerves and generate an axonal or central neuronal reflex to the paranasal sinuses and lead to an inflammatory response within these sinuses.

Clinical Association

Many studies have demonstrated a close clinical association between rhinosinusitis and allergic rhinitis. Patients with rhinosinusitis have been noted to have a higher incidence of allergy than the general population and, conversely, both adult and pediatric allergic patients tend to have a higher incidence of rhinosinusitis. Savolainen studied the prevalence of allergy in young adults with acute maxillary sinusitis confirmed with radiographs and sinus aspirates (39). Allergy was diagnosed by a combination of positive skin test, allergic symptoms, and nasal secretion eosinophilia, and the allergic subjects were compared to an age-matched control group without any sinusitis symptoms in whom no sinus radiographs were obtained. Out of 224 patients with confirmed acute maxillary sinusitis, 56 (25%) were allergic and another 14 (6.3%) had probable allergy, defined as a marked positive skin test to at least two allergens without accompanying symptoms. Of 103 control patients, only 17 (16.5%) had definite allergy, while three (2.9%) had probable allergy. The difference between the groups was statistically significant. Another early study conducted by Rachelefsky et al. assessed the incidence of sinus disease in children referred for allergy evaluation (40). Seventy children (3 to 16 years old) with confirmed atopy, 60 of whom had allergic rhinitis and bronchial asthma and 10 of whom had allergic rhinitis only, had sinus radiographs performed. Thirty-seven patients (53%) had some sinus abnormality, 15 (21%) of whom had complete opacification of one or more sinuses. Furthermore, other studies report that up to 54–84% of adults with chronic rhinosinusitis had allergic rhinitis symptoms or positive allergy tests (41,42), and there was a 25–75% concordance of these two diseases in children (43).

On the other hand, clinical studies have shown that patients with allergic rhinitis have a higher prevalence of rhinosinusitis than the general population. Over 50% of children with perennial allergic rhinitis have abnormal sinus radiographs (40). In a separate study, patients with chronic rhinosinusitis and allergic rhinitis had significantly more severe sinus CT scan scores than those without allergic rhinitis (44). One should remember, however, that the severity of CT scores has generally not been shown to correlate with severity of patient symptoms (45–47).

In children, a positive correlation between allergic rhinitis and rhinosinusitis has also been shown. Abnormal sinus radiographs have been demonstrated in more than 50% of allergic children; more specifically, up to 53% of children with seasonal allergic rhinitis had abnormal sinus radiographs during the allergy season (40,48). Huang studied the frequency of sinusitis in children with perennial allergic rhinitis and seasonal allergic rhinitis (49). This study found that 46% of children with perennial allergic rhinitis had two or more episodes of sinusitis annually, while only 4% of children with seasonal allergic rhinitis had as many sinusitis episodes, regardless of the season. Although there was no control group cited, this study does raise the possibility that perennial allergic rhinitis is more strongly associated with rhinosinusitis than seasonal allergic rhinitis, perhaps because of the more chronic nature of perennial disease.

Improving Rhinosinusitis Through Treatment of Allergic Rhinitis

The mainstay of treatment of acute rhinosinusitis remains antibiotic therapy. Adjunctive therapies have previously included local and systemic decongestants, though these have not been consistently proven to be helpful. Intranasal corticosteroids have also been studied as an adjunct in the treatment of rhinosinusitis. Meltzer et al. first looked at the effect of flunisolide in addition to antibiotics in the treatment of acute rhinosinusitis in adults more than a decade ago (50). They found a small but significant improvement in symptoms for patients who, in addition to a 21-day course of antibiotics, used intranasal flunisolide when compared to intranasal placebo. When antibiotics were discontinued, patients remained on either intranasal flunisolide or placebo for an additional four weeks. During that phase of the study, patients who had received placebo were more likely to have a recurrence of their rhinosinusitis than those who had received flunisolide. The recurrences tended to be more severe and occurred earlier than in the flunisolide group.

A similar study using intranasal mometasone or placebo in addition to a 21-day course of amoxicillin-clavulanate potassium in adults with acute rhinosinusitis has been completed recently (51). The diagnosis of acute rhinosinusitis was based on symptoms and evidence of mucosal thickening, opacification, or air-fluid level in at least one sinus on coronal CT scan. CT scans were performed before treatment and after the 21-day antibiotic course. Compared to the patients receiving intranasal placebo, symptoms of headache, facial pain, and congestion were significantly improved over the 21-day period in the mometasone group. Other reported symptoms of rhinorrhea, postnasal drip, and cough were also improved in the mometasone group compared to placebo, but the changes were not statistically significant. Repeat CT scores were lower for patients who received mometasone, with 49% of the mometasone group having a score of zero compared to only 30% of the placebo group. This difference was not statistically significant. The dose of mometasone used in this study was 400 µg bid, which is eight times higher than that normally used in the treatment of allergic rhinitis. One of the limitations of both studies mentioned above is that neither substratified their subjects according to their allergic status. It is, therefore, unclear whether the use of intranasal corticosteroids had a differential benefit for patients with concomitant allergic rhinitis as opposed to nonallergic patients.

The use of intranasal corticosteroids has also been studied in the pediatric population as an adjunct to antibiotic therapy for acute sinusitis. Eighty-nine patients (ages 1 to 15 years) with acute rhinosinusitis, diagnosed by history and in most cases a positive Waters' X-ray (performed in 79 of 89 patients), were randomized in a double-blind fashion to receive a 3-week course of either budesonide or placebo nasal spray in addition to amoxicillin/clavulanate (52). The budesonide group showed significant improvement in cough and nasal discharge scores at the end of the second week when compared to placebo. The placebo group did have a significant decrease in the cough and nasal discharge scores, but these were documented over weeks two and three, instead of dropping precipitously during the second week of treatment as in the budesonide group.

There are no studies to date evaluating the use of intranasal or systemic corticosteroids in pediatric patients with chronic rhinosinusitis. In adults, the effectiveness of intranasal and, in a separate study, intrasinus corticosteroids in chronic rhinosinusitis patients has been evaluated. The first study compared fluticasone to placebo spray in 22 patients with CRS (53). The group recorded symptom and endoscopic scores and also performed acoustic rhinometry and middle meatal swabs at the start of the trial and at 8 and 16 weeks. There were no significant differences found for any of these measures between the groups. The study was limited, however, because follow-up time was short, the number of subjects was small, and it was unclear whether antibiotics were used. The authors did emphasize the fact that the use of intranasal corticosteroids did not increase patients' risk of developing an acute infection, indicating that the probable downregulation of cytokines by corticosteroids may help prevent exacerbations of chronic rhinosinusitis. Larger studies need to be done in this area. The second study evaluated intrasinus instillation of budesonide versus placebo in 26 patients with chronic rhinosinusitis who had persistent symptoms after undergoing endoscopic sinus surgery (54). The patients all had skin-test-confirmed perennial allergic rhinitis and were randomized to instill budesonide or placebo into the maxillary sinus for three weeks. Eleven of 13 budesonide patients had a greater than 50% symptom improvement that lasted 2 to 12 months, but only 4 of 13 placebo patients had a greater than 50% symptom improvement that lasted less than two months, which was reported as a significant difference.

These studies provide evidence that adding intranasal steroids to antibiotics provides some benefit over antibiotics alone. Most of the benefit, however, seems to be related to improvement of nasal symptoms. Further studies should be done to determine whether the addition of intranasal corticosteroids can shorten the length of antibiotics needed or decrease the recurrence rate and to specifically look at the usefulness of adding intranasal steroids to the treatment of rhinosinusitis in allergic patients.

To evaluate the role of antihistamines in the treatment of rhinosinusitis, Braun et al. compared the use of loratadine and placebo in 139 allergic patients with acute episodes of rhinosinusitis (55). All patients received amoxicillin-clavulanate (2 g/day) for 14 days as well as prednisone at 40 mg/day for four days followed by 20 mg/day for four days. The patients were randomized to receive either loratadine (10 mg/day) or placebo starting the same day as the other medications and continuing through 28 days. Symptom scores, including rhinorrhea, nasal obstruction, sneezing, nasal itching, and cough, were reported daily by the patients and physician-assessed symptoms were recorded at the beginning and end of the treatment period. At the end of 28 days, there was a significant reduction in symptom scores in the patients taking loratadine. In the loratadine group, rhinorrhea at day 14 and nasal obstruction at day 28 were significantly improved compared to the placebo group. The results from this study support the benefit of using an antihistamine as an adjunct to antibiotic therapy to treat rhinosinusitis. However, very little data exist about the role of antihistamines in the treatment of rhinosinusitis. Other studies should be done to confirm these results and to investigate the role of other second-generation, non-sedating antihistamines or other anti-inflammatory medications in acute rhinosinusitis.

SUMMARY

Allergy and rhinosinusitis have similar pathophysiological mechanisms and are closely related clinical entities. Preliminary studies suggest that adjunctive therapies including intranasal steroids and antihistamines may be useful in the treatment of rhinosinusitis through treatment of the underlying allergic disease. More research into the pathophysiology of the relationship between allergic rhinitis and sinusitis will hopefully lead to the development of new venues for therapeutic intervention aimed at ameliorating the conditions of millions of children suffering from these disease entities.

REFERENCES

1. Slavin RG. Changing prevalence of allergic rhinitis and asthma. JAMA 1997; 289:1849–1854.
2. Aitken M, Taylor JA. Prevalence of clinical sinusitis in young children followed up by primary care pediatricians. Arch Pediatr Adolesc Med 1998; 152:244–248.
3. Skoner DP. Allergic rhinitis: definition, epidemiology, pathophysiology, detection, and diagnosis. J Allergy Clin Immunol 2001; 108:S2–S8.

4. Arrighi HM, Maier WC, Redding GJ, Morray RN, Llewellyn CE. The impact of allergic rhinitis in Seattle school children (abstract). J Allergy Clin Immunol 1995; 95:192.

5. Siegel SC. Clinical aspects. In: Mygind N, Naclerio RM, eds. Allergic and non-allergic rhinitis. Copenhagen, Denmark: Munksgaard; 1993:174–183.

6. Wright AL, Holberg CJ, Martinez FD, Halonen M, Morgan W, Taussig LM. Epidemiology of physician-diagnosed allergic rhinitis in childhood. Pediatrics 1994; 94:895–901.

7. Baroody FM. Allergic rhinitis: Broader disease effects and implications for management. Otolaryngol Head Neck Surg 2003; 128:616–631.

8. Cunningham MJ, Chiu EJ, Landraf JM, Gliklich RE. The health impact of chronic recurrent rhinosinusitis in children. Arch Otolaryngol Head Neck Surg 2000; 126:1363–1368.

9. Simons FE. Learning impairment and allergic rhinitis. Allergy Asthma Proc 1996; 17:185–189.

10. Juniper EF, Howland WC, Roberts NB, Thompson AK, King DR. Measuring quality of life in children with rhinoconjunctivitis. J Allergy Clin Immunol 1998; 101(2 Pt 1):163–170.

11. Roberts G, Hurley C, Lack G. Development of a quality-of-life assessment for the allergic child or teenager with multisystem allergic disease. J Allergy Clin Immunol 2003; 111(3):491–497.

12. Bousquet J, Bullinger M, Fayol C, Marquis P, Valentin B, Burtin B. Assessment of quality of life in patients with perennial allergic rhinitis with the French version of the SF-36 Health Status Questionnaire. J Allergy Clin Immunol 1994; 94:182–188.

13. Marshall PS, Colon EA. Effects of allergy season on mood and cognitive function. Ann Allergy 1993; 71:251–258.

14. Arrighi HM, Cook CK, Redding GJ. The prevalence and impact of allergic rhinitis among teenagers. J Allergy Clin Immunol 1996; 97(1 Pt 3):430.

15. Baroody FM, Naclerio RM. Allergic rhinitis. In: Rich RR, Fleisher TA, Shearer WT, Kotzin B, Schroeder HW, eds. Clinical Immunology, Principles and Practice. 2nd ed. Mosby International Limited, 2001:48.1–48.13.

16. Naclerio RM. Allergic rhinitis. N Engl J Med 1991; 325:860–869.

17. Baroody FM, Ford S, Proud D, Kagey-Sobotka A, Lichtenstein L, Naclerio RM. Relatioship between histamine and physiological changes during the early response to nasal antigen provocation. J Appl Physiol 1999; 86:659–668.

18. Bascom R, Pipkorn U, Lichtenstein LM, Naclerio RM. The influx of inflammatory cells into nasal washings during the late response to antigen challenge. Effect of systemic steroid pretreatment. Am Rev Respir Dis 1988; 138:406–412.

19. Bascom R, Wachs M, Naclerio RM, Pipkorn U, Galli SJ, Lichtenstein LM. Basophil influx occurs after nasal antigen challenge: effects of topical corticosteroid pretreatment. J Allergy Clin Immunol 1988; 81:580–589.

20. Lim MC, Taylor RM, Naclerio RM. The histology of allergic rhinitis and its comparison to cellular changes in nasal lavage. Am J Respir Crit Care Med 1995; 151:136–144.

21. Bascom R, Pepkorn U, Proud D, Dunnette S, Gleich GJ, Lichtenstein LM, Naclerio RM. Major basic protein and eosinophil-derived neurotoxin

concentrations in nasal-lavage fluid after antigen challenge; effect of systemic corticosteroids and relationship to eosinophil influx. J Allergy Clin Immunol 1989; 84:338–346.

22. Okuda M, Ohtsuka H, Kawabori S. Basophil leukocytes and mast cells in the nose. Eur J Respir Dis Suppl 1983; 128:7–15.

23. Nouri-Aria KT, O'Brien F, Noble W, Jabcobson MR, Rajakulasingam K, Durham SR. Cytokine expression during allergen-induced late nasal responses: IL-4 and IL-5 mRNA is expressed early (at 6 hr) predominantly by eosinophils. Clin Exp Allergy 2000; 30:1709–1716.

24. Cameron L, Hamid Q, Wright E, Nakamura Y, Christodoulopoulos P, Muro S, Frenkeil S, Lavigne F, Durham S, Gould H. Local synthesis of epsilon germline gene transcripts, IL-4, and IL-13 in allergic nasal mucosa after ex vivo allergen exposure. J Allergy Clin Immunol 2000; 106:46–52.

25. Wachs M, Proud D, Licktenstein, Kagey-Sobotka A, Norman PS, Naclerio RM. Observations on the pathogenesis of nasal priming. J Allergy Clin Immunol 1989; 84(4 Pt 1):492–501.

26. Walden SM, Proud D, Lichtenstein LM, Kagey-Sobotka A, Naclerio RM. Antigen-provoked increase in histamine reactivitiy: observations on mechanisms. Am Rev Respir Dis 1991; 144(3 Pt 1):642–648.

27. Baroody FM, Hughes CA, McDowell P, Hruban R, Zinreich SJ, Naclerio RM. Eosinophilia in chronic childhood sinusitis. Arch Otolaryngol Head Neck Surg 1995; 121:1396–1402.

28. Driscoll PV, Naclerio RM, Baroody FM. CD4+ lymphocytes are increased in the sinus mucosa of children with chronic sinusitis. Arch Otolaryngol Head Neck Surg 1996; 122:1071–1076.

29. Hamilos DL, Leung DY, Wood R, Meyers A, Stephens JK, Barkans J, Meng Q, Cunningham L, Bean DK, Kay AB, Hamid Q. Chronic hyperplastic sinusitis: association of tissue eosinophilia with mRNA expression of granulocyte-macrophage colony-stimulating factor and interleukin 3. J Allergy Clin Immunol 1993; 92: 39–48.

30. Suzuki M, Watanabe T, Suko T, Mogi G. Comparison of sinusitis with and without allergic rhinitis: characteristics of paranasal sinus effusion and mucosa. Am J Otolaryngol 1999; 20:143–150.

31. Hamilos DL, Leung DY, wood R, Cunningham L, Bean DK, Yasruel Z, Schotman E, Hamid Q. Evidence for distinct cytokine expression in allergic versus nonallergic chronic sinusitis. J Allergy Clin Immunol 1995; 96:537–544.

32. Naclerio RM, DeTineo ML, Baroody FM. Ragweed allergic rhinitis and the paranasal sinuses: a computed tomographic study. Arch Otolaryngol Head Neck Surg 1997; 123:193–196.

33. Crystal-Peters J, Neslusan CA, Smith MW, Togias A. Health care costs of allergic rhinitis-associated conditions vary with allergy season. Ann Allergy Asthma Immunol 2002; 89:457–462.

34. Gwaltney JM Jr, Hendley JO, Phillips CD, Bass CR, Mygind N, Winther B. Nose blowing propels nasal fluid into the paranasal sinuses. Clin Infect Dis 2000; 30:387–391.

35. Adkins TN, Goodgold HM, Hendershott L, Slavin RG. Does inhaled pollen enter the sinus cavities? Ann Allergy Asthma Immunol 1998; 81:181–184.

36. Stammberger H. Endocopic endonasal surgery-concepts in treatment of recovering rhinosinusitis. Part I: Anatomic and pathophysiological considerations. Otolaryngol Head Neck Surg 1986; 94:143–147.
37. Braunstahl GJ, Kleinjan A, Overbeek SE, Prins JB, Hoogsteden HC, Fokkens WJ. Segmental bronchial provocation induces nasal inflammation in allergic rhinitis patients. Am J Respir Crit Care Med 2000; 161(6):2051–2057.
38. Braunstahl GJ, Overbeek SE, KleinJan A, Prins JB, Hoogsteden HC, Fokkens WJ. Nasal allergen provocation induces adhesion molecule expression and tissue eosinophilia in upper and lower airways. J Allergy Clin Immunol 2001; 107:469–476.
39. Savolainen S. Allergy in patients with acute maxillary sinusitis. Allergy 1989; 44:116–122.
40. Rachelefsky GS, Goldberg M, Katz RM, Boris G, Gyepes MT, Shapiro MJ, Mickey MR, Finegold SM, Siegel SC. Sinus disease in children with respiratory allergy. J Allergy Clin Immunol 1978; 61:310–314.
41. Benninger M. Rhinitis, sinusitis and their relationships to allergies. Am J Rhinol 1992; 6:37–43.
42. Emanuel IA, Shah SB. Chronic rhinosinusitis: allergy and sinus computed relationships. Otolaryngol Head Neck Surg 2000; 123:687–691.
43. Furukawa CT. The role of allergy in sinusitis in children. J Allergy Clin Immunol 1992; 90:515–517.
44. Ramadan HH, Fornelli R, Ortiz AO, Rodman S. Correlation of allergy and severity of sinus disease. Am J Rhinol 1999; 13:345–347.
45. Jones NS. CT of the paranasal sinuses: a review of the correlation with clinical, surgical and histopathological findings. Clin Otolaryngol 2002; 27:11–17.
46. Mudgil SP, Wise SW, Hopper KD, Kasales CJ, Mauger D, Fornadley JA. Correlation between presumed sinusitis-induced pain and paranasal sinus computed tomographic findings. Ann Allergy Asthma Immunol 2002; 88:223–226.
47. Krouse JH. Computed tomography stage, allergy testing, and quality of life in patients with sinusitis. Otolaryngol Head Neck Surg 2000; 123:389–392.
48. Shapiro GG. Role of allergy in sinusitis. Pediatr Infect Dis 1985; 4:S55–S59.
49. Huang SW. The risk of sinusitis in children with allergic rhinitis. Allergy Asthma Proc 2000; 21:85–88.
50. Meltzer EO, Orgel HA, Backhaus JW, Busse WW, Cruce HM, Metzger WJ, Mitchell DQ, Selner JC, Shapiro GG, van Bavel JH, Basch C. Intranasal flunisolide spray as an adjunct to oral antibiotic therapy for sinusitis. J Allergy Clin Immunol 1993; 92:812–823.
51. Meltzer EO, Charous BL, Busse WW, Zinreich SJ, Lorber RR, Danzig MR. Added relief in the treatment of acute recurrent sinusitis with adjunctive mometasone furoate nasal spray. The Nasonex Sinusitis Group. J Allergy Clin Immunol 2000; 106:630–637.
52. Barlan IB, Erkan E, Bakir M, Berrak S, Basaran MM. Intranasal budesonide spray as an adjunct to oral antibiotic therapy for acute sinusitis in children. Ann Allergy Asthma Immunol 1997; 78:598–601.
53. Parikh A, Scadding GK, Darby Y, Baker RC. Topical corticosteroids in chronic rhinosinusitis: a randomized, double-blind, placebo-controlled trial using fluticasone propionate aqueous nasal spray. Rhinology 2001; 39:75–79.

54. Lavigne F, Cameron L, Renzi PM, Planet JF, Christodoulopoulos P, Lamkioued B, Hamid Q. Intrasinus administration of topical budesonide to allergic patients with chronic rhinosinusitis following surgery. Laryngoscope 2002; 112:858–864.

55. Braun JJ, Alabert JP, Michel FB, Quiniou M, Rat C, Cougnard J, Czorlewski W, Bousquet J. Adjunct effect of loratadine in the treatment of acute sinusitis in patients with allergic rhinitis. Allergy 1997; 52:650–655.

8

Immune Deficiency/Disorders and Pediatric Sinusitis

Gary Kleiner

Department of Pediatrics and Division of Immunology and Infectious Diseases,
University of Miami School of Medicine, Miami, Florida, U.S.A.

INTRODUCTION

Physicians who care for patients with recurrent sinusitis are often surprised by the frequency with which there is a complaint of repeated infections. Most often the complaint is without foundation as the symptoms are from an allergic rather than an infectious cause. Most patients with recurrent infections do not have an identifiable immunodeficiency disorder. A major reason for the apparent high rate of recurrent infections is excessive exposure of infants or children to infectious agents in out-of-home childcare and other group settings. Within this group of patients, however, several with primary immunodeficiency (PID) will be found. The approaches to proper diagnosis and treatment have changed over the years as more information is gained about them. It is therefore important that the physician remains current on the rapidly expanding knowledge about these genetically determined diseases. In addition, pediatricians must have a high index of suspicion if defects of the immune system are to be diagnosed early enough for appropriate treatment to be instituted before there is irreversible damage.

Immunodeficiency diseases are characterized by unusual susceptibility to infection. It has been over 50 years since Bruton discovered agammaglobulinemia in 1952 (1); more than 70 other PID syndromes have been described (2). These disorders may involve one or more components of the immune system including T, B, and NK lymphocytes, phagocytic cells, and complement proteins. Most are recessive traits, some of which are caused by mutations in genes on the X-chromosome, others in genes on autosomal chromosomes (Table 1). Often these diseases have associated autoimmune or allergic manifestations. Knowledge of the particular pathogen involved as well as the anatomic site affected in a given patient can provide clues as to the most likely type of defect. Patients with B-cell, phagocytic cell, or complement defects have recurrent infections with encapsulated bacterial pathogens. By contrast, patients with T-cell defects have problems with opportunistic infections with viral and fungal agents. They often develop failure to thrive shortly after these symptoms occur. Excessive use of antibiotics by primary care physicians has altered the textbook presentation of many of these conditions.

In contrast to acquired immunodeficiency disorders, genetically deter-mined immunodeficiency is rare (2). The B-cell defects far outnumber those affecting T-cells, phagocytic cells, or complement proteins. Selective IgA deficiency is the most common, with reported incidences ranging as high as 1 in 200 (3). The PID is diagnosed more often in childhood, when it occurs predominantly in males, than in adult life, when it occurs slightly more often in females than in males. A committee of the World Health Organization (WHO) has published several versions of a classification of PID diseases over the past three decades, with the most recent having been reported in 1997 (2).

Evaluation of immune function should be initiated for children with clinical manifestations of a specific immune disorder or with unusual, chronic, or recurrent infections such as (1) two or more systemic or serious bacterial infections (sepsis, osteomyelitis, or meningitis), (2) three or more serious respiratory or documented bacterial soft tissue infections (e.g., cellu-litis, draining otitis media, or lymphadenitis) within one year, (3) infections occurring at unusual sites (e.g., liver or brain abscess), (4) infections with unusual pathogens (e.g., *Aspergillus, Serratia marcescens, Nocardia,* or *Burkholderia cepacia*), and (5) infections with common childhood pathogens with unusual severity.

Some immunodeficiency diseases are accompanied by excessive pro-duction of immunoglobulin E (IgE) antibodies. The routine use of anti-biotics has masked the infection susceptibility of many of these diseases. As a result, allergic or autoimmune problems may be the presenting illnesses of patients with these conditions. Patients with PID have increased incidences of malignancy, particularly in those defects that involve defective B- or T-cell function (4). Whether this is attributable to defective immune elimination of tumor cells or to increased susceptibility of infection with agents associated with malignancy is unknown.

Table 1 Major Primary Immune Deficiency Disorders

Chromosome	Gene product	Disorder	Functional deficiency
2p11	K chain	K chain deficiency	Absence of immunoglobulins with K chain
6p21.3	Unknown	Selective IgA deficiency CVID	Low IgA; low concentrations of all immunoglobulins in CVID
12p13	Activation-induced cytidine deaminase	Autosomal recessive hyper IgM	Failure to produce IgG, IgA, and IgE antibodies
14q32.3	Immunoglobulin heavy chains	B-cell negative agammaglobulinemia	Lack of B-cells in μ chain deletions
20	CD40	Autosomal recessive hyper IgM	Failure to produce IgG, IgA, and IgE antibodies
22q11.22	Unknown	DiGeorge syndrome	Low numbers of T-cells
Xq13.1	Common γ chain	Severe combined immune deficiency	Absence of T, B, and NK function
Xq22	Bruton tyrosine kinase	XLA	Lack of B-cells
Xq25	SLAM-associated protein (SH2D1A)	X-linked lymphoproliferative disease	Lack of anti-EBNA and long-lived T-cell immunity, low immunoglobulins
Xq26	CD154 (CD40 ligand)	X-linked hyper IgM	Failure to produce IgA, IgA, and IgE antibodies
X28	NEMO	Anhidrotic ectodermal dysplasia with immunodeficiency	Hyper IgM or IgG subclass and antipolysaccharide antibodies

Abbreviations: NEMO, nuclear factor essential modulator; XLA, X-linked agammaglobulinemia; CVID, common variable immune deficiency; EBNA, Epstein-Barr virus nuclear antigen.

PRIMARY IMMUNE DEFICIENCIES ASSOCIATED WITH SINUSITIS

X-Linked Agammaglobulinemia

X-linked agammaglobulinemia (XLA) was the first recognized human host defect, having been discovered by Colonel Ogden Bruton in 1952 (1). Most patients with this or other antibody deficiency syndromes are identified because they have recurrent infections with encapsulated bacterial pathogens (5). Because of passive immunity from maternally transmitted IgG antibodies, boys with XLA usually remain well during the first few months of life. Early in life, they may develop mucous membrane infections (e.g., conjunctivitis and otitis) because of the lack of secretory IgA. Thereafter, they are highly susceptible to infections with organisms such as pneumococci, streptococci, and *Haemophilus influenzae* (6). They may also experience infections with other high-grade pathogens such as meningococci, staphylococci, *Pseudomonas* organisms, and various *Mycoplasma* species. Since XLA patients have a profound deficiency of antibodies of all isotypes, the infections may be systemic (e.g., meningitis or septicemia) or involve mucous membrane surfaces (sinusitis, pneumonia, otitis, conjunctivitis, gastrointestinal, or urinary tract infections), joints (septic arthritis), or skin (cellulitis, abscesses). Growth and development are usually normal despite chronic or recurrent bacterial infections, unless bronchiectasis or persistent enteroviral infections develop. Except for the hepatitis and enterovirus, viral infections are usually handled normally. Various echovirus and coxsackievirus also have caused chronic, progressive, and eventually fatal central nervous system infections in many patients (7,8).

Concentrations of all serum immunoglobulins are extremely low. Tests for antibodies to blood group substances and for antibodies to vaccine antigens (e.g., diphtheria, tetanus, and pneumococci) help to distinguish XLA from other B-cell defects because antibody formation is profoundly impaired in XLA. Few, if any, circulating B-cells can be detected by flow cytometry in these patients. The tonsils, adenoids, and peripheral lymph nodes are very small because of the absence of germinal centers. Circulating T-cells and natural killer (NK) cells are relatively increased in XLA. Both T and NK function are normal. The molecular defect of XLA was simultaneously discovered by two groups of investigators in 1993 (9,10). The genetic defect is an intracellular signaling tyrosine kinase (Btk). Thus far, all males with known XLA have had low or undetectable Btk mRNA and kinase activity. Over 250 mutations have been described (11). Female carriers of XLA can be identified by the finding of nonrandom X-chromosome inactivation in their B-cells or by the detection of the mutated gene.

A condition that resembles XLA phenotypically (i.e., there is an absence of circulating B-cells) occurs in some agammaglobulinemic females (12). The molecular basis for this autosomal recessive defect has recently been shown to be mutation in the mu heavy chain gene on chromosome 14 (13).

Except in patients who develop persistent enteroviral infections, or lymphoreticular malignancy (with an incidence as high as 6% having been reported), the overall prognosis for patients with XLA is reasonably good if intravenous immune globulin (IVIG) replacement is instituted early. Systemic infection can be prevented by administration of IVIG at a dose of 400 mg/kg every three to four weeks (14). Despite this therapy, however, many patients go on to develop persistent enteroviral infections or crippling sinopulmonary disease because no effective means exists for replacing secretory IgA at the mucosal surface. Chronic antibiotic therapy is usually necessary in addition to the IVIG infusions for effective management of XLA patients with pansinusitis or bronchiectasis.

X-Linked Immunodeficiency with Hyper IgM

These patients lack IgG, IgA, and IgE antibodies and are susceptible to encapsulated bacterial organisms (15). Unlike patients with XLA, however, those with hyper IgM sometimes have lymphoid hyperplasia. Coexistent neutropenia, autoimmune disease, and the fact that the problem lies with the T-cells explains the occurrence of *Pneumocystis carinii* pneumonia in some patients. Concentrations of serum IgG, IgA, and IgE are very low, whereas the serum IgM is either normal or, more frequently, elevated and polyclonal. There is an increased frequency of autoantibody formation (15). Hemolytic anemia and thrombocytopenia may occur and transient, persistent, or cyclic neutropenia is common. Normal numbers of B-cells are seen in circulation. The defective gene product is a surface molecule called CD40 ligand (CD154) on the surface of activated T-cells (16), which interacts with CD40 on B-cells (17). Mutations in the gene encoding CD154 in X-linked hyper IgM patients results in a lack of signaling of their B-cells by their activated T-cells. The B-cells fail to undergo isotype switch and produce only IgM. Of further importance to effective immune responses, the lack of stimulation of CD40 also results in these patients' B-cells not up regulating co-stimulatory molecules CD80 and CD86. The failure of this pathway results in a propensity for tolerogenic T-cell signaling. Not all males with hyper IgM have a mutation in the gene encoding CD154 (18), and there are several examples in females (19). The treatment of this condition is the same as that for XLA, that is, monthly IVIG infusions. The prognosis is guarded; there is increased incidence of both autoimmunity and malignancy in this syndrome.

Common Variable Immune Deficiency

Common variable immune deficiency (CVID) is a syndrome characterized by hypogammaglobulinemia with phenotypically normal B-cells. It is also known as acquired hypogammaglobulinemia because of a generally later age of onset of infections. The CVID patients may appear clinically similar to those with XLA in the kinds of infections experienced and bacterial etiologic agents involved (20). In contrast to XLA, the sex distribution in CVID is almost equal, the age of onset is later, and infections are less severe.

Most patients have no identified molecular diagnosis. The CVID likely consists of several different genetic defects. Several putative mutations have been described, but there is no "one" mutation. Since CVID occurs in first-degree relatives of patients with selective IgA deficiency and some patients with IgA deficiency may become hypogammaglobulinemic, these diseases may have a common genetic basis. Despite normal numbers of circulating B-cells, blood B lymphocytes do not differentiate normally into immunoglobulin-producing cells when stimulated. In some patients, defective T-cell functional help to B-cells has been described.

The serum immunoglobulin and antibody deficiencies in CVID may be as profound as in XLA. Patients with CVID often have autoantibody formation and normal-sized or enlarged tonsils and lymph nodes, and approximately 25% have splenomegaly. The CVID has also been associated with a sprue-like syndrome, with or without nodular follicular lymphoid hyperplasia of the intestine (21); thymoma; alopecia areata; hemolytic anemia; and gastric atrophia. Lymphoid interstitial pneumonia, B-cell lymphomas, amyloidosis, and noncaseating sarcoid-like granulomas of the lungs, spleen, skin, and liver also occur. Treatment consists of IVIG and frequent antibiotics.

Selective IgA Deficiency

An isolated absence (<10 mg/dL) of serum IgA is the most common well-defined immunodeficiency disorder, with a frequency of approximately 1/200 healthy blood donors. The basic genetic defect is unknown. Phenotypically normal B-cells are present. The occurrence of IgA deficiency in both males and females and in members of successive generations of families suggests autosomal dominant inheritance with variable expressivity. This defect also commonly occurs in pedigrees containing individuals with CVID. The IgA deficiency and CVID are associated with certain drugs (phenytoin, D-penicillamine, gold, and sulfasalazine), suggesting that environmental factors may trigger the disease.

Infections occur predominantly in the respiratory, gastrointestinal, and urogenital tracts. Bacterial agents responsible are the same as in other antibody deficiency syndromes. Serum concentrations of other immunoglobulins are usually normal in patients with selective IgA deficiency. Serum antibodies to IgA are reported in as many as 44% of patients with selective IgA deficiency. If these antibodies are of the IgE isotype, they can cause severe anaphylactic reactions after intravenous administration of blood products containing IgA. For this reason, only washed blood products should be given. Many IVIG preparations contain sufficient IgA to cause anaphylactic reactions.

Transient Hypogammaglobulinemia of Infancy

After birth, the serum level of IgG in an infant diminishes with the decline of maternally derived IgG antibodies, reaching a nadir at three to four months of age, and then rises as an infant's own IgG production gradually increases. Transient hypogammaglobulinemia of infancy (THI) is an extension of this physiologic hypogammaglobulinemia beyond six months of age. Children have normal B- and T-cell numbers, and have normal T-cell function. These patients are able to synthesize normal tetanus and diphtheria antibodies, as well as normal isohemagglutinin titers, despite having depressed total IgG. The condition is thought to represent the extremes of normal variability of the immune system. The THI children may have increased frequency of otitis media, sinusitis, and pneumonias. Infections respond to appropriate antimicrobial therapy. In almost all cases, IVIG therapy is not indicated.

IgG Subclass Deficiencies

Some patients have deficiencies of one or more of the four subclasses of IgG despite normal or elevated total IgG serum concentrations. Most patients with absent or very low concentrations of IgG_2 also have IgA deficiency. Some patients with IgG_2 deficiency may have an evolving pattern of immunodeficiency, such as CVID. The biological significance of the numerous moderate deficiencies of IgG subclasses is difficult to assess, particularly because commercial laboratory measurement of IgG subclasses is problematic. The most important issue is a patient's *functional* ability to make specific antibodies to protein and polysaccharide antigens. The IVIG should not be administered to patients with IgG subclass deficiency unless they are shown to have a deficiency of antibodies to a broad array of antigens.

Screening for Immune Deficiency

An ear, nose, and throat (ENT) physician who deals with pediatric sinusitis should be knowledgeable in the workup of children. The screening tests selected for immunologic evaluation should be broadly informative, reliable, and cost-effective. Patients with deficiencies of antibodies, phagocytic cells, or complement have encapsulated bacterial infections. Children with defects in antibody production, phagocytic cells, or complement proteins may grow and develop normally despite their recurrent infections unless they develop bronchiectasis from repeated lower respiratory tract infections. By contrast, patients with deficiencies in T-cell function usually develop opportunistic infections early in life and fail to thrive.

The initial evaluation of immunocompetence includes a thorough history, physical examination, and family history. Most immunologic defects can be excluded at minimal cost with the proper choice of screening tests (Table 2). A complete blood count and differential and erythrocyte sedimentation rate

Table 2 Initial Immunologic Testing of the Child with Recurrent Infections

---

Complete blood count, manual differential, and erythrocyte sedimentation rate (ESR)
Absolute lymphocyte (normal count makes T-cell defect unlikely)
Absolute neutrophil [normal count precludes congenital or acquired neutropenia
  and leukocyte adhesion deficiency (elevated counts)]
Platelet count (normal excludes Wiskott–Aldrich)
ESR (normal result indicates chronic bacterial or fungal infection unlikely)

Screening test for B-cell defects
IgG, IgA, IgM, Isohemagglutinins, blood type, antibody titers to tetanus, diptheria,
  H. influenzae, and *S. pneumoniae.*

Screening tests for T-cell defects
Absolute lymphocyte count
Candida albicans intradermal skin test: 0.1 mL of a 1:1000 dilution for patients older
  than 6 years, 0.1 mL of a 1:100 dilution for patients younger than 6 years

Screening test for phagocytic cell defects
Absolute neutrophil count
Respiratory burst assay

Screening test for complement deficiency
CH50, AH50

(ESR) are the most cost-effective screening tests. If the ESR is normal, chronic bacterial or fungal infection is unlikely.

A functional assessment of a child's immune system is much more informative merely measuring quantitative immunoglobulins. In most cases, referral to a pediatric clinical immunologist is warranted if screening tests are abnormal. In addition to standard allergy questions and testing (dust mite, aeroallergen RASTs, or skin testing), cystic fibrosis must be excluded.

In most cases, measurement of blood type and isohemaglutinins (in children older than one year) is helpful (AB blood type lacks isohemaglutinins). Children in which a B-cell defect is suspected should have total immunoglobulins, tetanus, diphtheria, *Hemophilus* B, and pneumococcal antibodies assessed. It is important to request 12 serotypes of pneumococcal antibodies; almost all commercial labs will perform this. If less than six pneumococcal titers are depressed, it is useful to immunize with the polysaccharide pneumococcal 23 valent vaccine and reassess titers four weeks later. It is important to utilize the same laboratory for both measurements. Patients with poor responses and recurrent sinusitis may benefit from prophylactic antibiotics and IVIG. In some cases of selective antibody deficiency, IVIG is administered for a one-year trial period. If there is concern about a severe T-cell defect or a complicated patient, it is usually beneficial to initially involve a clinical immunologist. More specialized T-cell function and antibody (bacteriophage phiX174) testing may be required. There are several patient support groups for PID that are helpful, especially the Jeffrey

Model Foundation and Immune Deficiency Foundation. Early diagnosis and intervention can usually prevent long-term sequelae from occurring in these rare diseases.

REFERENCES

1. Bruton OC. Agammaglobulinemia. Pediatrics 1952; 9:722–728.
2. Group WS. Primary immunodeficiency diseases: report of a WHO scientific group. Clin Exp Immunol 1997; 109(1):1–28.
3. Clark JA, Callicoat PA, Brenner NA. Selective IgA deficiency in blood donors. Am J Clin Pathol 1983; 80:210–213.
4. Penn I. Lymphoproliferative diseases in disorders of the immune system. Cancer Detect Prev 1990; 14:415–422.
5. Ochs HD, Smith CIE. Reviews in molecular medicine: X-linked agammaglobulinemia—a clinical and molecular analysis. Medicine 1996; 75:287–299.
6. Lederman HM, Winkelstein JA. X-Linked agammaglobulinemia: an analysis of 96 patients. Medicine 1985; 64:145–156.
7. McKinney RE, Katz SL, Wilfert CM. Chronic enteroviral meningoencephalitis in agammaglobulinemic patients. Rev Infect Dis 1987; 9:334–356.
8. Wilfert CM, Buckley RH, Mohanakumar T, Griffith JF, Katz SL, Whisnant JK, Eggleston PA, Moore M, Treadwell E, Oxman MN, Rosen FS. Persistent and fatal central nervous system echovirus infections in patients with agammaglobulinemia. N Engl J Med 1977; 296:1485–1489.
9. Tsukada S, Saffran DC, Rawlings DJ, Parolini O, Allen RC, Klisak I, Sparkes RS, Kubagawa H, Mohandas T, Quan S. Deficient expression of a B-cell cytoplasmic tyrosine kinase in human X-linked agammaglobulemia. Cell 1993; 72:279–290.
10. Vetrie D, Vorechovsky I, Sideras P, Holland J, Davies A, Flinter F, Hammarstrom L, Kinnon C, Levinsky R, Bobrow M. The gene involved in X-linked agammaglobulinemia is a member of the src family of protein tyrosine kinases. Nature 1993; 361:226–233.
11. Vihinen M, Iwata T, Kinnon C, Kwan SP, Ochs HD, Vorechovsky I, Smith CI. BTKbase, mutation database for X-linked agammaglobulinemia. Nucleic Acids Res 1996; 24:160–165.
12. Conley ME, Sweinberg SK. Females with a disorder phenotypically identical to X-linked agammaglobulinemia. J Clin Immunol 1992; 12:139–143.
13. Yel L, Mingeishi Y, Coustan-Smith E, Buckley RH, Trubel H, Pachman LM, Kitchingman GR, Campana D, Rohrer J, Conley ME. Mutations in the mu heavy chain gene in patients with agammaglobulinemia. N Engl J Med 1996; 335:1486–1493.
14. Buckley RH, Schiff RI. The use of intravenous immunoglobulin in immunodeficiency diseases. N Engl J Med 1991; 325:110–117.
15. Notarangelo LN, Duse M, Ugazio AG. Immunodeficiency with hyper IgM. Immunodef Rev 1992; 3:101–121.
16. Noelle RJ, Roy M, Shepherd DM, Stamenkovic I, Ledbetter JA, Aruffo A. A 39-kDa protein on activated helper T cells binds CD40 and transduces a signal for cogante activation of B cells. Proc Natl Acad Sci USA 1992; 89:6550–6554.

17. Allen RC, Armitage RJ, Conley ME, Rosenblatt H, Jenkins NA, Copeland NK, Bedell MA, Edelhoff S, Disteche CM, Simoneaux DK. CD40 ligand gene defects responsible for hyper IgM syndrome. Science 1993; 259:990–993.

18. Conley ME, Larche M, Bonagura VR, Lawton AR, Buckley RH, Fu SM, Coustan-Smith E, Herrod HG, Campana D. Hyper IgM syndrome associated with defective CD40-mediated B-cell activation. J Clin Invest 1994; 94: 1404–1409.

19. Oliva A, Quinti I, Scala E, Fanales-Belasio E, Rainaldi L, Pierdominici M, Giovannetti A, Paganelli R, Aiuti F, Pandolfi F. Immunodeficiency with hyper-immunoglobulinemia M in two female patients not associated with abnormalities of CD40 or CD40 ligand expression. J Allerg Clin Immunol 1995; 96: 403–410.

20. Cunningham-Rundles C. Clinical and immunologic analysis of 103 patients with common variable immunodeficiency. J Clin Immunol 1989; 9:22–33.

21. Washington K, Stenzel TT, Buckley RH, Gottfreid MR. Gastrointestinal pathology in patients with common variable immune deficiency and X-linked agammaglobulinemia. Am J Surg Pathol 1996; 20:1240–1252.

9

Cystic Fibrosis and Sinusitis

Craig S. Derkay

Departments of Otolaryngology-Head and Neck Surgery and Pediatrics, Eastern Virginia Medical School, The Children's Hospital of the King's Daughters, Norfolk, Virginia, U.S.A.

Scott A. Schraff

Department of Otolaryngology-Head and Neck Surgery, Eastern Virginia Medical School, Norfolk, Virginia, U.S.A.

INTRODUCTION

Since being discovered in 1936, cystic fibrosis (CF) has become the most common fatal inherited disease affecting Caucasians. The disease primarily affects the lung (pulmonary disease is the most common cause of morbidity and mortality), but head and neck manifestations are common. Chronic or recurrent sinusitis and/or nasal polyposis can often be the presenting symptom.

In the past 20 years, advances in molecular genetics have led to a better understanding of the disease and, as a result, those afflicted are being identified earlier in life and receiving better treatment. Life expectancy has dramatically increased as median survival has jumped from less than one year in 1930 to 14 years in 1969 to 28 years in 1994. A genetic marker now exists that allows prenatal identification of those afflicted (1). Today, those identified with CF in the first year are projected to live to 40 or more years with aggressive treatment, and 40% of the CF population is age 18 and older (2–4) (Fig. 1). According to the CF Foundation's National Patient Registry, the median age of survival for CF patients is about 33 years.

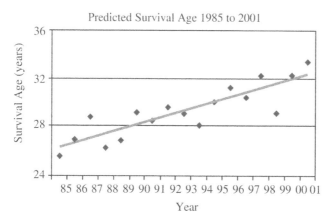

Figure 1 CF survival trend. *Abbreviation*: CF, cystic fibrosis.

CF presents many challenges for the pediatric otolaryngologist. Typically, the pediatric otolaryngologist is asked to address sinus disease and nasal polyposis. It has been shown that otitis media is not significantly more common in CF children compared with non-CF pediatric patients. However, there are both pulmonary and extrapulmonary manifestations that impact management. In this chapter we will review the epidemiology, genetics, pathophysiology, and clinical manifestations of CF-related sinus disease. We will also discuss the medical and surgical management of CF and the implications for the sinus surgeon.

EPIDEMIOLOGY AND GENETICS

CF is an autosomal recessive disease causing exocrine gland dysfunction that afflicts approximately 23,000 people in the United States. The incidence is about one in 3,200 Caucasian births with a gene frequency of about one in 20 (1,5). African Americans and those of Asian descent are affected much less frequently, with an incidence of one in 15,300, and one in 32,000, respectively (6). About 1,000 new cases of CF are diagnosed each year and about 80% of patients are diagnosed by age three. Those diagnosed early in life present with meconium ileus, pulmonary problems, or failure to thrive. The median and mean ages of diagnosis are six months and three years, respectively (1). However, patients with more mild disease may not be discovered to have CF until later in life. More than 10 million Americans are unknowing, asymptomatic carriers of the defective CF gene and nearly 10% of newly diagnosed cases are age 18 or older (1).

CF is caused by a genetic defect in the long arm (region 31) of chromosome 7 (7q31). The protein product of this gene is a c-AMP-mediated chloride channel called CF transmembrane conductance regulator (CFTR).

The genetic alteration results in a deficiency in this transmembrane regulator that causes a decrease in chloride permeability across apical membranes of epithelial cells. Researchers have identified over 1000 CFTR mutations, but the exact phenotypical manifestations of the genetic alterations to 7q31 are not well understood. The most common mutation is ΔF508, which causes a deletion of phenylalanine on the CFTR gene. In the United Kingdom, this accounts for approximately 70% of the mutations and is one of the most common mutations in Sweden (4,7). The majority of genetic screening programs use the ΔF508 mutation for their screening, which can detect about 87% of the CF mutations (6). However, some recommend testing a panel of genetic mutations based on the local prevalence of different mutations (8). DNA analysis is helpful in those patients in whom prior CF testing is equivocal or in couples with a family history of CF. This can be particularly important in preconceptual planning for such couples. In addition, in utero amniocentesis or chorionic villi sampling is available for couples desiring prenatal diagnosis (6).

Five broad categories of CFTR mutations have been described (4,9,10): class-I mutations cause CFTR synthesis defects resulting in absent production; class-II, which includes ΔF508, results in abnormal production of CFTR; class-III is characterized by normal production and trafficking of protein, but disrupted regulation at the cell membrane; class-IV has expression at the cell membrane but abnormal chloride conductance; and class-V has decreased splicing of normal CFTR. Classes I–III are associated with more severe phenotypic disease compared with classes IV and V.

In addition to the CFTR mutations, several other molecular events have been identified. Increased transmembrane sodium conductance due to a greater number of sodium channels has been described. In addition, there are an increased number of ATPase-dependent sodium/potassium pumps at the basal lateral surface of the respiratory epithelial cell. These alterations cause an influx of sodium from the extracellular matrix across the apical membrane of epithelial cells (11). This results in passive movement of water from the extracellular matrix into the cell, causing increased mucous viscosity and impaired mucociliary clearance due to desiccation of extracellular fluid.

PATHOPHYSIOLOGY

Epithelial cells of numerous organs, such as the lung, pancreas, and gastrointestinal tract, are affected in CF. While the lung is the primary organ affected, chronic sinusitis and nasal polyposis are the most common otolaryngological manifestations of CF. Of the paranasal sinuses, the ethmoid and maxillary sinuses are most commonly involved. There is a higher incidence of hypoplastic or aplastic sinuses in CF patients compared with non-CF patients (12–14). The frontal and sphenoid sinuses are not present at birth and frequently fail to develop in CF patients (15). It is believed that chronic inflammation and obstruction prevent pneumatization of these developing sinus cavities (16).

Similar to the tracheobroncial tree, the nasal cavity and paranasal sinuses are lined by pseudostratified ciliated epithelium. This epithelial layer acts as a barrier to inhaled microscopic foreign debris. It is believed that the cilia are embedded in two separate mucous layers that lie superficial to the respiratory epithelium (17). The more superficial of the layers is the gel layer, which is a rather viscous, mucous layer that helps entrap inhaled foreign particles. Beneath the gel layer but above the epithelium lies the sol layer, a more fluid layer that bathes the cilia. Ionic composition between these two layers and the epithelium is crucial for normal ciliary motion and mucociliary clearance.

In CF, mucociliary clearance is decreased despite normal ciliary structure and function. As described earlier, a deficiency in CFTR causes a decrease in chloride permeability across apical membranes of epithelial cells. This leads to an influx of sodium and water into cells. As a result, the extracellular matrix of exocrine secretions becomes more viscous. Although ciliary beat frequency does not change, the abnormal chloride conduction and sodium exchange result in impaired mucous clearance. The abnormal ionic composition also destroys the delicate balance between the gel, sol, and epithelial layers leading to mucous thickening (18).

In addition, it is believed that factors related to bacterial toxins also play a role in reducing clearance. A study on the bacterial content of the maxillary sinus found bacterial colonization in 95% of CF patients (19). Colonization is multimicrobial; however, CF patients suffer from *Pseudomonas* infection more often than non-CF patients. Bacterial toxins such as homolysin and pyocyanin produced by *Pseudomonas* contribute to impaired mucociliary clearance. In vitro studies have shown pyocyanin to slow ciliary beating and cause epithelial disruption (20).

Bacterial infection also causes inflammation resulting in goblet cell hyperplasia, squamous cell-metaplasia, and loss of ciliated cells (21). Individuals with CF have higher concentrations of interleukin-8 (IL-8) and other pro-inflammatory mediators in their sinuses and lungs (4,22). Mucous stasis results in retention of secretions and impaired gas exchange within the sinuses. As the partial pressure of carbon dioxide (CO_2) rises, a hypoxic environment is created in which infection can flourish. Subsequent inflammation causes a decrease in sinus ostial patency. This results in a vicious cycle causing further damage to the sinus cilia and epithelium (15).

In addition to thickening of secretions and sinonasal mucosa, nasal polyposis is common in CF patients. Although some believe allergy may play a role in the development of nasal polyps in CF patients (23), most agree the incidence of allergy is not greater in CF patients compared with non-CF patients (24,25). The exact etiology of nasal polyps is unclear; however, polyps found in CF patients differ histologically compared with those found in non-CF, atopic patients. CF polyps have a thin basement membrane and lack submucosal hyalinization and eosinophils. In addition, the mucous glands contain an abundance of acid mucin. Atopic polyps, in contrast, demonstrate a thick basement membrane, eosinophilia, and neutral mucin (21).

There are several theories used to explain the pathophysiology of nasal polyp development in CF patients. One theory, proposed by Rulon et al. (26) and supported by histological studies (27), suggests that inspissated nasal mucosa secretions cause dilation of the mucous glands. This, in turn, causes capillary and venous congestion that leads to stromal edema and mucosal prolapse with subsequent polyp formation. Another theory is based on infection or allergy-induced chronic inflammation that causes vasodilation, epithelial damage, and lamina propria prolapse (28).

CLINICAL MANIFESTATIONS

CF affects many organ systems (Table 1) and patients tend to present with a variety of symptoms including salty skin, persistent cough, wheezing or shortness of breath, failure to thrive despite an excessive appetite, and greasy, bulky stools. Overall, the number of CF patients who complain of sinus symptoms is relatively small at about 10% (29,30). This may be due to patient acclimation to the numerous symptoms that accompany CF and an unhealthy baseline status (31).

The clinical symptoms of sinusitis in the CF patient are similar to those found in non-CF patients; however, CF patients tend to have more severe disease. Symptomatic patients tend to be older children and teenagers, which

Table 1 Systemic Effects of Cystic Fibrosis

Organ system	Clinical manifestations
Head and neck	Sinusitis, nasal polyposis, and obstruction
Pulmonary	Impaired mucociliary clearance, hemoptysis, recurrent infections, bronchiectasis, bronchospasm, and poor pulmonary reserve
Cardiovascular	Cor pulmonale and clubbing
Gastrointestinal	Cirrhosis, colelithiasis, pancreatitis and pancreatic dysfunction, bowel obstruction, portal hypertension, meconium ileus, rectal prolapse, and malabsorption
Genito-urinary	Infertility
Nutritional	Vitamin deficiencies (A, D, E, and K)

may be due to a young child's inability to verbalize complaints (23,30). Postnasal drainage, purulent rhinorrhea, facial pain, halitosis, headache, and snoring are typical, with the most common complaint being nasal obstruction (25,32). Headache is usually reported more often in older patients and anosmia is reported in 12–71% (31,32). These symptoms are caused by the CF-related mucous stasis and nasal polyposis. However, anatomical abnormalities of the nose and paranasal sinuses, such as a deviated septum or inferior turbinate hypertrophy, can exacerbate the disease process.

Despite the low number of symptomatic patients, the prevalence of sinus disease in CF patients is close to 100%, and imaging studies reveal opacification of the maxillary and ethmoid sinuses in virtually all patients. Mucoceles have also been reported in pediatric CF patients (31,33,34). Given the rarity of mucocele findings in children, the presence of mucocele in a child should raise suspicion for CF (33). Anterior rhinoscopy usually shows edematous, and erythematous nasal mucosa with abundant secretions and polyposis also is fairly common, typically multiple and bilateral. Literature reports of polyposis incidence vary from 6% to 86% of patients; however, most report an incidence of about 10% (25,27,30,35–37). Most patients will develop polyps between the ages of 5 and 20 (25,30,38). Undiagnosed children with milder forms of the disease may first present to the otolaryngologist with polyp disease sequelae such as nasal obstruction, septal deviations, proptosis, or hypertelorism. Nasal polyps in a pediatric patient should raise suspicion for CF. It is recommended that all children with polyp disease should be screened for CF with a sweat chloride test, especially if there is a history of repeated lung infections.

Studies have shown that CF patients with nasal polyposis are more likely to have *Pseudomonas* colonization of their lower airways than patients without polyps (7,19). Despite colonization with more virulent bacteria, few CF patients develop serious sinus-related complications such as orbital and brain abscesses or osteomyelitis (39).

The increased viscosity of mucous in CF patients leads to both pulmonary and non-pulmonary disease. CF patients suffer life-long recurrences of pulmonary disease. Tenacious secretions and mucous plugging cause atelectasis resulting in bronchitis, pneumonia, abscess, empyema, pneumothorax, pulmonary hypertension, or respiratory failure. CF-related exocrine dysfunction also affects the gastrointestinal tract. Pancreatitis and pancreatic insufficiency are not uncommon. Pancreatic dysfunction can also lead to diabetes and nutritional deficiencies due to malabsorption of fat-soluble vitamins. Stasis of secretions can result in colelithiasis, biliary cirrhosis, and eventual portal hypertension. Meconium ileus, fecal impaction, volvulus, and rectal prolapse are intestinal manifestations. Infertility due to failure of vas deferens development in men and tubal stasis of secretions in women has been reported (5) and more than 95% of men with CF are sterile (2).

DIAGNOSIS

The diagnosis of CF can be confirmed by both laboratory test and clinical disease. Newborn screening has markedly improved identification and is based on elevated levels of serum immunoreactive trypsinogen. Newborn screening has also shown other benefits, as those identified early in life are less likely to suffer from malnutrition and growth retardation (40). Genetic testing for ΔF508 can also be performed. However, in many instances, family history may not be revealing and the diagnosis is not made until clinical symptoms arise. Usually, repeated pulmonary infections or sino-nasal disease lead to a suspicion of CF. The diagnosis is usually made with an abnormally high sweat chloride value (3). Sweat, an exocrine secretion of the skin, has an abnormally high chloride concentration (greater than 60 mEq/L) in CF patients and is the basis of the sweat test. It is recommended that patients with a borderline sweat test should undergo genetic testing (41).

MEDICAL MANAGEMENT

Medical management of CF patients continues to evolve and provides many challenges for the clinician. From an otolaryngologic standpoint, management of sinus disease often parallels treatment for pulmonary disease. The primary treatment modalities revolve around anti-inflammatory and antimicrobial medications.

Ideally, medical management involves controlling sinus disease and polyposis. It is presumed that control of sinus disease in these patients will improve pulmonary function and, hopefully, reduce pulmonary disease. Saline and nasal steroid sprays used for daily nasal hygiene have typically been the backbone of medical management, with oral steroids and antibiotics reserved for acute exacerbations.

Saline sprays are used to help mechanically debride the nasal cavities and decrease congestion. Buffered (3%) saline is preferred to physiologic (0.9%) saline due to its hypertonicity. It is felt that this hypertonic solution may help decongest nasal mucosa osmotically and has been shown to improve mucociliary clearance (42,43).

Nasal steroids have been shown to be clearly beneficial in CF patients. While polyp response rates to nasal steroid sprays have been variable in the past, a recent prospective, double-blinded, and randomized trial demonstrated that betamethasone nasal drops result in a statistically significant reduction in nasal polyp size compared to a placebo (44). Oral glucocorticoids also are typically used, but their use is tempered by the side effects, such as hypothalamic-pituitary-adrenal axis suppression, growth retardation, Cushing's disease, glucose intolerance, water retention, increased gastric acid secretion, and impaired wound healing. Unpleasant side effects led to the discontinuation of the largest controlled trial on their use. In addition, the benefits of oral steroids are short-lived and do not persist once the medication is discontinued (4).

Antibacterial nasal sprays have also been used with mixed results. In theory, such sprays should help decrease bacterial load, and inhaled tobramycin has been used successfully to treat *Pseudomonas* pulmonary disease. Clinical trial results show that this reformulated version of the common antibiotic improved lung function in people with CF and reduced the number of hospital days (45,46). A recent clinical trial on azithromycin showed that patients with CF who took the antibiotic experienced an almost 50% reduction in hospitalizations, a significant improvement in lung function, and weight gain (2). However, a study using tobramycin and saline administered by a large-particle nebulizer reduced pain but increased nasal congestion (47). There also is the concern that daily use of antimicrobial nasal sprays will select for resistant bacteria.

However, a promising topical preparation called dornase alfa has been shown to improve nasal symptoms in CF patients. Dornase alfa, recombinant human deoxyribonuclease I, acts by decreasing inflammation and mucous viscosity, thus increasing mucociliary clearance. When administered to CF patients by jet nebulizer, it has been shown to improve forced expiratory volume in one second. A recent study (48) demonstrated a reduction in nasal mucosal edema, polyps, and need for revision surgery in a small cohort of CF patients treated after functional endoscopic sinus surgery.

While *Streptococcus pneumoniae*, *Haemophilus influenza*, and *Moraxella catarrhalis* are the typical bacteria found in non-CF patients, *Staphylococcus aureus* and *Pseudomonas aeruginosa* have a particular affinity for the respiratory mucosa in CF patients. One study (37) showed that 89% of CF patients had cultures positive for *Pseudomonas* while none of the non-CF patients demonstrated its presence. *Pseudomonas* is particularly problematic due to its biofilm production, which enhances its antibiotic resistance. To prevent the development of biofilms and reduce bacterial load, many clinicians recommend extended courses of high dose anti-pseudomonal antibiotics (49).

Macrolides have recently been discovered to possibly have anti-inflammatory effects that are beneficial to CF patients. IL-8 is a potent chemotactic and neutrophil-activating factor that is believed to play an important role in inflammation. It is highly expressed in nasal polyps and the nasal mucosa of patients with chronic rhinosinusitis. Several studies have demonstrated that macrolides reduce IL-8 and neutrophil concentration as well as modulate immune-complex reaction against *Pseudomonas* biofilm. They have also been shown to reduce nasal polyp size (50–53).

Sputum, middle meatus, and tracheal aspirate cultures can be used to guide antimicrobial therapy; however, these usually do not accurately correlate with the organism colonizing the sinuses (19,54). Despite lack of U.S. Food and Drug Administration approval for use in the pediatric population due to potential joint maldevelopment, quinolones are being used due to the prevalence of *Psuedomonas* (5). Aminoglycoside and other broad-spectrum antibiotics, such as piperacillin, ceftazidime, cefsulodin, and imipenem, have been frequently used in the past; however, renal, cochlear, and vestibular toxicities must be closely monitored.

We recommend aggressive, individually tailored medical treatment when CF patients present with sinusitis. In addition, maintenance nasal care is mandatory during times of quiescent disease. Hypertonic saline irrigation (3–7%), used two to three times a day, and a nasal steroid spray should be used daily. During flare-ups of acute disease, oral antibiotics with antipseudomonal coverage should be added to the nasal hygiene regimen for a minimum of three to four weeks. A short course of oral steroids can be given. Antihistamines and decongestants should be avoided in CF patients because these can cause mucous thickening and worsen disease. Broad-spectrum intravenous or oral fluoroquinolone antibiotics may be needed for those with persistent disease, polyposis, or sinus-induced pulmonary complications. Typically, CF patients harbor resistant organisms due to frequent antibiotic use to treat airway disease, and surgical management should be considered in patients with recalcitrant disease.

SURGICAL MANAGEMENT

Surgical management of sinusitis in CF patients is reserved for those who have failed medical management, have polyposis, or are awaiting lung transplantation. CF patient comorbidities related to lung and hematological abnormalities, as well as anatomical variances, present challenges for the sinus surgeon. Fortunately, the advent of endoscopic sinus surgery and power instruments has greatly facilitated surgical management of sinus disease and polyposis.

While timing, indications, and extent of surgery can be controversial in non-CF pediatric patients, it is generally agreed that CF patients deserve special consideration, especially regarding preoperative work-up (Table 2). CF patients who present with either frequent exacerbation of lung disease, polyposis, or radiological evidence of sinusitis along with clinical symptoms (nasal obstruction, facial pain, headache, and fevers) refractory to medical management merit surgical intervention. Nasal obstruction and the resulting increase in pulmonary effort is particularly concerning given the lack of pulmonary reserve in CF patients (55). It should be noted, however, that abnormal radiographic findings are common in CF patients, but are not always accompanied by symptoms.

The preoperative imaging for CF patients is similar to non-CF patients; however, particular attention should be focused on CT findings (Fig. 2). Paranasal sinus development in CF patients has been shown to be characteristically different compared with controls who have non-CF

Table 2 Preoperative Work-Up

All cases
CT scan (image-guidance system protocol, if available)
Serum electrolyte analysis
Complete blood count
Coagulopathy panel
Blood glucose level
Liver function test
Chest x-ray
Pulmonary function test
Sputum culture and sensitivity
When indicated
Arterial blood gas analysis
Electrocardiogram
Echocardiogram

Source: From Refs. 6, 59.

inflammatory sinonasal disease (13). CF patients have a higher incidence of hypoplastic or aplastic sinuses, especially the frontal and sphenoid sinuses, and have fewer pneumatization variants, such as Haller or Agger Nasi cells. Typically, these patients have medial bowing of the medial wall of the maxillary sinus as well as resorption of the uncinate process (32). It is hypothesized that these bony changes are caused by osteitis or a pressure-induced phenomenon caused by polyps and inspissated mucous (32,56).

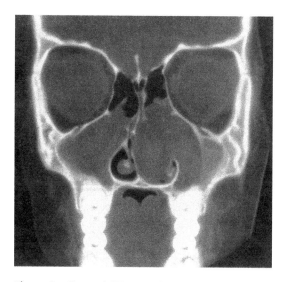

Figure 2 Coronal CT scan of CF patient with sinusitis. *Abbreviations*: CT, computed tomography; CF, cystic fibrosis.

Other anatomical abnormalities, such as maxillary and ethmoid sinus hypoplasia, place the orbit at risk during surgery. In maxillary sinus hypoplasia, the orbit is enlarged and the lateral nasal wall is more laterally located. In ethmoid sinus hypoplasia, the lamina papyracea is more medial and often found medial to the lateral wall of the maxillary ostium. Furthermore, the fovea ethmoidalis is often lower in CF children compared with non-CF children and, when combined with other CF-related abnormalities, exposes these patients to a greater risk of intracranial injury or cerebrospinal fluid leak (13). However, recent advances in image-guided technology and the use of nasal endoscopes (Fig. 3) have greatly reduced the risks and complications of sinus surgery in CF patients. Endoscopic sinus surgery combined with an image-guidance system allows surgical precision to less than 2 mm (57) and should be considered if the equipment is readily available.

In addition to CT variances, the sinus surgeon must be wary of hematological abnormalities in CF patients. Nutritional deficiencies and coagulopathies are common in these patients. Frequently, CF can involve the liver and lead to impaired processing of Vitamin K as well as elevated prothrombin (PT) and partial thromboplastin times (PTT). These deficiencies need to be corrected preoperatively and monitored closely in the perioperative period. Pancreatic and intestinal involvement can greatly diminish the absorption of fat-soluble vitamins, which can have nutritional and hematological consequences.

These patients also deserve special consideration from an anesthesia standpoint. In children and teenagers with CF, the most common reason for anesthesia is sinus surgery (58). In the past, CF patients, due to poor lung function, had tolerated anesthesia poorly. However, as medical management of pulmonary disease has improved, the anesthetic risks have subsequently declined. Only about 5% of patients undergoing routine types of ear, nose,

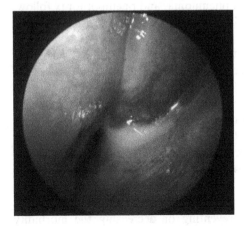

Figure 3 Nasal endoscopy of CF patient with sinusitis.

or throat surgery suffer minor postoperative complications (58). However, in patients with moderate to severe pulmonary disease, preoperative pulmonary function studies should be obtained. CF patients typically demonstrate an obstructive pattern with an increased functional residual capacity and decreased vital capacity, FEV1, and peak expiratory flow rate. Fibrosis, secretions and bronchospasm can cause ventilation problems. An indicator of advanced disease is increased levels of arterial CO_2, which are usually low to normal in CF patients (58,59).

Preoperative patients should be given anti-reflux medications to prevent pulmonary irritation due to gastroesophageal reflux. Opioids should be avoided due to problems with constipation. It is recommended that all routine pulmonary medications, such as inhalers and corticosteroids, should be continued and given on the morning of surgery (59). Preoperative consultation with the patient's pulmonologist is recommended since some patients will need "tuning-up" from a pulmonary standpoint prior to undergoing general anesthesia.

Intraoperatively, the choice of anesthetic agent is very important. Sevoflurane should be used given its bronchodilatory properties, and ketamine, isoflurane, and desflurane should be avoided. These agents have little bronchodilatory effect and can cause increased pulmonary secretions. Muscle relaxants can be used, but sparingly. It should be noted that aminoglycosides can potentiate the effect of neuromuscular blockers (6). Propofol is a good choice as a short-acting sedative. Stress dose steroids should also be considered in patients who take daily maintenance oral steroids.

Postoperatively, the head of bed should be elevated to 30° and the patient admitted to the post-anesthetic care unit for aggressive respiratory therapy. The extent of surgery and CF severity will determine whether the patient should be admitted to the hospital. These patients are at risk for respiratory depression, obstruction, pneumonia, and pneumothorax following endotracheal intubation (58). Stool softeners and laxatives can be used to alleviate constipation.

Sinus disease can be particularly problematic for the CF patient awaiting lung transplantation. The sinuses can act as a pathogen reserve that can seed the lungs in the post-transplant patient. To avoid this, all CF transplant patients need to be aggressively managed, both medically and sometimes surgically. There is controversy regarding prophylactic sinus surgery in pretransplant patients. Those in favor believe surgery will lower the sinus bacterial load, thus decreasing the chance of infection in the post-transplanted, immunocompromised patient. Others, however, have shown that pretransplant surgery confers no benefit and does not affect transplant success rates (3). A recent consensus statement stated that the benefit of sinus surgery toward preventing or decreasing the morbidity and mortality in the post-transplant patient is unknown (60).

Unfortunately, transplantation is not curative and does not have any effect on the extrapulmonary manifestations of disease. Patients continue to suffer from sinusitis and other *Pseudomonas* infections (61). One-year survival is about 70–80%, with a 5-year survival rate of about 30–45% (4). Due to organ shortages, about 40% of those awaiting transplantation die before a suitable lung donor can be found (6).

The objectives of sinus surgery in the CF patient are similar to those in a non-CF patient: relief of nasal obstruction by removing polyps and obstructing structures to improve sinus ventilation and drainage while preserving key anatomical landmarks. Prior to surgery, imaging studies are a must. A fine cut sinus CT with coronal views is a minimum requirement for sinus surgery in these patients. Given the anatomical abnormalities that are relatively common in CF patients, we recommend using an image-guidance system with the corresponding CT scans. A chest x-ray and preoperative blood work consisting of a complete blood count to assess hemoglobin and platelet levels as well as a coagulation study (PT, PTT, and INR) are recommended. Abnormalities should be corrected before proceeding with surgery. All CF patients should have their pulmonary function maximized, and pulmonary function tests are recommended in all patients with moderate and severe disease.

Some believe preoperative hospital admission is warranted to maximize pulmonary function in these patients (25,56); however, we have found that only a select few patients warrant preoperative admission. Some studies (30,62) have shown that blood loss is no different in the CF patient compared to non-CF patients; however, Duplechain et al. (37) reported a slightly higher blood loss in CF patients. In general, we do not believe that routine typing and crossing of blood is necessary. If nasal obstruction in the face of polyposis is the only complaint, some advocate office-based polypectomy in older patients. However, many argue that simple polypectomy is inadequate and that proper endoscopic surgery that addresses maxillary and ethmoid sinus disease and polyposis is the minimum surgical requirement (12,25,62). It has been shown that this technique results in reduced recurrence rates compared to simple polypectomy. Cepero et al. (30) reported a reduction in polyp recurrence from 61% for simple polypectomy to 13% when ethmoidectomy was done in conjunction with polypectomy. Crocket et al. (23) agree and reported recurrence rates of 89% and 35% for simple polypectomy versus a combined procedure. Also, most pediatric patients do not tolerate in-office nasal procedures.

Typically, the frontal and sphenoid sinuses are poorly developed and not involved, but when involved should be adequately drained and ventilated. Some advocate frontal sinus obliteration due to high recurrence of thick tenacious mucous. However, like medical management, surgery should be tailored to the individual needs of each patient, taking into account comorbidities and outcome objectives.

Surgery is quite efficacious in reducing patient symptoms. Nishioka et al. (63) have shown that patients have a statistically significant reduction in nasal obstruction and discharge, while smell and activity tolerance are improved. Sinus surgery has also been shown to decrease the severity of asthma attacks and hospitalizations and reduce the number of medications required by CF patients (64).

Postoperative care should consist of saline irrigation several times daily and topical steroid sprays should be restarted several days after surgery. Antibiotics are not necessarily employed unless intraoperative findings indicate indolent infection, and then therapy should be tailored to culture results.

CONCLUSIONS

Sinus disease in the CF-patient continues to be a sometimes difficult entity for the pediatric otolaryngologist. The pathophysiology and anatomical variations found in CF patients present many challenges. Usually patients are referred to otolaryngologists after failing medical management for their pulmonary and/or sinus disease. Thus, the otolaryngologist is asked to provide expertise regarding medical and usually surgical management of this disease. Awareness of the possible pitfalls and complications of surgical intervention in CF patients is instrumental in diminishing the morbidity of disease and improving quality of life.

In addition, the diagnosis of CF carries an emotional and economic burden that requires a multidisciplinary team approach. In addition to the otolaryngologist, this team should consist of a geneticist, pulmonologist, gastroenterologist, social worker, and nutritionist as well as primary care doctor to coordinate patient care. Parents and family members should be put in contact with CF support groups and given information, both of which can be obtained at the CF Foundation, Bethesda, MD (www.CFF.org).

Hopefully, with continued understanding of the molecular biology and pathophysiology of disease, new medications and management strategies will continue to evolve. The future of CF management will most likely incorporate gene therapy, with the hope that normal copies of CFTR can be delivered to the upper and lower airway in an attempt to reduce morbidity and mortality, and possibly cure CF.

REFERENCES

1. White R, Woodward S, Leppert M, O'Connell P, Hoff M, Herbst J, Lalouel JM, Dean M, van de Woude G. A closely linked genetic marker for cystic fibrosis. Nature 1985; 318:382–384.
2. Cystic Fibrosis Foundation. National Cystic Fibrosis Registry Annual Data Report. Bethesda, MD: Cystic Fibrosis Foundation, 2001.

3. Varlotta L. Management and care of the newly diagnosed patient with cystic fibrosis. Curr Opin Pulm Med 1998; 4:311–318.

4. Doull IJ. Recent advances in cystic fibrosis. Arch Dis Child 2001; 85:62–66.

5. Hulka GF. Head and neck manifestations of cystic fibrosis and ciliary dyskinesia. Otolaryngol Clin North Am 2000; 33:1333–1341.

6. Karlet MC. An update on cystic fibrosis and implications for anesthesia. AANA J 2000; 68:141–148.

7. Henriksson G, Westrin KM, Karpate F, Wikstrom AC, Stierna P, Hjelte L. Nasal polyps in cystic fibrosis. Chest 2002; 121:40–47.

8. Bobadilla JL, Macek M Jr, Fine JP, Farrell PM. Cystic fibrosis: a worldwide analysis of CFTR mutations—correlation with incidence data and application to screening. Hum Mutat 2002; 19:575–606.

9. Zeitlin PL. Novel pharmacologic therapies for cystic fibrosis. J Clin Invest 1999; 103:447–452.

10. Quinton PM. Cystic fibrosis: a disease of electrolyte transport. FASEB J 1990; 4:2709–2717.

11. Bernstein JM. The molecular biology of nasal polyposis. Curr Allergy Asthma Rep 2001; 1:262–267.

12. Eggesbo HB, Sovik S, Dolvik S, Eiklid K, Kolmannskog F. CT Characterization of developmental variations of the paranasal sinuses in cystic fibrosis. Acta Radiol 2001; 42:482–493.

13. Gentil V, Isaacson G. Patterns of sinusitis in cystic fibrosis. Laryngoscope 1996; 106:1005–1009.

14. Ledesma-Media J, Osman M, Girdany B. Abnormal paranasal sinuses in patients with cystic fibrosis of the pancreas. Pediatr Radiol 1980; 9:61–64.

15. Hui Y, Gaffney R, Crysdale WS. Sinusitis in patients with cystic fibrosis. Eur Arch Otorhinolaryngol 1995; 252:191–196.

16. Davidson T, Murphy C, Mitchell M, Smith C, Light M. Management of chronic sinusitis in cystic fibrosis. Laryngoscope 1995; 105:354–358.

17. Sleigh M, Blake J, Liron N. The propulsion of mucus by cilia. Am Rev Respir Dis 1988; 137:726–741.

18. Rutland J, Cole P. Nasal mucociliary clearance and ciliary beat frequency in cystic fibrosis compared with sinusitis and bronchiectsis. Thorax 1981; 36: 654–658.

19. Shapiro ED, Milmoe GJ, Wald ER, Rodnan JB, Bowen AD. Bacteriology of the maxillary sinuses in patients with cystic fibrosis. J Infect Dis 1982; 146: 589–593.

20. Wilson R, Pitt T, Taylor G, Watson D, MacDermot J, Sykes D, Roberts D, Cole P. Pyocyanin and 1-hydroxyphenazine produced by *Pseudomonas aeruginosa* inhibit the beating of human respiratory cilia in vitro. J Clin Invest 1987; 79:221–229.

21. Gysin C, Alothman GA, Papsin BC. Sinonasal disease in cystic fibrosis: clinical characteristics, diagnosis and management. Pediatr Pulmonol 2000; 30:481–489.

22. Sobol SE, Christodoulopoulos P, Manoukian JJ, Hauber HP, Frenkiel S, Desrosiers M, Fukakusa M, Schloss MD, Hamid Q. Cytokine profile of chronic sinusitis in patients with cystic fibrosis. Arch Otolaryngol Head Neck Surg 2002; 128:1295–1298.

23. Crocket DM, McGill FJ, Healy GB, Friedman EM, Salkeld LJ. Nasal and paranasal sinus surgery in children with cystic fibrosis. Ann Otol Rhinol Laryngol 1987; 96:367–372.

24. Lee AB, Pitcher-Wilmott RW. The clinical and laboratory correlates of nasal polyps in cystic fibrosis. Int J Pediatr Otorhinolaryngol 1982; 4:209–214.

25. Stern RC, Boat TF, Wood RE, Matthews LW, Doershuk CF. Treatment and prognosis of nasal polyps in cystic fibrosis. Am J Dis Child 1982; 136: 1067–1070.

26. Rulon JT, Brown HA, Logan GB. Nasal polyps and cystic fibrosis of the pancreas. Arch Otolaryngol 1963; 78:192–199.

27. Schwachman H, Kulczycki LL, Mueller HL, Flake CG. Nasal polyposis in patients with cystic fibrosis. Pediatrics 1962; 30:389–401.

28. Tos M, Mogensen C, Thomsen J. Nasal polyps in cystic fibrosis. J Laryngol Otol 1977; 91:827–835.

29. King V. Upper respiratory disease, sinusitis, and polyposis. Clin Rev Allergy 1991; 9:143–157.

30. Cepero R, Smith R, Catlin F, Bressler K, Furuta G, Shandera K. Cystic fibrosis—an otolaryngologic perspective. Otolaryngol Head Neck Surg 1987; 97:356–360.

31. Nishioka G, Cook P. Paranasal sinus disease in patients with cystic fibrosis. Otolaryngol Clin North Am 1996; 29:193–204.

32. Brihaye P, Clement PA, Dab I, Despechin B. Pathological changes of the lateral nasal wall in patients with cystic fibrosis (mucovicidosi). Int J Pediatr Otorhinolaryngol 1994; 28:141.

33. Guttenplan M, Wetmore R. Paransal sinus mucocele in cystic fibrosis. Clin Pediatr 1989; 28:429–430.

34. Tunkel D, Naclerio R, Baroody F, Rosenstein B. Bilateral maxillary sinus mucoceles in an infant with cystic fibrosis. Otolaryngol Head Neck Surg 1994; 111:116–120.

35. Parsons DS. Sinusitis and cystic fibrosis. In: Lusk RP, ed. Pediatric Sinusitis. New York: Raven Press, 1992:65.

36. Schramm VL Jr, Effron MZ. Nasal polyps in children. Laryngoscope 1980; 90:1488–1495.

37. Duplechain KJ, White JA, Miller RH. Pediatric sinusitis: the role endoscopic sinus surgery in cystic fibrosis and other forms of sinonasal disease. Arch Otolaryngol Head Neck Surg 1991; 117:422–426.

38. Cuyler JP, Monaghan AJ. Cystic fibrosis and sinusitis. J Otolaryngol 1989; 18:173–175.

39. Ramsey B, Richardson MA. Impact of sinusitis in cystic fibrosis. J Allergy Clin Immunol 1992; 90:547–552.

40. Farrell PM, Kosorok MR, Rock MJ, Laxova A, Zeng L, Lai HC, Hoffman G, Laessig RH, Splaingard ML. Early diagnosis of cystic fibrosis through neonatal screening prevents sever malnutrition and improves long term growth. Pediatrics 2001; 107:1–13.

41. Wagener JS, Sontag MK, Accurso FJ. Newborn screening for cystic fibrosis. Curr Opin Pediatr 2003; 15:309–315.

42. Parsons D, van Leeuwen R. Management of sinusitis in children. Adv Otolaryngol Head Neck Surg 1997; 11:131–154.
43. Talbot A, Herr T, Parsons D. Mucociliary clearance and buffered hypertonic saline solution. Laryngoscope 1997; 107:500–503.
44. Hadfield PJ, Rowe-Jones JM, Mackay IS. A recent prospective treatment trial of nasal polyps in adults with cystic fibrosis. Rhinology 2000; 38:63–65.
45. Maclusky I, Gold R, Corey M, Levison H. Long-term effect of inhaled tobramycin in patients with cystic fibrosis colonized with *Pseudomonas aeruginosa*. Pediatr Pulmonol 1989; 7:42–48.
46. Ramsey B, Dorkin H, Eisenberg J, Gibson R, Harwood I, Kravitz R, Schidlow D, Wilmott R, Astley S, McBurnie M. Efficacy of aerosolized tobramycin in patients with cystic fibrosis. N Engl J Med 1993; 328:1740–1746.
47. Desrosiers MY, Salas-Prato M. Treatment of chronic rhinosinusitis refractory to other treatments with topical antibiotic therapy delivered by means of large-particle nebulizer: results of a controlled trial. Otolaryngol Head Neck Surg 2001; 125:265–269.
48. Raynor EM, Butler A, Guill M, Bent III JP. Nasally inhaled dornase alfa in the postoperative management of chronic sinusitis due to cystic fibrosis. Arch Otolaryngol Head Neck Surg 2000; 126:581–583.
49. Jaffe A, Francis J, Rosenthal M, Bush A. Long-term azithromycin may improve lung function in children with cystic fibrosis. Lancet 1998; 351:420.
50. Yamada T, Fujieda S, Mori S, Yammamoto H, Saito H. Macrolide treatment decreased the size of nasal polyps and IL-8 levels in nasal lavage. Am J Rhinol 2000; 14:143–148.
51. Takeuchi K, Yuta A, Sakakura Y. Interleukin-8 gene expression in chronic sinusitis. Am J Otolaryngol 1995; 16:98–102.
52. Suzuki H, Shimomura A, Ikeda K, Furukawa M, Oshima T, Takasaka T. Inhibitory effect of marcrolids on interleukin-8 secretion from cultured human nasal epithelial cells. Laryngoscope 1997; 107:1661–1667.
53. Hoiby, N. New antimicrobials in the management of cystic fibrosis. J Antimicrob Chemother 2002; 49:235–238.
54. Iaccocco VF, Sibinga M, Barbero G. Respiration tract bacteriology in cystic fibrosis. Am J Dis Child 1963; 106:115–124.
55. Adams GL, Hilger P, Warwick WJ. Cystic Fibrosis. Arch Otolaryngol 1980; 106:127–132.
56. Jaffe BF, Strome M, Khaw KT, Shwachman H. Nasal polypectomy and sinus surgery for cystic fibrosis—a 10-year review. Otolaryngol Clin North Am 1977; 10:81–90.
57. Olson G, Citardi MJ. Image-guided functional endoscopic sinus surgery. Otolaryngol Head Neck Surg 2000; 123:188–194.
58. Della Rocca, G. Anaesthesia in patients with cystic fibrosis. Curr Opin Anaesth 2002; 15:95–101.
59. Walsh TS, Young CH. Anaesthesia and cystic fibrosis. Anaesthesia 1995; 50:614–622.
60. Yankaskas FR, Mallory GB, The Consensus Committee. Lung transplantation in cystic fibrosis. Chest 1998; 113:1.

61. Kanj S, Tapson V, Davis R, Madden J, Browning I. Infections in patients with cystic fibrosis following lung transplantation. Chest 1997; 112:924–930.
62. Reilly JS, Kenna MA, Stool SE, Bluestone CD. Nasal surgery in children with cystic fibrosis: complications and risk management. Laryngoscope 1985; 95: 1491–1493.
63. Nishioka G, Barbero G, Konig P, Parsons D, Cook P, Davis W. Symptom outcome after functional endoscopic sinus surgery in patients with cystic fibrosis: a prospective study. Otolaryngol head Neck Surg 1995; 113:440–445.
64. Nishioka G, Cook P, Davis W, McKinsey J. Functional endoscopic sinus surgery in patients with chronic sinusitis and asthma. Otolaryngol Head Neck Surg 1994; 110:494–500.

10

Medical Treatment of Rhinosinusitis in Infants and Children

Joshua A. Gottschall and Michael S. Benninger

Department of Otolaryngology-Head and Neck Surgery, Henry Ford Hospital, Detroit, Michigan, U.S.A.

INTRODUCTION

Rhinosinusitis is inflammation of the mucosal linings of the nose and paranasal sinuses. It is a prevalent disease that accounts for a large portion of annual health care expenditures in the United States each year, representing the fifth most common diagnosis in children for which antibiotics are prescribed (1). In 1996, overall health care expenditures attributable to rhinosinusitis were estimated at $5.8 billion, of which $1.8 billion (30.6%) was for children 12 years and younger (2). This does not include out-of-pocket costs for patients who do not seek medical care, including cost for over-the-counter medications, and indirect costs caused by lost work productivity and care for sick children. More importantly, it is a source of significant morbidity and may be associated with infrequent, although occasionally severe, complications.

The most common predisposing factors leading to clinically significant bacterial rhinosinusitis in children are recent cold or upper respiratory infection (URI) and allergy. However, other factors may play an important role in the pathophysiology of rhinosinusitis. Important questions to consider include: Is the primary cause likely due to an infectious etiology and is the inflammation acute or chronic? In general, rhinosinusitis occurs when there is mucous stasis as a result of sinus outflow obstruction and impaired mucociliary function. An ideal environment for bacterial colonization is created which may lead to a bacterial rhinosinusitis. The term *rhinosinusitis* has largely supplanted *sinusitis* as a more appropriate descriptor since the former reflects a continuum of disease that involves not only the paranasal sinuses, but also the nasal cavities. In children, the nasopharynx and middle ear are often also involved as a result of diffuse upper airway inflammation or infection.

Accurate diagnosis through strict clinical criteria is essential in order to initiate an appropriate treatment plan. Controversy currently exists regarding the medical treatment of both acute and chronic rhinosinusitis. How is rhinosinusitis diagnosed? What are the definitions of acute, subacute, and chronic rhinosinusitis, and how are they best managed? Are antibiotics always indicated in their treatment? What is the definition of "maximal medical therapy"? What are the roles of adjuvant therapies such as nasal irrigations, topical corticosteroids, decongestants, and antihistamines? What role do vaccines play? When should surgery be considered? Many of these questions are heavily debated and remain to be answered. Although viral rhinosinusitis is most common, antimicrobial therapy forms the foundation of medical treatment for those children with suspected or confirmed bacterial rhinosinusitis. Most children with uncomplicated bacterial rhinosinusitis, however, will eventually improve with or without antibiotics. Thankfully, complications are infrequent. Thus a balance must be struck between the natural history of the disease, the expectations of the caregiver, and the consequences and costs of treatment.

DEFINITIONS

General definitions of rhinosinusitis have been developed for both the adult and pediatric age groups (3,4). Acute bacterial rhinosinusitis (ABRS) is defined as a bacterial infection of the paranasal sinuses lasting less than 30 days. In general, the symptoms resolve completely. Subacute bacterial rhinosinusitis is a bacterial infection of the paranasal sinuses lasting between 30 and 90 days with a similar presentation as seen in acute rhinosinusitis. Recurrent acute bacterial rhinosinusitis is defined as multiple episodes of bacterial infection of the paranasal sinuses, each lasting for at least 7 to 10 days but less than 30 days, and separated by intervals of at least 10 days during which the patient is asymptomatic. Chronic rhinosinusitis (CRS) has recently been redefined as a group of disorders characterized by inflammation of the mucosa of the nose and paranasal sinuses of at least 12 consecutive weeks' duration (5). Patients often have persistent residual respiratory symptoms such as rhinorrhea or nasal obstruction, and there may be persistent cough in children. Acute exacerbation of chronic rhinosinusitis occurs when individuals with CRS develop new acute respira-

Table 1 Rhinosinusitis: Definitions

Acute bacterial rhinosinusitis (ABRS): a bacterial infection of the nose and paranasal sinuses lasting less than 30 days

Subacute bacterial rhinosinusitis: a bacterial infection of the nose and paranasal sinuses lasting between 30 and 90 days. In general, these symptoms resolve completely

Recurrent acute bacterial rhinosinusitis: multiple episodes of bacterial infection of the nose and paranasal sinuses, each lasting for at least 7–10 days but less than 30 days and separated by intervals of at least 10 days during which the patient is asymptomatic

Chronic rhinosinusitis (CRS): a group of disorders characterized by inflammation of the mucosa of the nose and paranasal sinuses of at least 12 consecutive weeks' duration

Acute exacerbation of chronic rhinosinusitis: when individuals with chronic rhinosinusitis develop new acute respiratory symptoms

---

Source: Adapted from Refs. 3, 4, 6.

tory symptoms. When treated with antimicrobials, these new symptoms resolve, but the underlying chronic symptoms do not.

The diagnosis of both pediatric and adult rhinosinusitis is best made based upon clinical criteria (6), with a large portion of the diagnosis being defined by the duration of symptoms as acute, subacute, and chronic subtypes. The duration of symptoms that define acute, subacute, and chronic subtypes (Table 1) is supported by clinical symptoms and physical findings. Thus, the diagnoses are dependent upon establishing a time frame for the disease and then applying clinical criteria to assure the diagnosis.

CLINICAL PRESENTATION AND DIAGNOSIS

In the pediatric population, clinical diagnosis of rhinosinusitis can be quite challenging. Although the most accepted gold standard for the diagnosis of bacterial rhinosinusitis is sinus puncture with aspiration and culture (6), this is rarely required in uncomplicated cases of ABRS. The diagnosis of rhinosinusitis is therefore made by the clinical history and supported by findings on physical examination. However, the child is often unwilling or unable to participate in the history and physical examination. Thus, the account of the parent or caregiver is essential. Facial pain and general malaise may manifest as irritability or lethargy in infants. This may be the only presenting symptom in this age group. In older children, the presence of two major symptoms or one major and two minor symptoms would strongly support the diagnosis of ABRS (Table 2). They may present with symptoms of nasal congestion, purulent nasal discharge, daytime or nocturnal cough, facial pressure or pain, hyposmia or anosmia, and general malaise. They may

Table 2 Diagnosis of Rhinosinusitis in Children

Major factors	Minor factors
Facial pain/pressure	Headache/Irritability
Nasal obstruction/congestion	Fever
Nasal discharge/purulence	Halitosis
Hyposmia/anosmia	Fatigue
Cough (not due to asthma)	Dental pain
	Ear pain/pressure/fullness

Source: Adapted from Ref. 3.

also report nontender periorbital edema upon awakening, halitosis, fever, and headache. Rhinosinusitis is the second most common cause of chronic cough in children (7). Children presenting with a self-limiting viral URI or cold may be indistinguishable from those with bacterial rhinosinusitis. Thus differentiating between these two diagnoses is primarily based on the time of onset. Most viral URIs will begin to improve within seven days and completely resolve by 10 to 14 days. Symptoms worsening after seven days or persisting for 10 days or more are highly suggestive of bacterial rhinosinusitis (4,6). The color of the mucous will not readily differentiate a bacterial from a viral rhinosinusitis and distinguishing between purulent-appearing nasal secretions from an infected sinus versus colonized stagnant secretions from the nasal cavity or chronic adenoiditis may prove difficult.

Acute rhinosinusitis may occasionally present with moderate or severe symptoms including high fevers ($>39°C$) and purulent rhinorrhea with or without orbital and intracranial involvement. Hospitalization with empiric parenteral antibiotic therapy should be considered. Close observation with medical management for a period of 24 to 48 hours is reasonable with appropriate surgical intervention reserved for treatment failures or those with evidence of orbital or intracranial extension. Caution and early treatment should be instituted in any child with a toxic appearance or who has diabetes or is otherwise immunocompromised and meets the clinical criteria of acute rhinosinusitis. In such cases, selective middle meatal cultures or sinus tap cultures should be considered.

Patients with CRS often present with a history of failing multiple courses of antibiotics and may have had prior sinus surgery. The symptoms of CRS are similar to those of acute rhinosinusitis; however, symptoms tend to be mild and indolent with nasal congestion, rhinorrhea, and changes in smell being most common. These patients may also have bronchial hyperresponsiveness and a concurrent diagnosis of asthma. Effective management of rhinosinusitis in asthmatic children has been shown to result in improvement of their pulmonary function studies and overall course of asthma (8).

Radiographic studies are not routinely employed in the diagnosis of uncomplicated ABRS. Plain sinus radiographs are rarely helpful in the clinical setting and are the least accurate imaging method for evaluating the ethmoid sinuses where inflammatory disease is most prevalent (9). Computed tomography (CT) of the paranasal sinuses is usually reserved for cases refractory to medical therapy and where orbital or intracranial extension is suspected. CT of the paranasal sinuses is also recommended when sinus surgery is being considered. CT is superior to magnetic resonance imaging (MRI) for evaluation of bony anatomy. MRI may be useful in the evaluation of a suspected fungal sinusitis.

Intranasal examination with an otoscope or nasal speculum or endoscopic examination of the cooperative child may reveal purulent discharge in the middle meatus. This, in conjunction with the characteristic history, further supports a diagnosis of bacterial rhinosinusitis. Assessment of the nasopharynx may reveal large adenoid vegetations or a concurrent adenoiditis, both of which may produce symptoms of nasal congestion and rhinorrhea. A nasal foreign body must be considered in the case of foul unilateral purulent rhinorrhea.

When following strict clinical criteria, an accurate diagnosis of rhinosinusitis can be made. The medical treatment of the common cold and acute versus chronic bacterial rhinosinusitis differs significantly and thus reflects the importance of accurate diagnosis. Although the subtypes of rhinosinusitis are somewhat arbitrarily derived, they are useful in formulating a treatment plan.

CAUSATIVE FACTORS AND ASSOCIATED ILLNESSES

The pathophysiology of rhinosinusitis can be simplified to a common theme: mucous stasis due to osteomeatal obstruction and mucociliary dysfunction. Persistent obstruction results in decreased oxygen tension, reduced sinus pH, ciliary dysfunction, and negative pressure within the sinus cavity. With sneezing or nose blowing, transient opening of the sinus drainage pathways may allow inoculation of pathogenic bacteria in an otherwise sterile sinus cavity (10). An optimal environment for overgrowth is thereby created, resulting in bacterial rhinosinusitis. Children are susceptible to developing rhinosinusitis due to the relative antigenic naivete of their immune systems and immature sinonasal anatomy. They are much more prone to developing a viral URI than adults, predisposing to the development of bacterial rhinosinusitis. However, other etiologies and cofactors leading to rhinosinusitis must be considered. This is especially true in children with recurrent acute rhinosinusitis and CRS.

Upper Respiratory Infection

On average, children have six to eight URIs per year, with 5 to 10% progressing into ABRS (11). This number increases dramatically in an otolaryngology clinic, where up to 83% of patients presenting with an acute URI may have ABRS (12). The "common cold" is actually a viral rhinosinusitis (13). A viral URI is a self-limiting disease. However, mucosal edema with sinus ostia obstruction and derangement of normal ciliary function as a result of the virus may set the stage for a secondary bacterial infection. Respiratory viruses may have a direct cytotoxic effect on the cilia that may result in impaired mucociliary clearance long after resolution of the acute viral infection. Certain viruses, such as rhinovirus, also increase the adherence of pathogenic bacteria such as *Streptococcus pneumoniae* and *Hemophilus influenzae* in the nasopharynx, increasing the likelihood of bacterial colonization and infection (14). This is the most common cause of ABRS in children. As these patients enter adolescence, the frequency of both viral and bacterial rhinosinusitis gradually decreases.

Allergy

Allergy can play a significant role in children with recurrent acute and chronic rhinosinusitis. It may be the underlying etiology in failed antimicrobial therapy. All patients should be evaluated for allergies when taking the history, with a focus on both ingested (food) and inhalant (dust mite, mold, dander, and pollen) allergies (15). Symptoms such as nasal congestion, cough, and behavioral changes are seen in both allergic rhinitis and rhinosinusitis, and seasonal allergic rhinitis is often confused with acute rhinosinusitis, occasionally prompting inappropriate antibiotic therapy. Symptoms and signs consistent with allergies include sneezing, clear nasal secretions, itchy mucous membranes of the upper aerodigestive tract, conjunctivitis, and "allergic shiners." Patients may have the characteristic supratip crease caused by wiping the nose with the palm of the hand, also known as the "allergic salute." There may be a history of sinusitis during the allergy season. The tendency to have allergies is genetically determined and therefore is reflected in the family history. If one parent has had a history of allergy problems, any child in that family has a 20 to 40% chance of having allergic disease. If both parents have allergy problems, children have a 50 to 70% chance of having allergic manifestations at some time in their life (16,17). In 13% of children with a negative allergy history, skin testing is nevertheless positive. This has prompted some to advocate formal allergy testing in all cases of CRS who fail medical treatment and prior to proceeding with surgery (18). Appropriate allergy skin testing or in vitro tests [radioallergosorbent test (RAST), enzyme-linked immunosorbent assay (ELISA), and IgE] may be performed. In vitro tests for allergy are useful in young children.

Role of the Adenoid

An enlarged adenoid pad, with or without chronic adenoiditis, may produce symptoms indistinguishable from rhinosinusitis. Chronic nasal obstruction produces mucous stasis in the nasal cavities, especially in young children who are unable to blow their noses. This mucous may become locally infected and produce purulent anterior rhinorrhea. Nasal congestion results in the typical "adenoid facies" with persistent open-mouth-breathing posture. Diagnosis may be confirmed by anterior rhinoscopy of the decongested nose, office endoscopy, or lateral neck radiograph. Similar to the rationale behind adenoidectomy for the treatment of recurrent suppurative otitis media, the adenoid pad may serve as a bacterial reservoir predisposing to rhinosinusitis. There is evidence to suggest that adenoidectomy alone provides symptomatic improvement in 79% of children with CRS (19). We advocate adenoidectomy as an initial surgical intervention prior to endoscopic sinus surgery in children with CRS refractory to medical treatment.

Extraesophageal Reflux (EER)

EER has been shown to play an important role in chronic and acute inflammatory disorders of the airway. Double-lumen pH probe studies confirm that acid from the stomach does, in fact, reach the nasopharynx in children with chronic sinus disease (20,21). Children seldom complain of the classic symptoms of gastroesophageal reflux such as heartburn, indigestion, regurgitation, and sour taste in the mouth, and it is estimated that as many as 50% of individuals have "silent" reflux. The gold standard for the evaluation of reflux disease is double-lumen pH probe monitoring. However, reflux may be assessed by a variety of methods including an upper gastrointestinal series, technetium scintigraphy, bronchoscopy with telescopic visualization, and bronchoalveolar lavage for lipid-laden macrophages. Empiric antireflux therapy may be instituted as well. Bothwell et al. retrospectively reviewed 30 children with CRS refractive to medical therapy (22). All were considered candidates for endoscopic sinus surgery. All 30 were treated for reflux including counseling, H2 mockers, prokinetic agents, and proton pump inhibitors. Two patients required Nissen fundoplication. Although they responded to antireflux therapy, two patients underwent surgery for contact point release. Of the remaining 28 patients, 89% avoided sinus surgery after a two-year follow up.

Anatomic or Structural Abnormalities

Although the presence of a deviated septum, choncha bullosa, paradoxical middle turbinate, uncinate hypoplasia, enlarged infraorbital cells, and others have not been definitively shown to cause rhinosinusitis, they may potentiate an infection or may delay resolution of normal mucous drainage and aeration as a result of impaired mucociliary clearance. Medical management aimed at improving the nasal airway and the sinus drainage pathways include topical nasal steroids and decongestants. However, surgical correction may be necessary.

Humoral Immunity Deficiencies

Impaired primary or secondary humoral immunity must be considered in children with recurrent acute rhinosinusitis and CRS who fail to respond to conservative management or fail to improve, even temporarily. The most common of these include IgG subclass deficiency, IgA deficiency, and common variable deficiency. The indication for immune function testing has not been clearly defined. These children present with multiple upper and lower respiratory tract infections. In addition to rhinosinusitis, they may present with recurrent pneumonia, bronchitis, and otitis media. The diagnosis of immunodeficiency is usually made by serum immunoglobulin quantization.

Cystic Fibrosis

Any child with a history of chronic sinusitis with nasal polyposis must be evaluated for cystic fibrosis. Cystic fibrosis is the most common life-threatening autosomal recessive disorder in Caucasians with an incidence of 1:3200 newborns in the United States. It is less common in African Americans (1:15,000) and Asian Americans (1:31,000). It presents as a progressive obstructive exocrine insufficiency, which manifests as pulmonary and pancreatic insufficiency. Nasal polyposis and sinusitis are seen in varying degrees of severity in nearly all patients. In addition to the clinical presentation, a sweat chloride concentration greater than 60 mmol/L is diagnostic for cystic fibrosis (23).

Disorders of Ciliary Motility

Primary ciliary dyskinesia is an autosomal recessive condition characterized by chronic sinusitis, bronchiectasis, and infertility. Situs inversus occurs in 50% of cases (Kartagener syndrome). It has an estimated incidence of one in 20,000 live births. The clinical phenotype is caused by defective ciliary function associated with a range of ultrastructural abnormalities including absent dynein arms, absent radial spokes, and disturbed ciliary orientation (normal is the $9 + 2$ microtubule orientation) (24). The molecular and genetic basis is unknown. The saccharin test, which measures the time taken for a pellet of saccharin placed on the inferior turbinate to be tasted (normal <30 min), is very difficult to perform properly in children (25). Confirmation of the diagnosis ideally requires nasal brushings or biopsy which is available only at specialized centers.

Environmental Exposures

Attendance at day care facilities is associated with a higher incidence of URIs and otitis media. The National Institute of Child Health and Human Development (NICHD) Early Child Care Research Network reported that children in large-group care during the preschool years were about twice as likely to have a respiratory tract illness and approximately 1.5 times as likely to have a reported ear infection (26). Secondary or passive exposure to cigarette smoke is known to cause increased rates of otitis media and URIs in children. There is growing evidence that secondary smoke exposure may be an important factor in the development of acute rhinosinusitis and CRS as well as chronic rhinitis in children (27).

TREATMENT OVERVIEW

Antimicrobial therapy remains the primary focus in the medical treatment of acute rhinosinusitis. In 1986, Wald et al. conducted a randomized trial comparing the effectiveness of amoxicillin and amoxicillin-clavulanate therapy compared to placebo in the treatment of children with clinical and radiographic diagnosis of ABRS (28). On the third day of treatment, 83% of children receiving antibiotics were cured or improved compared to 51% of the children in the placebo group. On the tenth day of treatment, 79% of children receiving antibiotics were cured or improved compared to 60% of children receiving placebo. They demonstrated approximately 50 to 60% of children will improve gradually without the use of antimicrobials; however, the recovery of an additional 20 to 30% is delayed substantially compared with children who receive appropriate antibiotics.

In contrast, Garbutt et al. challenged the notion that antibiotics are beneficial in children diagnosed with acute rhinosinusitis in 2001 (29). Children with a clinical diagnosis of acute rhinosinusitis were randomized to receive standard dose amoxicillin, amoxicillin-clavulanate, and placebo. Day 14 improvement rates were 79%, 81%, and 79%, respectively. There were no differences in the observed outcome measures of timing or frequency of recovery.

In 1997, the Agency for Healthcare Policy and Research (AHCPR) contracted an expert panel to prepare an evidence-based review of the world's literature related to the diagnosis and treatment of uncomplicated, community-based rhinosinusitis (30). They conducted a meta-analysis reviewing over 9000 articles from the literature. Their key findings were that clinical criteria-based diagnosis is the most cost-effective, while sinus radiograms are not cost-effective in the initial management strategy. Antibiotics were found to reduce the incidence of clinical failures by one-half in comparison to no treatment (30).

Currently, the American Academy of Pediatrics Subcommittee on Management of Sinusitis and Committee on Quality Improvement as well as the Sinus and Allergy Health Partnership (SAHP) recommend the use of antibiotics in the treatment of acute sinusitis after completing a review of the literature and conducting a consensus poll of its respective members (4,6). In 2002, Morris and Leach conducted a meta-analysis of available randomized, controlled trials which compared antibiotics versus placebo or standard therapy (nasal irrigations) (31). The evidence contained within this review supports the notion that antibiotics increase rates of clinical cure or improvement in children with rhinosinusitis. This was based upon the results of six small, randomized, controlled trials incorporating a total of 562 children.

Although antibiotics remain the primary treatment of rhinosinusitis in children, unnecessary antibiotic-prescribing practices may be contributing to increasing rates of antibiotic resistance. Antibiotics prescribed for a viral illness may do nothing more than result in gastrointestinal side effects and hold the potential for serious side effects including allergy, systemic toxicity, and anaphylaxis. The axiom that antibiotics will do no harm is unjustified since the overuse of antibiotics is the principle cause of progressive antibiotic resistance. The overwhelming cost of prescription medications also adds merit to the argument for judicious prescribing practices.

The overall goal of therapy for rhinosinusitis is to reestablish the normal sinonasal drainage pathways, eradicate pathogenic organisms, prevent suppurative complications, and improve general well-being. These goals must be considered along with the knowledge that as in otitis media, the majority of cases of acute rhinosinusitis will resolve with or without antibiotics.

MICROBIOLOGY OF ACUTE AND CHRONIC RHINOSINUSITIS

The microbiology of ABRS in children has been shown to be similar to that of adults (32). In 2000, a review of bacterial isolation studies was conducted by the SAHP. In children with ABRS, *S. pneumoniae* is isolated in approximately 35 to 42% of aspirates, whereas *H. influenzae* and *Moraxella catarrhalis* are each isolated in 21 to 28%. Other organisms recovered include *Streptococcus pyogenes* and anaerobes, both of which account for 3 to 7% (Fig. 1) (6). Culture results of children with subacute bacterial rhinosinusitis show a similar organism profile as that found in ABRS (33).

Bacteriologic studies of children with CRS are less certain than those conducted in children with acute rhinosinusitis. Due to differences in the definition of CRS and variations in methods of collection, a wide variability of pathogenic bacteria has been identified. In 1991, Muntz and Lusk (34) cultured 204 ethmoid bullae in children operated on for CRS. The most common organisms isolated were α-hemolytic *Streptococcus* (23%), *S. aureus* (19%), *S. pneumoniae* (7%), *H. influenzae* (7%), and *M. catarrhalis* (7%). Anaerobes are more frequently encountered in children with CRS than acute rhinosinusitis. This may be explained by the low-oxygen tension of chronically obstructed sinuses resulting in a more favorable growth environment for anaerobes. Although not universally accepted, Brook (35) strongly emphasizes the role of anaerobes in chronic sinusitis in children. In a series of 37 culture-positive pediatric patients, anaerobic species were recovered in 100% of cases. The most commonly isolated anaerobes were *Prevotella*, *Peptostreptococcus*, and *Bacteriodes*. In 1988, Otten and Grote (36) studied

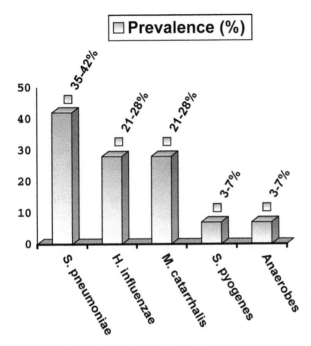

Figure 1 Ranges and prevalence of the major pathogens associated with ABRS in children. *Source*: Adapted from SAHP Ref. 6. *Abbreviation*: ABRS, acute bacterial rhinosinusitis.

CRS in children, which they defined as the presence of purulent nasal discharge for more than 3 months. Sinus aspiration yielded positive cultures in 91% of cases. *S. pneumoniae* and *H. influenzae* were found in the majority of cases (60%). In 1989, Tinkleman and Silk (37) found that in 35 children with CRS, the most common isolates were *H. influenzae*, *S. pneumoniae*, and *M. catarrhalis*. Finally, in patients with acute exacerbations of chronic sinusitis, the usual microorganisms associated with acute sinusitis (*S. pneumoniae*, *M. catarrhalis*, and *H. influenzae*) are seen most often (32). The use of vaccines may be shifting the distribution of pathogens. Close observation of these trends is necessary to determine whether or not prescribing behaviors should follow.

ANTIMICROBIAL MANAGEMENT OF RHINOSINUSITIS

Acute Rhinosinusitis

Antimicrobial therapy forms the foundation of treatment in children with suspected or culture-confirmed ABRS. Numerous antibiotic choices are available; however, the efficacy of a particular agent against the usual offending organisms must be considered. Since up to 70% of ABRS cases are caused by either *S. pneumoniae* or *H. influenzae*, empiric antibiotic therapy should be directed at these organisms (10). Of these, *S. pneumoniae* is more likely to result in more severe disease and suppurative complications such as orbital or intracranial extension. Several factors should be considered in the selection of an antibiotic for ABRS. These include severity of disease, rate of progression of the disease, recent antibiotic therapies, and community resistance rates of the suspected pathogen. Other factors that may influence antibiotic selection include medication allergy or intolerance, cost, taste, available preparations, and frequency of dosing. Compliance with therapy is a major factor that will influence treatment success. Available antibiotics for use in children with rhinosinusitis include β-lactams (penicillins and cephalosporins), augmented β-lactams, macrolides (erythromycin, clarithromycin, and azithromycin), lincosamides (clindamycin), and folate inhibitors. Although the fluoroquinolones, particularly the newer respiratory fluoroquinolones, provide excellent coverage for both *S. pneumoniae* and *H. influenzae* infections, they are currently not approved for use in children younger than 18 years. Tetracyclines are contraindicated for use in children younger than eight years due to risk of tooth enamel discoloration.

According to the guidelines of the SAHP (Table 3), appropriate therapies for children with mild disease who have not received antibiotics in the past four to six weeks include amoxicillin (45–90 mg/kg/day) with or without clavulanate, cetpodoxime proxetil, and cefuroxime axetil. In patients with significant allergy to penicillins and cephalosporins, doxycyline (>8 years old), azithromycin, clarithromycin, erythromycin, or TMP/SMX may be used (6). For children who have received a prior antibiotic in the past four to six weeks or have moderate disease, double dose amoxicillin (80–90 mg/kg/day) with or without clavulanate should be used if this agent is selected. Also, clindamycin may be considered if *S. pneumoniae* is identified as a pathogen. Patients with moderate sinus disease and who have received antibiotics, amoxicillin with clavulanate (80–90 mg/kg/day) would be the first line choice. Combination therapy is an alternative, which would include amoxicillin (80–90 mg/kg/day) or clindamycin for gram-positive coverage, plus cefixime, cepodoxime proxetil, or TMP/SMX for gram-negative coverage.

According to the SAHP, the terms mild and moderate disease reflect the symptom complex, the degree of discomfort of the patient, and the time course of the infection. A child, who is otherwise healthy, with 10 days of persistent anterior and posterior rhinorrhea and fatigue is considered to have mild disease. This same patient with worsening symptoms, including fever and maxillary or frontal tenderness that worsens with bending over, is considered to have moderate disease. These definitions are by no means strict; the determination of the severity of disease requires clinical judgment on a case-by-case basis.

Table 3 SAHP Guidelines for Antibiotic Treatment in Children with Mild/ Moderate ABRS

Symptom severity	
Mild	Amoxicillin (45–90 mg/kg/day)
	Amoxicillin/clavulanate
	(45–90 mg/kg/day)
	Cefpodoxime proxetil
	Cefuroxime axetil
	For β-lactam allergic:
	TMP/SMX
	Doxycyline
	Azithromycin
	Clarithromycin
	Erythromycin
Mild with antibiotic use in past 4–6 weeks	Amoxicillin (80–90 mg/kg/day)
Moderate	Amoxicillin/clavulanate (80–90 mg/kg/day)
	Cefpodoxime proxetil
	Cefuroxime axetil
	For β-lactam allergic:
	Azithromycin
	Clarithromycin
	Erythromycin
	TMP/SMX
	Clindamycin
Moderate with antibiotic use in past 4–6 weeks	Amoxicillin/clavulanate (80–90 mg/kg/day) or combination therapy (amoxicillin 80–90 mg/kg/day or clindamycin + cefixime, cefpodoxime proxetil, or TMP/SMX)
	For β-lactam allergic:
	TMP/SMX + clindamycin

Abbreviations: SAHP, Sinus and Allergy Health Partnership; ABRS, acute bacterial rhinosinusitis. *Source*: From Ref. 6

The predicted efficacy of each antibiotic in the treatment of children with ABRS has been calculated by the SAHP: >90% (amoxicillin/clavulanate and high-dose amoxicillin), 80–90% [(cefpodoxime proxetil, cefixime-based upon *H. influenzae* and *M. catarrhalis* coverage only), (cefuroxime axetil, clindamycin-based on gram-positive coverage only), azithromycin, clarithromycin, erythromycin, and TMP/SMX], 70–80% (cefprozil), and 60–70% (cefaclor and loracarbef) (6). The predicted efficacy of cefaclor and loracarbef is slightly better than placebo (49.6%) and thus would not be a good choice in the management of ABRS in children.

Uncomplicated ABRS, as previously defined, may be managed most appropriately with amoxicillin in either standard (45 mg/kg/day) or high (90 mg/kg/day) dose. Amoxicillin is the most suitable choice in the initial management of non-penicillin allergic children due to its proven efficacy, safety profile, low cost, and tolerability. All but highly resistant *S. pneumoniae* will respond to conventional doses of amoxicillin, but given the safety profile of high-dose amoxicillin and gradually rising resistance rates, there does not seem to be any compelling reason to use standard dose amoxicillin. *S. pneumoniae* resistance to penicillins has been documented to be as high as 30% (4,6). Double-dose amoxicillin (90 mg/kg/day) will improve coverage of highly resistant strains of *S. pneumoniae*. In cases of mild, uncomplicated rhinosinusitis and absence of *risk factors*, approximately 88% of children with ABRS will respond to amoxicillin (6). Risk factors associated with increased rates of resistant *S. pneumoniae* and *H. influenzae* include attendance at day care, prior antimicrobial treatment within past four to six weeks, and age less than two years. Although most of these will still respond to high-dose amoxicillin, the physician should also consider treatment with high-dose amoxicillin-clavulanate (80–90 mg/kg/day).

Selection of a β-lactamase resistant drug is indicated if the infection is due to *H. influenzae* or *M. catarrhalis*, since 40% and nearly 98%, respectively, are likely to be β-lactamase positive (4,6). In general, *M. catarrhalis* is expected to be largely a self-limited disease, not necessarily requiring antibiotic therapy, so treatment directed at *S. pneumoniae* or *H. influenzae* should be the primary goal. The addition of clavulanic acid results in irreversible binding of β-lactamase and restoration of the activity of amoxicillin. Cefuroxime axetil and Cefpodoxime proxetil have potent activity against most strains of *H. influenzae*.

First-generation cephalosporins are rarely used in the treatment of bacterial rhinosinusitis due to lower activity against gram-negative organisms. Second-and third-generation cephalosporins have good spectrum of activity against the most common pathogens, and may be considered in patients with allergy to penicillins, although some cross-class reactivity can occur. Although cefuroxime-axetil, cefpodoxime, and cefixime are potent against most strains of *H. influenzae*, they are not active against penicillin-resistant *S. pneumoniae*. Ceftriaxone has good activity against both *H. influenzae* and *S. pneumoniae*. Cefaclor is susceptible to β-lactamase and is a poor choice overall. Clarithromycin and azithromycin may also be used. Penicillin, cephalexin, and tetracycline should not be used because these drugs do not cover the major organisms that cause acute rhinosinusitis (10). An alternative is the combination of erythromycin (30–50 mg/kg/day) and sulfisoxazole (150 mg/kg/day). Sulfisoxazole is added because erythromycin alone does not adequately cover *H. influenziae* (38).

Treatment durations recommended for uncomplicated acute rhinosinusitis include a 5- to 14-day course depending on the antibiotic, with a

10-day course most commonly recommended (6,39,40). Although there is no evidence that longer therapy increases the likelihood of a clinical response, some advocate that treatment can be prolonged for one month if symptoms have improved but have not resolved completely. This is not recommended for uncomplicated ABRS. However, the effect of short-course, high-dose amoxicillin therapy 90 mg/kg/day for five days compared to 40 mg/kg/day for 10 days is comparable (41). This regimen showed improved compliance to treatment and suggests a reduction of resistant pneumococcal selection. If symptoms are unchanged at 72 hours, or worsen at any time, reevaluation is necessary. Switching the antibiotic to one that is β-lactamase stable is appropriate in this situation. Others recommend extending treatment for an additional seven days after resolution of symptoms (1,11).

Chronic Rhinosinusitis

"The CRS is a group of disorders characterized by inflammation of the mucosa of the nose and paranasal sinuses of at least 12 consecutive weeks' duration (5)." This definition identifies CRS as a group of inflammatory disorders, which may or may not be related to an infectious etiology. Although pediatric CRS has not been clearly defined, a similar definition would be expected to apply.

The treatment of CRS is very controversial, largely because of the various potential etiologies and associated conditions. Whether or not antibiotics or antifungal medications are indicated has been widely debated, although selected patients might benefit from such treatment. Most patients respond well to treatment with topical intranasal cortico steroids, allergy therapy where appropriate, or short bursts of systemic corticosteroids. This is particularly true in patients who have chronic symptoms and develop acute exacerbations with worsening symptoms and increase in purulent nasal drainage. In such cases, antibiotics may be indicated.

Although it is commonly recommended that antibiotic treatment for CRS may include a protracted three-to-six-week course of β-lactamase-stable antibiotic, there are no scientific data supporting this. Acute exacerbations of chronic sinusitis would seem to benefit from antibiotics directed at *S. pneumoniae*, *H. influenzae*, *S. aureus*, and anaerobes. Culture-directed therapy should be strongly considered. This may be performed as an office procedure with a cooperative child, but more often requires sedation or a general anesthetic. The maxillary sinus is the most easily accessible. A trocar is inserted into the maxillary sinus via the inferior meatus, and material is aspirated for culture. The risk of contamination of the specimen with organisms representing the nasal flora may lead to misleading results. Quantitative cultures with recovery of bacteria in a density of $>10^4$ colony-forming-units/mL is considered representative of a true infection (11). The difficulty in obtaining sinus puncture and aspirate and the growing evidence that selective middle meatal endoscopically guided cultures may be as accurate have prompted many otolaryngologists to prefer obtaining such cultures over the more difficult sinus tap (42). Although nasopharyngeal cultures are not very predictive of sinus pathogens in the adult, they do correlate better in children. Despite this, selective middle meatal cultures or sinus taps are preferred if the pathogen needs to be definitively identified.

High-dose amoxicillin-clavulanate (90 mg/kg/day) or a second generation cephalosporin would be appropriate if antimicrobial therapy is considered in children with CRS. Clarithromycin would be an alternative in highly penicillin-allergic patients. Clindamycin at 30–40 mg/kg/day in three divided doses would be an alternative in addition to providing good anaerobic coverage.

The difficulty of successful medical treatment of children with CRS "is less likely to be a failure to prescribe the correct agent then it is a reflection of the fact that the process causing the chronic symptoms is not caused by bacterial agents" (32).

ADJUVANT THERAPIES

General Treatment Measures

The goal of treatment of both acute and chronic rhinosinusitis, in addition to sterilization of sinus contents, is the reestablishment of normal mucociliary clearance. This is accomplished in part by a number of general treatment measures directed at establishing a more normal nasal environment through moisturization, humidification, and the reduction of swelling. A number of adjuvant therapies in addition to antimicrobials have gained wide acceptance despite lack of case-controlled trials proving their efficacy as compared to antibiotics alone or placebo.

Nasal Saline Irrigations

In addition to moisturizing the nasal cavities, saline irrigation clears purulent drainage and crusts and serves to decongest the nasal mucosa due to its hypertonicity. The low cost and low risk of this treatment and the symptomatic relief it provides to the patient argue for its routine use in both acute and chronic rhinosinusitis. Saline irrigations have been shown to reduce the symptoms of both allergic and non-allergic rhinitis and they are likely to be beneficial in rhinosinusitis as well (10).

Humidification

Systemic hydration and use of portable humidifiers may be valuable in the treatment regimen for rhinosinusitis. A dry nasal environment results in more viscous nasal secretion which may interfere with mucociliary transport. Controversy exists as to whether warm or cool humidification is preferable. In most patients, humidification can help to control symptoms.

Care must be taken to keep the humidifier clean. Patients with mold allergies may actually have a worsening of their rhinosinusitis, since excessive humidification may increase inflammation (10).

Mucolytic Agents

In addition to humidification, the addition of a mucolytic agent such as guaifenesin, a component of many decongestants and expectorants, serves to thin mucous. This will theoretically assist in restoring mucociliary clearance and promote clearing of stagnant secretions. This may be particularly important in disorders of mucociliary clearance and disorders in which there is a reduction or thickening of glandular secretions such as in cystic fibrosis (43).

Decongestants

Decongestants result in shrinking of nasal mucosa through vasoconstriction acting through α-adrenergic receptors located in the sinonasal mucosa. This would be expected to help reduce obstruction of sinus drainage pathways and improve ventilation. Thus decongestants may have a role in the treatment of rhinosinusitis. Oxymetazoline hydrochloride applied topically will provide rapid decongestion of nasal mucosa; however, extended use beyond three to five days may result in rebound rhinitis and habituation. Bende et al. suggested that topical decongestants may actually have a detrimental effect by actually increasing inflammation of sinonasal mucosa (44). In this study, histological sections of rabbit sinuses obtained after induction of sinusitis and treatment with topical oxymetazoline were actually found to have a significantly greater degree of inflammation than sections of untreated sinuses on the opposite side. This may be due to the interference of the normal defense mechanisms during bacterial-induced rhinosinusitis, possibly by decreased mucosal blood flow. Despite these reservations, topical decongestants will usually reduce symptoms and speed recovery in patients with rhinosinusitis (10). Systemic decongestants may also be used to treat patients with rhinosinusitis. The effects are similar to topical decongestant, but the likelihood of systemic side effects and their relative contraindications in some patients may limit their use. The role of systemic decongestants in the treatment of pediatric rhinosinusitis is unclear.

Antihistamines

Both sedating and the newer non-sedating antihistamines have been routinely used in the symptomatic treatment of allergies and allergic rhinitis. Since allergy is frequently seen in patients with rhinosinusitis, antihistamines may be beneficial in controlling not only allergy symptoms, but rhinosinusitis itself. However, due to the anticholinergic side effects common to all antihistamines, drying and dehydration of nasal secretions may actually have a negative effect on mucociliary transport by increasing viscosity of mucous. First-generation antihistamines such as diphenhydramine and cetirizine have the additional and often unwanted side effect of increased sedation as a result of central nervous system penetration. Second-generation antihistamines such as fexofenadine and loratadine have less sedation.

Topical Nasal Steroids

Nasal steroids are beneficial in the long-term treatment of allergic and non-allergic rhinitis and CRS. Their use in the management of CRS in children is not supported in the literature. However, reduction of nasal mucosal edema and inflammation has a theoretical benefit and is commonly used as in conjunction with antibiotics in the treatment of CRS. When used as an adjunct to antibiotic therapy, topical nasal steroids have been shown to improve symptoms, decrease volume of inflammatory cells, and aid in the regression of radiographic abnormalities (10). A trial of topical intranasal steroid sprays is usually recommended prior to surgical intervention. Concerns related to potential growth suppression in children have largely been dismissed with growing evidence of the safety of the newer generation steroid sprays and the lowering of the indicated ages for some of the products (45).

Vaccinations

Children with chronic and recurrent rhinosinusitis may benefit from vaccination against the most common bacterial pathogens. Conjugated protein to *H. influenza* B is currently part of the routine vaccination regimen in infants and children. However, these patients continue to be susceptible to non-typeable *Hemophilus* sp. Pneumovax raises an IgG_2 response, which is protective against *S. pneumoniae*. Post-immunization titers obtained two months after immunization allow assessment of the normal 4- to 6-fold increase in titers (1). Vaccinations may play an important role in the reduction or prevention of bacterial rhinosinusitis.

WHEN DO WE OPERATE?

At times, an acute process causing sepsis or threatening to involve the surrounding anatomy, such as the orbit, meninges, and brain, may precipitate early surgical intervention. Patients with severe acute rhinosinusitis characterized by high fevers ($>39°C$), toxic appearance, and suspected orbital or intracranial extension should be hospitalized and treated aggressively with intravenous antibiotics such as ceftriaxone or ampicillin/sublactam. If no improvement is seen in 24 to 48 hours for cellulitis, or if frank orbital (Fig. 2) or intracranial suppuration is seen, prompt surgical drainage is indicated. Thankfully, these consequences of rhinosinusitis are infrequent.

The decision to proceed to surgery in patients with mild to moderate chronic symptoms is less clear. Pediatric functional endoscopic sinus surgery

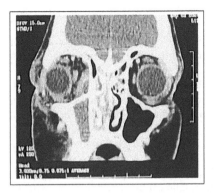 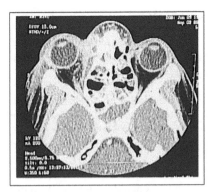

Figure 2 Subperiosteal abscess in a 15-year-old child with severe ABRS.

is effective at managing disease recalcitrant to medical therapy, but it is rarely, if ever, a cure. The long-term effects on facial growth in children undergoing functional endoscopic sinus surgery are uncertain; however, animal studies do suggest we proceed with caution. Failure of medical management including an appropriate antimicrobial, topical nasal steroid, and nasal hydration for a period of six months would be a reasonable guide. At our institution, an adenoidectomy would be performed prior to endoscopic sinus surgery.

Rhinosinusitis is not primarily a consequence of a bacterial overgrowth, but a result of impaired mucocilliary transport and aeration. Thus, addressing the underlying cause of the transport dysfunction ultimately will provide better long-term control of this disease and the avoidance of unnecessary treatments and surgeries.

CONCLUSION

The definition of maximum medical therapy is the selection of the appropriate antibiotic based upon an accurate clinical diagnosis. However vague, this definition reflects how little is truly understood about the pathophysiology and management of this disease. Thus "failing maximal medical treatment" is a great axiom with no real scientific meaning (46). The role of adjuvant therapies is uncertain, although theoretical and anecdotal reports support their use. This is particularly true for intranasal steroids and saline irrigations. The current trend is to reserve surgery as the last resort after maximal medical therapy is exhausted. There has been a significant shift in the last decade from an initial emphasis on surgical treatment of chronic sinusitis in children and adults to a more recent emphasis on maximizing medical treatment with antibiotics and conservative surgery.

REFERENCES

1. Nyquist AC, Gonzales R, Steiner JF, Sande MA. Antibiotic prescribing for children with colds, upper respiratory tract infections, and bronchitis. JAMA 1998; 279:875–877.
2. Ray NF, Baraniuk JN, Thamer M, Rinehart CS, Gergen PJ, Kaliner M, Josephs S, Pung YH. Healthcare expenditures for sinusitis in 1996: contributions of asthma, rhinitis, and other airway disorders. J All Clin Immunol 1999; 103:408–414.
3. Lanza DC, Kennedy DW. Adult rhinosinusitis defined. Otolaryngol Head Neck Surg 1997; 117:S1–S7.
4. American Academy of Pediatrics. Subcommittee on Management of Sinusitis and Committee on Quality Improvement. Clinical practice guideline: management of sinusitis. Pediatrics 2001; 108(3):798–808.
5. Benninger MS, Ferguson BJ, Hadley JA, Hamilos DL, Jacobs M, Kennedy DW, Lanza DC, Marple BF, Osguthorpe JD, Stankiewicz JA, et al. Adult chronic rhinosinusitis: definitions, diagnosis, epidemiology, and pathophysiology. Otolaryngol Head Neck Surg 2003; 129(3):S1–S32.
6. Sinus and Allergy Health Partnership. Antimicrobial treatment guidelines for acute bacterial rhinosinusitis. Otolaryngol Head Neck Surg 2000; 123(suppl 1): S1–S32.
7. Holinger LD. Chronic cough in infants and children. Laryngoscope 1986; 96:316–322.
8. Tsao CH, Chen LC, Yen KW, Huang JL. Concomitant chronic sinusitis treatment in children with mild asthma. Chest 2003; 123:757–764.
9. Zinreich SJ. Report of the rhinosinusitis task force committee meeting, rhinosinusitis: radiologic diagnosis. Otolaryngol Head Neck Surg 1997; 117(3): S27–S34.
10. Benninger MS, Anon J, Mabry RL. The medical management of rhinosinusitis. Otolaryngol Head Neck Surg 1997; 117:S41–S49.
11. Wald ER. Sinusitis. Pediatr Rev 1993; 14(9):345–351.
12. Savolainen S, Pietola M, Kiukaanniemi H, Lappalainen E, Salminen M, Mikkonen P. An ultrasound device in the diagnosis of acute maxillary sinusitis. Acta Otolaryngol Suppl (Stockh) 1997; 529:148–152.
13. Gwaltney JM, Phillips CD, Miller RD, Riker DK. Computed tomographic study of the common cold. N Engl J Med 1994; 330(1):25–30.
14. Fainstein V, Musher DM, Cate TR. Bacterial adherence to pharyngeal cells during viral infection. J Infect Dis 1980; 141(2):172–176.
15. Goldsmith AJ, Rosenfeld RM. Treatment of pediatric sinusitis. Pediatr Clin North Am 2003; 50:413–426.
16. Gungor A, Corey JP. Pediatric sinusitis: a literature review with emphasis on the role of allergy. Otolaryngol Head Neck Surg 1997; 116:4–15.
17. Cook PR, Nishioka GJ. Allergic rhinosinusitis in the pediatric population. Otolaryngol Clin North Am 1996; 29:29–56.
18. Parsons DS. Chronic sinusitis: a medical or surgical disease? Otolaryngol Clin North Am 1996; 29(1):1–9.

19. Vandenberg SF, Heatley DG. Efficacy of adenoidectomy in relieving symptoms of chronic sinusitis in children. Arch Otolaryngol Head Neck Surg 1997; 123: 675–678.
20. Contercin P, Narcy P. Nasopharyngeal pH monitoring in infants and children with chronic rhinopharyngitis. Int J Pediatr Otolaryngol 1991; 22:249–256.
21. Phipps CD, Wood WE, Gibson WS, Cochran WJ. Gastroesophageal reflus contributing to chronic sinus disease in children. Arch Otolaryngol Head Neck Surg 2000; 126:831–836.
22. Bothwell MR, Parsons DS, Talbot A, Barbero GJ, Wilder B. Outcome of reflux therapy on pediatric chronic sinusitis. Otolaryngol Head Neck Surg 1999; 121:255–262.
23. Rosenstein BJ, Cutting GR. The diagnosis of cystic fibrosis: a consensus statement. J Pediatr 1998; 132(4):589–595.
24. Meeks M, Walne A, Spiden S, Simpson H, Mussaffi-Georgi H, Hamam HD, Fehaid EL, Cheehab M, Al-Dubbagh M, Polak-Charcon S, Blau H, O'Rawe A, Mitchinson HM, Gardiner RM, Chung E. A locus for primary ciliary dyskinesia maps to chromosome 19q. J Med Genet 2000; 37(4):241–244.
25. Bush A, O'Callaghan C. Primary ciliary dyskinesia. Arch diseases of childhood 2002; 87(5):363–364.
26. Bradley RH. National Institute of Child Health and Human Development (NICHD) Early Child Care Research Network. Child care and common communicable illnesses in children aged 37–54 months. Arch Pediatr Adolesc Med 2003; 157(2):196–200.
27. Benninger MS. The impact of cigarette smoking and environmental tobacco smoke on nasal and sinus disease: a review of the literature. Am J Rhinol 1999; 13(6):435–438.
28. Wald ER, Chiponis D, Ledesma-Medina J. Comparative effectiveness of amoxicillin and amoxicillin-clavulanate potassium in acute paranasal sinus infections in children: a double-blinded, placebo-controlled trial. Pediatrics 1986; 77:795–800.
29. Garbutt JM, Goldstein M, Gellman E, Shannon W, Littenberg B. A randomized, placebo-controlled trial of antimicrobial treatment for children with clinically diagnosed acute sinusitis. Pediatrics 2001; 107(4):619–625.
30. Benninger MS, Sedory Holzer SE, Lau J. Diagnosis and treatment of uncomplicated acute bacterial rhinosinusitis: summary of the agency for health care policy and research evidence-based report. Otolaryngol Head Neck Surg 2000; 122(1):1–7.
31. Morris P, Leach A. Antibiotics for persistent nasal discharge (rhinosinusitis) in children. The Cochrane Lib 2003; 1:1–26.
32. Wald ER. Microbiology of acute and chronic sinusitis in children and adults. Am J Med Sci 1998; 316(1):12–20.
33. Wald ER, Byers C, Guerra N, Casselbrant M, Beste D. Subacute sinusitis in children. J Pediatr 1989; 115:28–32.
34. Muntz HR, Lusk RP. Bacteriology of the ethmoid bullae in children with chronic sinusitis. Arch Otolaryngol Head Neck Surg 1991; 117:179–181.
35. Brook I. Microbiology and management of sinusitis. J Otolaryngol 1996; 25(4):249–256.

36. Otten FWA, Grote JJ. Treatment of chronic maxillary sinusitis in children. Int J Pediatr Otorhinolaryngol 1988; 15:269–278.
37. Tinkleman DG, Silk HJ. Clinical and bacteriologic features of chronic sinusitis in children. Amer J Dis Child 1989; 143:938–941.
38. Arjmand EM, Lusk RP. Management of recurrent and chronic sinusitis in children. Am J Otolaryngol 1995; 16(6):367–382.
39. Clement PAR, Bluestone CD, Gordts F, Lusk RP, Otten FWA, Goossens H, Scadding GK, Takahashi H, Van Buchem FL, Van Cauwenberge P, et al. Management of rhinosinusitis in children. Int J Pediatr Otorhinolaryngol 1999; 49:S95–S100.
40. Lusk RP, Stankiewicz JA. Pediatric rhinosinusitis. Otolaryngol Head Neck Surg 1997; 117(3):S53–S57.
41. Schrag SJ, Pena C, Fernandez J, Sanchez J, Gomez V, Perez E, Feris JM, Besser RE. Effect of short-course, high-dose amoxicillin therapy on resistant pneumococcal carriage. JAMA 2001; 286(1):49–56.
42. Benninger MS, Applebaum PC, Denneny JC, Osguthorpe JD, Stankiewicz J, Zucker D. Maxillary sinus puncture and culture in the diagnosis of acute rhinosinusitis: the case for pursuing alternative culture methods. Otolaryngol Head Neck Surg 2002; 127:7–12.
43. Davidson TM, Murphy C, Mitchell M, Smith C, Light M. Management of chronic sinusitis in cystic fibrosis. Laryngoscope 1995; 105:354–358.
44. Bende M, Fukami M, Arfars KE, Mark J, Stierna P, Intaglietta M. The effect of oxymetazoline nose drops on acute sinusitis in the rabbit. Ann Otol Rhinol Laryngol 1996; 105:222–225.
45. Benninger MS, Ahmad N, Marple BF. The safety of intranasal steroids. Otolaryngol Head Neck Surg 2003; 129:739–750.
46. Baroody FM. Pediatric Sinusitis, editorial. Arch Otolaryngol Head Neck Surg 2001; 127:1099–1101.

11

Pediatric Endoscopic Sinus Surgery

Ramzi T. Younis

Department of Pediatrics, University of Miami, Miami, Florida, U.S.A.

INTRODUCTION

In the past 20 years, the technique of endoscopic sinus surgery has developed as the primary surgical procedure for nasal and sinus problems. The main objective behind this surgery is the reestablishment of the physiological drainage and ventilation of the paranasal sinuses. Pediatric endoscopic sinus surgery (PESS) is performed very conservatively in children who display persistent, debilitating, and refractory chronic rhinosinusitis (CRS) despite appropriate therapy. Complicated acute rhinosinusitis is certainly one main reason for sinus surgery. Additionally, children with more serious or debilitating conditions such as immunodeficiency, cystic fibrosis, fungal infections, and tumors can have sinusitis that necessitates surgical treatment using PESS. Although CRS has been one of the main indications for PESS, surgery may be required in fewer instances. Other procedures and treatment with consideration of age, contributory factor, and comormibidity may be helpful prior to PESS. Like chronic serous otitis media, CRS in children may diminish greatly as the child gets to be seven or eight years old. Thus, children with CRS may grow out of their disease (1–3).

The role of PESS in CRS continues to evolve. In the early 1990s, the trend of endoscopic sinus surgery seemed to follow a pattern similar to adult surgery. CRS was one of the main indications in all age groups. Nevertheless these endoscopic techniques were being attempted in a variety of other nasal and sinus conditions such as choanal atresia, congenital sinonasal malformations,

CSF leaks, meningoceles, and angiofibroma. Time, improved training, and experience have allowed PESS to become a very popular procedure in the pediatric age group. However, concerns and skepticism grew due to its wide range of application in infants and children. In 1996, a group of specialists in pediatric sinusitis met in Brussels and created a consensus document (4). Ironically, CRS was considered a possible indication but not "absolute."

PESS remains the procedure of choice for resistant sinus conditions. Rhinosinusitis is a complex and challenging disease in children that may be governed by a variety of factors and conditions. During the past decade, a number of important advances have helped change the role and perspective of endoscopic sinus surgery in pediatric CRS. These include increased knowledge of the natural pathophysiological progression of the disease process, change in the importance of aggressively treating sinusitis, increasing interest in the role of adenoidectomy, and the role of better instrumentation and research. PESS is the last resort in the management of rhinosinusitis. Endoscopic sinus surgery is usually considered after all other measures have been exhausted. These may include maximal medical therapy, control of contributory factors, and adenoidectomy.

PEDIATRIC RHINOSINUSITIS

CRS is the number one chronic illness in the United States according to the National Center for Disease statistics (5). Pediatric sinusitis is estimated to complicate 5% to 10% of upper respiratory tract infections (URI) in early childhood (6). Children average six to eight URIs per year, which makes sinusitis a very prevalent problem in the pediatric age group. Subsequently, chronic pediatric rhinosinusitis carries a substantial impact on the quality of life (7,8) and an immense financial burden on the children who are already suffering its symptoms. About 5.8 billion dollars were spent in 1996 on sinus-related problems, 1.8 billion (31%) for children under 12 (9). The impact includes days off from school, number of physician visits, parental days off from work, and potential behavioral problems. Thus, early recognition with optimal medical and surgical management is warranted (7,10).

Sinusitis, an inflammatory process of the mucosal lining of the paranasal sinuses, is a multifunctional, dynamic process commonly seen in children. Prolonged inflammation can produce a characteristic cellular and cytokine response, resulting in irreversible mucosal changes (11). The exact incidence of sinusitis in children is not known. In pediatric patients, sinusitis often is the sequel of a URI or allergic disease (6,12). However, various etiologic factors can predispose children to sinusitis. These factors range from an inflammatory process to a systemic disorder.

In children, sinusitis is a unique entity that requires thorough investigation and treatment. The initial symptoms and radiological findings of sinusitis in children differ from those of adults. In adults, the diagnosis may be based on clinical findings and confirmed radiologically. However, in children, symptoms may vary from an annoying cough of little consequence to a serious complication with substantial morbidity and mortality. Additionally, x-ray findings may be somewhat confusing. Ostensibly, asymptomatic children may have abnormal findings on plain x-rays (13), and clinically symptomatic children may have normal results on x-rays.

Sinusitis in children may have been misdiagnosed because some physicians have believed that the sinuses are not sufficiently developed to be of clinical importance, especially in young children. Additionally, the diagnosis of URI, allergic disease, and adenoiditis may be confused with sinusitis. Subsequently, the reported incidence of CRS in children may be inaccurate.

Selection of a therapeutic modality is as difficult as the diagnosis. With the introduction of various chemotherapeutic agents, surgical techniques, and decreased anesthetic risks, the therapeutic spectrum has widened. However, as a rule, optimal medical treatment should be exhausted before surgical intervention is considered.

Many theories have been proposed regarding the exact function of the paranasal sinuses, but none has met with universal acceptance. Among these theories are that the sinuses may humidify and warm inspired air, impart resonance to the voice, and act as shock absorbers (14).

The normal physiology of the paranasal sinuses is maintained by continuous clearance of secretions, which can be achieved by the coordination of three essential sinus components: patent sinus ostia, functioning ciliary apparatus, and normal sinus secretions. The sinuses continuously secrete mucus into the sinus cavity. The ciliary beat moves the mucus toward the patent ostia, thereby avoiding stagnation. The mucus is then moved through the ostia into the nose and nasopharynx. Once sinonasal secretions are in the nasopharynx, they are either swallowed or expectorated. Conditions that interfere with one or more of these elements may predispose patients to sinusitis.

Ostial Obstruction

As early as the nineteenth century, Caldwell stressed the functional relationship between the ostia of the anterior ethmoid, frontal, and maxillary sinuses (15). He also recognized that maxillary sinusitis may be secondary to other diseases in the region. In 1916, Schaeffer agreed with this theory (16). In 1966, Proctor stated that the ethmoid sinuses were the primary cause of problems involving the sinuses (17). Additionally, he noted that infection usually begins in the ethmoids, and persistent infection usually results in ineffective treatment. Better diagnostic techniques using high-resolution coronal computerized tomography (CT) and direct visualization with fiberoptic telescopes led to the rediscovery of this entity.

Obstruction of sinus ostia is the major cause of sinus infection. When ostial obstruction occurs, the continuously secreted mucus remains in the sinus cavity. Stagnant secretions form an excellent medium for bacterial growth. Gas exchange within the sinus also is impaired when the ostium is completely obstructed. The entrapped oxygen is absorbed by the mucosa, leading to hypoxia, which results in further exudation and exacerbation of the sinus infection. Pooling of secretions, mucosal edema, and decreased oxygen tension also hinder mucociliary clearance.

Numerous factors may compromise ostial patency. The key to understanding the pathophysiology of sinusitis is the ostiomeatal complex. The ostiomeatal complex is the region of the middle meatus where the pathway of mucociliary flow converges from the frontal, maxillary, and ethmoid sinuses. It consists of the infundibulum, hiatus semilunaris, ethmoid bulla, and anterior wall of the middle turbinate. Obstruction of the ostiomeatal complex prevents mucociliary clearance of the sinuses, thus leading to sinusitis.

Narrowing or obstruction of the ostiomeatal complex is caused by various factors. Massive enlargement of an air cell within the middle turbinate (concha bullosa) may result in narrowing of the middle meatus. In one study, the incidence of this variation was more than twice as common in patients with sinusitis than in the general population (18). Similarly, marked lateral convexity of the middle turbinate (paradoxical middle turbinate) may result in obstruction of the ostiomeatal complex. Enlargement of the bulla ethmoidalis may lead to narrowing of the hiatus semilunaris. Marked rotation of the uncinate process also may cause narrowing of the ostiomeatal complex. Septal deviation may be a contributing factor as well.

Viral URI and allergic inflammatory diseases are the most common predisposing causes of acute sinusitis in children (12). Patent sinus ostia is found in only 20% of children with acute rhinitis (19). Allergy also plays a significant role in sinusitis.

An inflammatory process, whether infectious or allergic, can result in thickening of the sinonasal mucosa, capillary dilatation, and inflammatory exudate. Subsequently, ostial obstruction occurs with stasis of secretions and secondary bacterial infection. These events can result in mucociliary dysfunction and interfere with other protective functions.

In contrast to adults, adenoidal hypertrophy is a major contributing factor of the development of sinusitis in children. Markedly enlarged adenoids obstruct drainage of the sinonasal secretions into the naso-oropharynx, resulting in sinus infections. Adenoids involute during puberty and generally are not a causative factor of sinusitis in adults.

Mucociliary Dysfunction

The sinuses and the posterior two-thirds of the nasal cavity are covered by pseudostratified ciliated columnar epithelium. The cilia beat at a frequency of 1000 strokes/min to propel the mucous blanket toward the natural ostia (19). The mucous blanket is made up of two layers: the superficial gel layer, which is viscid, and the sol layer, which is serous. The consistency of each layer is essential for the well being of the sinuses. The viscid layer traps larger particulate matter such as bacteria and other debris. The serous medium surrounds the body of the cilia and is essential for efficient ciliary beat. The tips of the cilia touch the superficial layer of mucus during forward movement and discard debris from the sinus.

The ciliary apparatus and sinus secretions are an integral system that cannot be separated. The mucociliary system forms a local sinonasal defense mechanism consisting of the ciliary beat, mucous blanket, lysozymes, secretory IgA, and other surface enzymes. Alterations in ciliary function, number, morphology, or mobility may cause sinusitis. Similarly, any change in the quality or quantity of mucus may result in a secondary sinus infection. Ciliary dysfunction may be caused by various factors. A simple viral infection can have a direct, but temporary, cytotoxic effect on the cilia (19). Systemic anomalies, such as immotile cilia syndrome or Kartagener's syndrome, may cause ciliary dysfunction. Dry or cold air or topical medications may cause ciliary dysfunction. When ciliary dysfunction occurs, mucous secretions and debris remain in the sinus cavity and form a medium for bacterial growth.

Changes in mucous secretions may cause ostial obstruction or ciliary dysfunction resulting in sinusitis. In cases of cystic fibrosis, the quality of mucus is changed; it is thick and viscid, which obstructs the sinus ostium and decreases the efficiency of ciliary beat. An inflammatory process can increase the quantity of secretion and delay ciliary function. Disorders of the mucociliary apparatus or compromised ostiomeatal complex/ostial patency often result in sinusitis.

DIAGNOSIS OF RHINOSINUSITIS

Rhinosinusitis is classified into four categories based on the duration of symptoms rather than severity: acute (symptoms last up to two weeks but not more than four weeks), subacute (symptoms last two to four weeks but not more than three months), chronic (symptoms last more than three months), and recurrent (frequent attacks of acute sinusitis).

The diagnosis of sinusitis in children is more difficult than in adults. Clinical and radiologic findings in children vary and are not well established. The precise diagnosis is often difficult to make because of the overlap of symptomatology with other common pediatric conditions such as viral URI, adenoiditis, adenoidal hypertrophy, allergy, and gastroesophageal reflux. Additionally, preschool children attending daycare will pose a more challenging issue due to the higher rate of URI, immature immune system, and tendency of many physicians to prescribe antibiotics. The diagnosis usually is based on a combination of clinical presentation, history, physical examination, laboratory results, and radiologic findings.

Clinical Presentation

Symptoms of sinusitis vary in pediatric patients. In general, children who present with either prolonged or severe symptoms of URI may have sinusitis (20). The majority of cases of uncomplicated URI last five to seven days. The most common clinical presentations of sinusitis in children are nasal discharge and daytime cough lasting more than 10 days without improvement (20).

Persistence of symptoms of URI for more than 10 days suggests a complication. The quality of nasal discharge and cough has no diagnostic significance. Nasal discharge may be thin, clear, or purulent, and the cough may be dry or productive. The cough usually is present during the day and becomes worse at night (20). Nighttime cough is a common residual symptom and does not suggest sinus infection. Low-grade fever and fetid breath also may be present. Facial pain rarely is noted, and intermittent periorbital swelling may occasionally occur.

Severe URI is a less common clinical manifestation of sinusitis in children. Children usually present with high-grade fever (39°C), copious purulent nasal discharge, and occasional periorbital edema and pain. Periorbital swelling is intermittent, more prominent in the early morning and absent during the day. Children older than five years may complain of fullness behind or above the eyes. Isolated headache is not a common complaint of acute sinusitis in children (20).

Of children with acute sinusitis, 80% present with cough and nasal discharge (21,22). Chronic sinusitis is distinguished from acute sinusitis by the duration of symptoms. In cases of chronic sinusitis, respiratory symptoms of nasal obstruction, nasal discharge, night and day cough, and postnasal drip persist beyond four weeks. Systemic diseases such as immotile cilia syndrome, Kartagener's syndrome, cystic fibrosis, immunodeficiency, and congenital cyanotic heart disease may predispose patients to develop sinusitis. Additionally, a significant number of patients with asthma may have associated sinusitis (23,24).

The most common symptoms of sinusitis in children are: rhinorhea (77%), otitis media (61%), and cough (48%) (25). In contrast, adults usually present with long standing history of nasal congestion, rhinorrhea, postnasal drip, chronic cough, and headaches (26). In a recent study of 202 patients undergoing PESS, Ramadan noted that nasal discharge was most frequent (75%), followed by cough (73%), nasal congestion (72%), and headache (72%) (10). Chronic mucopurulent rhinorrhea, a common symptom compatible with chronic sinusitis, may affect 20% of the pediatric population (27,28), which makes the clinical diagnosis a difficult task. The clinical diagnosis of CRS may be complicated in children due to several factors. These confusing issues include: (a) children may not be able to express their symptoms or concerns, (b) we rely primarily on parents and caregivers who themselves may have a range of expectations and worries, (c) pediatric patients may have a significant overlap with other conditions associated with sinusitis, e.g., allergic rhinitis, URI, and chronic adenoiditis, and (d) physicians have a tendency to treat symptoms, which may confound the overall presentation and management.

Physical Examination

The nose is the only area of the sinonasal system readily available for examination. However, it does not accurately reveal the status of the sinuses. Moreover, effective nasal examination of pediatric patients is often challenging. Children with acute sinusitis have nasal or postnasal mucopurulent discharge. The nasal mucosa is erythematous and boggy, and the throat may be infected. However, none of these signs differentiates rhinitis from sinusitis (20). Occasionally, periorbital edema or tenderness over the sinuses may be present. Malodorous breath can be suggestive of bacterial sinusitis in the absence of pharyngitis, dental infections, or a foreign body in the nose (20). Cervical lymph nodes rarely are enlarged or tender.

Anterior rhinoscopy may be helpful in diagnosing sinusitis. An otoscope provides visualization of the anterior nasal cavity. With adequate vasoconstriction, mucopurulent material may be seen emerging from the middle meatus, which is one of the most specific findings in acute sinusitis. Flexible and rigid endoscopy provides a more complete evaluation in older and cooperative children. Although a rigid endoscope provides superior evaluation compared with flexible endoscope, it can be used only in cooperative children and in patients whose nose is well anesthetized. Transillumination is not an effective diagnostic tool.

Initially, a complete examination should be performed if sinusitis is suspected. Cleft palate (29), adenotonsillar hypertrophy (30), and other systemic diseases must be ruled out as causative factors of sinusitis in children. At times, there may be no signs or symptoms directly related to the sinuses, and complications of sinusitis may be the initial symptoms. Bronchitis, laryngitis, otitis media, and periorbital cellulitis also are presenting symptoms. Up to 60% of children with chronic sinusitis have associated middle ear disease (31).

Laboratory Results

The diagnosis of acute bacterial sinusitis is best confirmed by a biopsy of the sinus mucosa. The biopsy demonstrates acute inflammation with bacterial invasion. However, a biopsy is rarely obtained in the office; instead, aspiration of sinus secretions is performed. Maxillary sinus aspirate is best performed via a transnasal route, with a needle directed beneath the inferior turbinate, requiring general anesthesia. Aspirate secretions should be submitted for gram stain, culture, sensitivity, and cell count. Sinus aspiration is not a routine diagnostic tool; it is reserved for pediatric patients with severe symptoms, immunodeficiency, or toxemia, or those in whom appropriate medical therapy has been ineffective.

Surface culture of the nose, throat, or nasopharynx of patients with acute sinusitis has no predictive value (12). A complete blood count as well as erythrocyte sedimentation rate may be of value in children with acute sinusitis (31). Nasal smears from children with acute sinusitis may reveal a large number of polymorphonuclear cells with intracellular bacteria. Although these findings are sensitive, they are not specific predictors of sinusitis. In contrast, the nasal smear in children with allergic rhinitis has a predominance of eosinophils (31).

RADIOLOGIC FINDINGS

Plain Radiography

Traditionally, plain sinus x-rays have been used to evaluate sinus disease. The standard radiographic projections include an anteroposterior (Caldwell) view for the frontal and ethmoid sinuses, an occipitomental (Waters') view for the maxillary sinus, and a lateral view with a submentovertex view for the sphenoid sinuses. A single Waters' view may be sufficient for the diagnosis of maxillary sinusitis in most patients.

Numerous reports have been published regarding the frequency of abnormal radiographic findings in asymptomatic children. Caffey noted variations in children that can lead to misinterpretation of plain x-rays and advised caution in interpreting the results of sinus x-rays in this patient population (13). In contrast, another study showed that abnormal maxillary sinus x-rays were rare in children younger than one year of age without recent symptoms and signs of respiratory tract infection (32,33).

The most reliable diagnostic x-ray findings of sinusitis in children are air fluid levels, uniform unilateral opacity, and thickened polypoid mucosa. Mucosal thickening of 4 mm or more in children is considered by some investigators to be a diagnostic criterion (33). However, it is not specific for bacterial sinusitis (22). In one study, when clinical signs and symptoms suggesting acute sinusitis were accompanied by abnormal results on maxillary sinus x-rays, 70% of sinus aspirates revealed bacteria (21). Normal x-ray results may only be suggestive and not diagnostic of healthy sinuses. Plain radiographs of the sinuses are not obsolete, but are easily accessible, economical, and can serve as an intial screening tool. They are especially valuable in acute sinusitis cases where an air-fluid level or a unilateral total opacification can be diagnostic.

Computerized Tomography

Given the health impact of pediatric sinusitis, the inaccuracy of plain radiographs, the significance of treatment expenditure incurred, and the fact that outcomes vary substantially between different diagnoses, it is of clinical and practical importance to be able to accurately diagnose pediatric chronic rhinosinusitis. CT has emerged as the diagnostic gold standard for CRS in general (27,34–36). Coronal and axial CT of the sinuses and appropriate bone windows is the most sensitive diagnostic tool for detecting chronic sinusitis. CT demonstrates disease that is not shown on routine x-rays. It helps in evaluating inaccessible structures and displays anatomic variations, thereby aiding in therapeutic planning. Studies of children with sinusitis found that plain x-rays both overestimated and underestimated the amount of sinus disease compared with findings on CT (37,38). In a recent study, Bhattacharyya and Fried (36) found that CT exhibited a good overall accuracy along with solid sensitivity and specificity of 85% and 59%, respectively. Also, in another study to determine diagnostic accuracy in 66 patients, Bhattacharyya et al. reported an excellent accuracy of CT scan to demonstrate pediatric CRS (27). In a survey of ASPO members, Sobol et al. reported that 95% of respondents use CT scans as the diagnostic modality of choice (39). Only 2% of respondents used plain radiographs and 1% used ultrasound or MRI (39). Computed tomography is widely believed to be extremely sensitive for mucosal inflammation in the sinuses; as a result, it is possible that CT can identify "incidental" mucosal findings that do not represent true sinus disease (27,40). This extreme sensitivity may lead to over diagnosis leading to false positive results. Computed tomography is not the ideal diagnostic tool for the detection of sinusitis. In a review of 210 patients who underwent functional endonasal sinus surgery (FESS), almost 20% of patients had more significant intraoperative findings than noted on CT (41). In a study of 31 adults with URI who underwent CT scan of the sinuses, Gwaltney et al. demonstrated CT evidence of sinusitis in 87%. Two weeks later, 79% showed CT resolution with no treatment (42). CT reflects the status of the sinuses at the time and date it was taken. Additionally, three-dimensional CT reconstruction is beneficial in illustrating the complex anatomy of the sinonasal area. However, such limitations as exposure to irradiation preclude its wide clinical use for the detection of inflammatory sinus disease.

No single diagnostic test for CRS in children can be used in isolation. Therefore, pediatricians and otolaryngologists need to rely on a combination of factors with more emphasis on objective measures such as CT scan and nasal endoscopy. Otolaryngologists in particular may need to rely more on CT scan to avoid unnecessary surgery, thus excluding patients who do not have true sinusitis.

Ultrasonography

Reports from Europe have shown that ultrasonography is both sensitive and specific for the diagnosis of maxillary sinusitis in adults and children (43,44). A study of 135 children noted a specificity of 98% and sensitivity of 87% with ultrasonography, compared with results from sinus aspirate. Ultrasonography is a nonionizing diagnostic tool. It is primarily used for the detection of retained secretions and not mucosal thickening. In the United States, more experience is required to assess the value of this tool, especially in pediatric patients.

Magnetic Resonance Imaging

The most recent advance in radiography is MRI. This modality has proved to be superior in demonstrating soft tissues; however, it is less effective in outlining bony architecture. The use and value of MRI in sinus disease have not been studied extensively. It may be of value in the diagnosis of extramucosal fungal sinus disease (18). Additionally, MRI is an important radiographic tool for differentiating between neoplasma and inflammatory diseases of the sinuses. It is an extremely valuable tool whenever intracranial pathology or involvement is suspected.

TREATMENT

The management of pediatric sinusitis has evolved rapidly over the past decade. The Subcommittee on Management of Sinusitis has nicely identified the clinical practice guidelines for pediatric sinusitis (10,45). Despite the fact that revolutionary changes have taken place in the surgical treatment of pediatric rhinosinus disorder, many issues remain unanswered. The surgical management for CRS in children lacks consensus and no scientific guidelines are available, contrary to medical treatment. Similarly, the surgical treatment of pediatric CRS is not uniformly identified. Typically, children who did not respond to medical treatment present for surgical management to improve their quality of life and control the disease process.

The current medical therapy recommended for CRS consists of nasal steroid spray and at least one four- to six-week course of a lactamase-resistant antibiotic such as amoxicillin/clavulinic acid, clindamycin, or second- and third-generation cephalosporins (41,46,47). Systemic antihistamines may be employed in children with symptomatic allergic rhinitis (48). Systemic decongestants may be prescribed, although never proven to be effective (49,50). No clear consensus even exists as to the recommended length of antibiotic therapy. Nevertheless, no randomized trials comparing medical versus surgical treatment or versus watchful observation have been published. Historically, surgical treatment of CRS consisted of intranasal surgery, nasoantral windows, or external approaches (10,51,52). After the introduction of PESS in 1989 (53) and the newer understanding of pediatric sinusitis, our surgical treatment options for chronic pediatric rhinosinusitis may be limited to PESS, adenoidectomy ± sinus lavage. Other procedures such septoplasty and turbinate reduction may have selected indications. Traditional surgeries such as external approaches or Caldwell-Luc have a very limited and reserved role.

SURGICAL MANAGEMENT

Surgical therapy is reserved for cases of chronic or recurrent sinusitis where maximal medical management has been ineffective. Surgery is undertaken to promote better drainage of the sinuses. Antral lavage, antral nasal windows, tonsillectomy, adenoidectomy, limited septoplasty, and partial turbinectomies have been used in the past as appropriate surgical modalities for treatment of children with sinusitis for whom traditional medical therapy was ineffective. Although these procedures have a role in the treatment of CRS, endoscopic sinus surgery remains the standard procedure of choice. The high success rate and low morbidity of endoscopic sinus surgery has been remarkable (54–61). Despite the fact that endoscopic sinus surgery has been widely accepted and popularized in adults, the enthusiasm is decreasing in children (54). Other alternatives or less invasive procedures with emphasis on accute diagnosis may be considered prior to PESS.

ADENOIDECTOMY

The adenoids may act as an obstructive barrier, inhibiting the appropriate drainage and secretions of the sino-nasal system. Additionally, the adenoids may act as a reservoir for bacteria (62,63). Thus one or both features of adenoids in children may result or contribute to sinusitis. This is not to mention that chronic infection/inflammation of the adenoids (adenoiditis) in children can easily mimic or compound pediatric sinusitis. The exact role of adenoids in pediatric sinusitis is not known and the success rate in the treatment is not clear. However, removal of the adenoids theoretically may allow better drainage and eliminate the source of infection. One of the initial pioneering studies to determine the role of adenoidectomy in pediatric sinusitis was published in 1995 by Rosenfeld (64), where he recommended a stepped treatment protocol for pediatric CRS. In this study, he recommended medical therapy as an initial step, with the next step adenoidectomy followed by PESS as a last resort, with success rates of 32%, 70%, and 89%, respectively. In a retrospective study of 48 children with CRS undergoing adenoidectomy, the author reported complete or near-complete resolution of symptoms in 58% of cases and some improvement in 21%, with only three cases requiring PESS (65). In another study comparing adenoidectomy versus PESS, Ramadan (54) demonstrated that 77% of children who underwent PESS had improved symptoms compared to 47% who underwent adenoidectomy. The overall success rate of adenoidectomy in the treatment of CSR is 50% (64–66). Adenoidectomy alone may be considered initially in children who are less than six years of age, have low-CT score, no asthma, and failed maximal medical therapy (10,64,65).

OTHER CONSIDERATIONS

The therapy of pediatric CRS remains controversial and may include a very wide spectrum ranging from PESS to minimal or no intervention. Recently, a step-wise protocol that includes intravenous (IV) antibiotic therapy was recommended by a study that included 70 patients with CRS which reported 89% resolution of symptoms following three to four weeks of IV therapy with selective adenoidectomy and oral antibiotic prophylaxis; 11% who failed required PESS (66). All patients had CT evidence of CRS and underwent maxillary sinus lavage with cultures. The authors concluded that their step-wise protocol with IV therapy may be a reasonable alternative to PESS (66–68).

Inferior meatal antrostomies has been shown to be ineffective for the management of CRS (69). However, this procedure may have limited application for lavage and obtaining cultures with or without adenoidectomy. Moreover, it may be beneficial in cases such as cystic fibrosis or immotile cilia syndrome where dependent drainage is desired.

External ethmoidectomy or frontal sinus trephination may have limited indications in acute sinusitis with complications or occasionally may be combined with PESS (70,71). Osteoplastic flap or transnasal ethmoidectomy/ Caldwell-Luc are rarely considered in the pediatric age group and reserved for special unusual cases with neoplasms (72,73).

Nasal turbinate surgery is very uncommon in children. It is occasionally required in allergic adolescent patients with hypertrophic inferior turbinate unresponsive to optimal therapy. Nasal turbinectomy is too aggressive in a child, but a limited submucous resection of the inferior third of the inferior turbinate may be extremely helpful. Similarly, septoplasty is reserved for adolescents with severely obstructive and symptomatic septal deviation. Consequently a limited septoplasty—possibly endoscopic—with preservation of bone may be warranted.

PEDIATRIC ENDOSCOPIC SINUS SURGERY

PESS was first introduced in adults in Europe (74) and became popular in the United States for the treatment of sinus disease (75). The philosophy behind PESS is the anterior ethmoids and ostiomeatal complex are usually the main problem areas behind sinusitis (74,76). PESS is used to reestablish normal sinus physiology. With this approach, diseased tissue is removed and normal tissue is left with minimal trauma. The first reports of PESS mirrored the success rate initially reported in the adult age group (41,55–61).

PESS is the most precise surgical modality for the treatment of chronic/recurrent sinusitis. Typical candidates for PESS are children with persistent sinusitis, despite "maximal conservative therapy." PESS using an endoscope is considered a more conservative approach than allowing children to become chronically ill or require several courses of medical treatment. The quality of life of children with CRS can improve significantly following PESS (7).

TECHNIQUE AND INSTRUMENTATION

Special instruments are available for PESS from many companies. If these instruments are unavailable or unaffordable, then adult instruments may be utilized in the majority of cases; otological instruments may also be useful. Tissue-sparing instruments are preferred, but if unavailable, mucosal-tearing with biting forceps can be diminished using a gentle twisting motion. Powered instruments (i.e., microdebriders and soft-tissue shavers) represent the newest advance in tissue-sparing. Setliff and Parsons were the first to report the use of shavers in 345 adult and pediatric patients who underwent endoscopic sinus surgery (77–79). Powered instruments offer precision in tissue resection while inherent continuous suction maintains a clear surgical field. Furthermore, one grasp with a biting forceps can inadvertently denude a large area of uninvolved mucosa. The potential advantages of soft tissue shavers may include less trauma, decreased bleeding, greater comfort, shorter surgical time, improved healing, and more rapid recovery (77–79). Micro-debriders may be used not only in CRS, but also in nasal polyps, nasal papillomas, scar tissues, septal deviation, choanal atresia, and adenoid removal (77). The most dramatic advantage has been in the case of nasal polyps. A 3.5 mm shaver is commonly used in the pediatric age group. It is not unusual to use a combination of a variety of adult, pediatric, and powered instruments in all cases. It is very important to emphasize that the use of powered instruments is no substitution for the careful approach of a knowledgeable and experienced sinus surgeon.

When used in children, PESS requires significant attention to detail. The technique is essentially the same for adults and children. However, in contrast to adults, PESS in children has certain characteristic differences in the indications, preoperative assessment, type of anesthesia, and postoperative follow-up.

Indications and Preoperative Preparations

No clear indications were maintained for PESS until September 1996, when an international consensus meeting consisting of ENT specialists, pediatricians, and microbiologists provided us with absolute and possible indications for PESS (4). Absolute indications included:

1. cystic fibrosis with complete nasal obstruction and massive nasal polyposis
2. antrochoanal polyp
3. mucocoeles or mucopyocoeles
4. intracranial complications
5. orbital abscess

6. traumatic injury to optic canal (endoscopic decompression)
7. dacrocystorhinitis due to sinusitis resistant to medical treatment
8. fungal sinusitis
9. meningoencephalocoeles (some)
10. neoplasms (some), including juvenile angiofibroma

The possible indications included CRS. The consensus committee decided that only CRS with frequent exacerbations and nonresponsive to optimal medical treatment (two to six weeks of oral antibiotic treatment or even parental antibiotics) and after exclusion of a noninfectious condition or systemic disease should be considered for surgery.

Preparations for FESS begin by obtaining a coronal and axial CT scan of the sinuses. In children, CT of the sinuses may form the only objective modality for the accurate assessment of the anatomy and the disease process. It provides an excellent guide for surgery and should be displayed in the operating room for reference.

The most important step in the immediate preoperative preparation of pediatric patients is to obtain optimal vasoconstriction. Maximal vasoconstriction can markedly improve visualization intraoperatively, which significantly reduces edematous nasal mucosa, thereby providing better visualization of the anatomical landmarks. Additionally, vasoconstriction minimizes intraoperative bleeding, enabling surgeons to proceed in an efficient manner.

Vasoconstriction begins preoperatively when patients are sprayed with a topical decongestant (oxymetazoline) on call to the operating room. The protocol for vasoconstriction is continued in the operating room. After administration of general anesthesia, the surgical site is injected with 2% lidocaine and 1:100,000 epinephrine using a dental carpel (1.8 mL/carpule) with a 27-gauge, 0.5-in. needle. About 2% lidocaine with 1:50,000 epinephrine also may be used but with extreme caution. Two to three carpules generally may be needed in children. Additionally, the selection of the anesthetic agent is critical when epinephrine is injected. The next step is to pack the nose with neurosurgical cottonoids soaked in a 4% cocaine solution or oxymetazoline. The packs should be left in place for at least 10 minutes. Strict adherence to this protocol results in optimal visualization and homeostasis.

Procedure

PESS in children is performed in the same manner as in adults. Storz–Hopkins rigid nasal endoscopes are used. The 0°, 4-mm telescope generally is used for the ethmoid and sphenoid sinuses if indicated, whereas the 30°, 4-mm telescope is employed for the frontal recess and the maxillary sinus. Despite the smaller anatomy in children, there is usually no difficulty in using 4-mm telescopes, even in young patients. The smaller telescopes (2.7 mm) are rarely used because they do not provide the depth of field and the degree of visualization obtained from the larger (4 mm) telescopes.

Increasingly, the 70° telescope is used for the identification and exploration of the frontal recess and maxillary sinus.

An initial intraoperative nasal examination is performed. The septum, middle turbinate, posterior nasal airway, and adenoids, if present, are assessed. Intraoperative nasal endoscopy may be the first adequate nasal examination in children, and it is an essential step in planning surgery. A planned surgical approach is especially important in children because it aids in reducing trauma and minimizes postoperative morbidity. Additionally, a nasal endoscopic examination may reveal certain abnormalities that were not readily identified on CT.

Occasionally, a deviated septum or a large middle turbinate may be present. In such cases, limited septoplasty or partial middle turbinectomy may be performed. This practice not only provides better exposure during PESS, but also facilitates aeration and drainage of the sinuses postoperatively.

The procedure begins by identifying the middle turbinate with a 4-mm, 0° Storz–Hopkins telescope. The turbinate is medialized using a freer elevator. The uncinate process is identified. In children, the uncinate process is located more anteriorly than it is in adults. The sinuses are then entered by performing an infundibulotomy. An incision is made using a sickle knife over the anterior border of the uncinate process, starting superiorly and ending over the poster inferior edge. The uncinate process is retracted medially and gently removed. Alternatively, a smallback-biting forceps may be placed into the hiatus semilunaris and the uncinate is removed from behind. If a microdebrider is present, it may be used in removing the uncinate and other steps in the procedure thereafter. The bulla ethmoidalis is exposed and entered by blunt dissection with a straight suction tip. The diseased mucosa and bony septa of the anterior ethmoids are then removed using straight-biting forceps. Subsequently, the anterior ethmoids are totally exenterated until the basal lamella is identified, which is also entered bluntly using a straight suction tip. The posterior ethmoids are cleared using straight-biting forceps. The fovea ethmoidalis, lamina papyracae, and middle turbinate are visualized at all times, being utilized as excellent anatomical landmarks. Continous correlation with CT imaging is also done to verify the diseased regions and anatomical landmarks.

Additionally, a navigator system—if available—can add another tool to identify diseased areas and provide precise anatomical guidance. Computer Assisted Navigation System (CANS) was used in children as a surgical control and not as a surgical guide. With increasing experience and accuracy of 1.1 mm, CANS has been progressively used as a real surgical guide in PESS. CANS may allow us to precisely limit our surgery to pathological regions (80–85). Its use has increased with experience, demonstrating its utility in a variety of conditions such as revision surgery, recurrent or initial naso pharyngeal angiofibroma, choanal atresia, cystic fibrosis, and tumor biopsies (80–85). CANS may be a useful guide for experienced surgeons and could be of help in teaching endoscopic sinus surgery to residents and fellows. It is not a substitute for experience and perfect endoscopic anatomical knowledge (83,84); it may be beneficial, yet it has not been proven to decrease risk of restenosis or surgical complication. Actually, CANS may encourage the surgeon—especially the inexperienced one—to take more risks, with the temptation to perform more surgery with a possibly higher chance of inadvertent mistakes. Additionally, the system is not perfect; it has sensitivity, accuracy, and calibration issues and concerns about its high costs. At the same time, the sinus surgeon needs to always be cognizant of the fact that CANS does not provide any protection or advantage in legal requirements or liability.

The frontal recess area is inspected by switching to a 30° telescope. Polypoid mucosa may be found invariably. The frontal recess is cleaned using a 45° up-biting forceps and a right-angle suction tip. It is further visualized and assessed using a 70° telescope. The maxillary sinus ostium is identified using a 30° telescope. The ostium is enlarged posteriorly. It is also enlarged anteriorly to a lesser extent, using side-biting forceps. Care should be taken not to injure the nasolacrimal duct anteriorly and the sphenopalatine artery posteriorly. The maxillary sinus mucosa is inspected closely using a 70° telescope; finally, it is copiously irrigated with saline.

In children, the sphenoid sinus is not entered unless there is evidence of disease on the CT scan of the sinuses. In the latter case, gentle dissection is made in the inferior medial aspect of the posterior ethmoids. Identification of the sphenoid sinus ostium may be made using a variety of telescopes; a small probe may act as a guide for localizing the sphenoid sinus cavity. The superior turbinate if present, should be identified, and may require partial resection to enhance opening the sphenoid sinus. Care should be taken to avoid potential injury to critical structures within the sphenoid sinus. Additionally, stripping the sphenoid sinus mucosa should be avoided to minimize the risk of injury to a dehiscent optic nerve or internal carotid artery.

The procedure lasts 45 to 60 minutes and blood loss ranges between 10 and 50 mL. Packing is not generally needed. Middle meatal stenting remains a controversial issue; various stent materials were used to prevent adhesions. Nonetheless, some of these stents may actually promote granulation tissue and thereby adhesions. We don't use or recommend using any stents; precise and delicate handling of tissue is more important than any stenting or packing. Patients are routinely discharged the same day.

Alternatively, a limited approach PESS has been described (86) and may be adopted. This approach entails partial opening of the bulla ethmoidalis, opening but not widening of the maxillary ostium; evacuation of anterior ethmoid is reserved for extensive disease. If disease exists in the posterior ethmoid, then a posterior ethmoid sinusotomy is mandatory to minimize the possibility of residual disease. In a review of 101 patients undergoing this limited approach, Chang et al. reported 90% improvement in the symptoms of these patients (86).

Postoperative Follow-Up

Postoperative management begins with maintaining patients on a steroid spray, nasal decongestant, saline nasal mist, and wide-spectrum oral antibiotic. This regimen is employed for six weeks. Patients are weaned off the steroid spray and other medications during the last two weeks of therapy. Follow-up may include nasal endoscopy performed two to three weeks postoperatively. In contrast to adults, nasal endoscopy in children is performed under general anesthesia. Blood, blood clots, crusting, eschar, and granulation tissues may cause further inflammation, infection, restenosis, scarring, and possibly failure.

Initially, second-look endoscopy (SLSE) after PESS was a common procedure performed routinely on every patient two to three weeks after PESS. In recent years, several authors pointed out that no definite benefits for routine SLSE but increased risks (87–89). The pros and cons of SLSE have been recently detailed by the author (90). SLSE is now currently indicated in selected cases such as patients with systemic disease (cystic fibrosis and immotile cilia), cases with strong clinical suspicion of poor nasal hygiene or high suspicion of recurrence, extensive sinonasal polyposis, revision refractory surgery, incomplete primary surgery, or young children who are unable to adequately care for their sinonasal system following PESS (86,90).

OUTCOMES AND PITFALLS

Endoscopic sinus surgery has been shown to play an important role in the surgical treatment of CRS in all age groups. Several published series of children undergoing PESS described positive outcomes ranging from 77% to 100% (41,55–61,91,92). However, the main drawbacks were retrospective chart review or caregiver surveys in all but one of these series! Also, to date, it has been difficult to establish pure objective measures for outcomes or a standardized format to assess PESS. In a recent meta-analysis study, Hebert and Bent reviewed eight published articles (832 patients), plus unpublished data on 50 patients. The positive outcomes for published, unpublished, and combined data were 88.4%, 92%, and 88.7%, respectively (91), with a major complication rate of 0.6%. Thus, the cumulative literature provides evidence that PESS is an effective and safe procedure for the treatment of CRS refractory to optimal medical therapy. In a prospective, nonrandomized study of 183 pediatric patients, Ramadan reported that of all variables studied, asthma, age, and cigarette smoke exposure were the only predictors of success (10). Children with asthma and smoking environment benefited the least from adenoidectomy alone (37%). PESS in conjunction with adenoidectomy gave the best outcomes, especially when looking at children with asthma who are exposed to smoke. Ramadan recommended adenoidectomy alone as an initial step for patients with low-CT score, no asthma, and six years old or younger. Children with asthma at any age and children older than 6 years with high CT scores after failure of repeated medical therapy and repeated positive scan will benefit from PESS and adenoidectomy simultaneously (96% success rate) (10).

Complications of PESS are similar to those reported in the adult age group. One of the biggest problems is synechia formation, restenosis, and failure. CSF rhinorrhea, meningitis, intracerebral bleeding or injury, blindness, extra ocular muscle impairment, intraobital hematoma, and carotid artery injury are extremely rare.

One of the major concerns that has been raised is the effect of PESS on facial development and growth. In the mid-1990s, two studies involving piglets demonstrated significant changes in facial growth (93–95). However, in two independent papers involving humans, there was no evidence to suggest any substantial risk of effects on facial growth as a result of sinus surgery (96,97) Bothwell et al. (96) compared two cohorts who had either sinus surgery or medical management at a young age. The patients were brought back 10 years later and evaluated by anthropometric measurements and facial plastic surgeons. Both quantitative and qualitative assessments could discern significant facial changes (96). It is the general consensus that PESS does significantly alter the facial growth in children.

CONCLUSION

Children with refractory sinusitis are potential candidates for PESS. Children with persistent sinusitis should be investigated for systemic disorders, e.g., Kartagener's syndrome, cystic fibrosis, and immunodeficiency. Additionally, evaluation of allergies should be performed by a pediatric otolaryngic allergist or pediatric allergist. Many children with asthma also have associated sinusitis that aggravates their asthmatic problems (98). Children who present with sinusitis are best managed by a team approach, including an otolaryngologist, allergist, pediatrician, family practitioner, pulmonologist, and infectious disease specialist.

Children with resistant chronic or recurrent sinusitis are best managed by PESS. PESS has proved to be a curative and safe procedure in children. PESS is a functional approach that attempts to correct disease of the ostiomeatal complex. The goal of PESS is to resume conditions that promote normal mucociliary clearance of the sinuses. Minimal symptomatology may return during the early postoperative period, probably resulting from edema and nonhealed tissue. Medical and allergic treatment should be continued, especially during the first six weeks postoperatively. Thereafter, medical treatment may be discontinued. However, allergy treatment should continue long enough to control inhalant allergens.

Serious complications of this procedure are rare, and the cure rate is high. Specialized training and instrumentation, CT, and multiple postoperative visits may be needed.

The role of surgery in the treatment of pediatric sinusitis is still in process of evolution. In a recent publication investigating when to operate in pediatric sinusitis, Lieser and Derkay (99) concluded that there is growing support in literature for adenoidectomy as a first-line of surgical intervention for CRS when maximal medical therapy fails. Maxillary aspiration or middle meatal cultures can be performed at the same sitting to facilitate directed antibiotic therapy. IV antibiotics seem to be a promising alternative to PESS, especially in younger or high-risk patients. Current literature continues to support PESS as a safe and effective procedure (99). A survey of ASPO members questioned the current trends in the management of pediatric sinusitis. The majority of respondents initially treat medically with oral antibiotics (95%), topical steroids (90%), and nasal saline spray (68%). About 55% perform adenoidectomy as part of the treatment of CRS with 81% performing the operation before PESS (39). About 87% currently perform PESS, 9% have stopped, 55% perform 10 to 25 cases per year, 25% less than 10, and only 5% perform more than 25 cases of PESS per year. The majority (66%) performed middle meatal antrostomy and anterior ethmoidectomy. About 6% use CANS routinely and 49% in selected cases, but 34% do not use it. When compared to three years earlier, only 47% of respondents performed approximately the same number of PESS, whereas 35% reported doing fewer cases annually, which means more than a third of the respondents are using more stringent criteria and performing less surgery than three years ago. About 72% of practitioners do not routinely perform SLSE. The majority of respondents reported more than 75% success rate for PESS and most of them reported no change in outcomes over the past three years (39). These are findings that support the continuous use and success of PESS over the years, which is also consistent with other reports (55–57).

In summary, we need to exhaust all and every means of diagnosis, prevention, and medical therapy before entertaining any surgical intervention. Adenoidectomy seems to be the initial reasonable procedure of choice. This is more justified in younger age group children with or without lavage and/or IV antibiotic treatment.

PESS remains the surgical procedure of choice for the ultimate treatment of pediatric sinusitis whenever everything else fails.

REFERENCES

1. Otten FW, Aarem AV, Grote JJ. Long-term follow up of chronic maxillary sinusitis in children. Int J Otolaryngol 1991; 22:81–84.
2. Parsons DS. Pediatric sinusitis. Otolaryngol Clin North Am 1996; 29:1–11.

3. Poole MD. Pediatric endoscopic sinus surgery: the conservative view. J Ear Nose Throat 1994; 73(4):221–227.

4. Clement PA. Pediatric endoscopic sinus surgery—does it have a future? Int J Pediatr Otorhinolaryngol 2003; 67(suppl 1):S209–S211.

5. Benson V, Marano MA. Current Estimates From the National Health Interview Survey, 1995. Hyattsville, MD: National Center for Health Statistics, 1998:5.

6. Wald ER. Sinusitis in children. N Engl J Med 1992; 326:319–323.

7. Cunningham JM, Chiu EJ, Landgraf JM, Gliklich RE. The health impact of chronic recurrent rhinosinusitis in children. Arch Otolaryngol Head Neck Surg 2000; 126(11):1363–1368.

8. Lieu JE, Piccirillo JF, Lusk RP. Prognostic staging system and therapeutic effectiveness for recurrent or chronic sinusitis in children. Otolayrngol Head Neck Surg 2003; 129(3):222–232.

9. Ray NF, Baraniuk JN, Thamer M, Rinehart CS, Gergen PJ, Kaliner M, Josephs S, Pung YH. Healthcare expenditures for sinusitis in 1996: contributions of asthma, rhinitis, and other airway disorders. J Allergy Clin Immunol 1999; 103(3 Pt 1):408–414.

10. Ramadan HH. Surgical management of chronic sinusitis in children. Laryngoscope 2004; 114(12):2103–2109.

11. Christodoulopoulos P, Cameron L, Durham S, Hamid Q. Molecular pathology of allergic disease. II: upper airway disease. J All Clin Immunol 2000; 105: 211–223.

12. Wald ER. Diagnosis and management of acute sinusitis. Pediatr Ann 1988; 17:629–638.

13. Caffey J. Pediatric X-Ray Diagnosis: A Textbook for Students and Practitioners in Pediatrics, Surgery, and Radiology. 7th ed. Chicago: Year Book, 1978.

14. Graney DO. Anatomy: Otolaryngology Head and Neck Surgery. St. Louis: Mosby, 1986.

15. Caldwell GW. The accessory sinuses of the nose: an improved method of treatment for suppuration of the maxillary antrum. NY Med J 1893; 58:526–528.

16. Schaefer JP. The genesis, development, and adult anatomy of the nasofrontal region in man. Am J Anat 1916; 0:125–143.

17. Proctor DF. The nose, paranasal sinuses, and pharynx. In: Walters W, ed. Lewis Walters Practice of Surgery. Hagerstown, MD: WF Prior, 1966:1–37.

18. Kennedy DW, Zeinreich SJ. Functional Endoscopic Surgery: Advances in Otolaryngology Head and Neck Surgery. Chicago: Year Book, 1989:1–26.

19. Wald ER. Epidemiology, pathophysiology, and etiology of sinusitis. Pediatr Infect Dis J 1985; 4(suppl 6):551–554.

20. Wald ER. Management of sinusitis in infants and children. Pediatr Infect Dis J 1988; 7:449–452.

21. Wald ER, Milmoe GJ, Bowen A, Ledesma-Medina J, Slamon N, Bluestone CD. Acute maxillary sinusitis in children. N Engl J Med 1981; 304(13):749–754.

22. Siegel JD. Diagnosis and management of acute sinusitis in children. Pediatr Infect Dis J 1987; 6:95–99.

23. Slavin RG, Cannon RE, Friedman WH, Palitang E, Sundaram M. Sinusitis and bronchial asthma. J Allergy Clin Immonol 1980; 66(3):250–257.
24. Slavin RG. Sinus disease and asthma. Ear Nose Throat J 1984; 63:48–56.
25. Kogutt MS, Swischuck LE. Diagnosis of sinusitis in infants and children. Pediatrics 1973; 52:121–124.
26. Sobol SE, Wright ED, Frenkiel S. One-year outcome analysis of functional endoscopic sinus surgery for chronic sinusitis. J Otolaryngol 1998; 27: 252–257.
27. Bhattacharyya N, Jones DT, Hill M, Shapiro NL. The diagnostic accuracy of computed tomography in pediatric chronic rhinosinusitis. Arch Otolaryngol Head Neck Surg 2004; 130(9):1029–1032.
28. Clement PAR, Gordts F. Epidemiology and prevalence of aspecific chronic sinusitis. Int J Pediatr Otorhinolaryngol 1999; 49(suppl 1):S101–S103.
29. Robinson HE, Zerlin GK, Passy VE. Maxillary sinus development in patients with cleft palates as compared to those with normal palates. Laryngoscope 1982; 92:183–189.
30. Dharam P. Sinus infections and adenotonsillitis in pediatric patients. Laryngoscope 1981; 91:997–1000.
31. Rachelefsky GS. Chronic sinusitis: the disease of all ages (editorials). Am J Dis Child 1989; 143:886–888.
32. Wald ER. The diagnosis and management of sinusitis in children: diagnostic considerations. Pediatr Infect Dis J 1985; 4(suppl 6):555–559.
33. Kovatch AL, Wald ER, Ledesma-Medina J, Chiponis DM, Bedingfield B. Maxillary sinus radiographs in children with nonrespiratory complaints. Pediatrics 1984; 73(3):306–308.
34. Zinreich J. Rhinosinusitis:radiologic diagnosis. Otolaryngol Head Neck Surg 1997; 117:S27–S34.
35. Lund VJ, Kennedy DW. Staging for rhinosinusitis. Otolaryngol Head Neck Surg 1997; 117:S35–S40.
36. Bhattacharyya N, Freid MP. The accuracy of computer tomography in the diagnosis of chronic sinusitis. Laryngoscope 2003; 113:125–129.
37. Lazar RH, Younis RT, Parvey LS. Comparison of plain radiographs, coronal CT, and interoperative findings in children with chronic sinusitis. Otolaryngol Head Neck Surg 1992; 107:29–34.
38. McAllister WH, Lusk RP, Muntz HR. Comparison of plain radiographs and coronal scans in infants and children with recurrent sinusitis. Am J Radiol 1989; 153:1259–1264.
39. Sobol SE, Samadi DS, Kazahaya K, Tom LW. Trends in the management of pediatric chronic sinusitis: survey of the American society of pediatric otolaryngology. Laryngoscope 2005; 115(1):78–80.
40. Bhattacharyya N. Do maxillary sinus retention cysts reflect obstructive sinus phenomena? Arch Otolaryngol Head Neck Surg 2000; 126:1369–1371
41. Lazar RH, Younis RT, Gross CW. Pediatric functional endonasal sinus surgery: review of 210 cases. Head Neck 1992; 14:92–98.
42. Gwaltney JM Jr, Phillips CD, Miller RD, Riker DK. Computed tomographic study of the common cold. N Engl J Med 1994; 330(1):25–30.

43. Revonta M, Suonpa J. Diagnosis of subacute sinusitis in children. J Laryngol Otol 1981; 95:133–140.
44. Revonta M, Kuuliola I. The diagnosis and follow-up of pediatric sinusitis: water's view radiography vs. ultrasonography. Laryngoscope 1989; 99:321–324.
45. Subcommittee on management of Sinusitis, Committee on quality improvement practice guideline: management of sinusitis. Pediatrics 2001; 108:798–808.
46. Arjmand EM, Lusk RP. Managementof recurrent and chronic sinusitis in children. Am J Otolaryngol 1995; 16:367–382.
47. Haltom JR, Cannon CR. Functional endoscopic sinus surgery in children. J Miss State Med Assoc 1993; 34(1):1–6.
48. Gungor A, Corey JP. Pediatric sinusitis: a literature review with emphasis on the role of allergy. Otolaryngol Head Neck Surg 1997; 116:4–15.
49. Hutton N, Wilson MH, Mellits ED, Baumgardner R, Wissow LS, Bonucelli C, Hotzman NA, DeAngelis C. Effectiveness of an antihistamine-decongestant combination for young children with the common cold: a randomized controlled clinical trial. J Pediatr 1991; 118(1):125–130.
50. Cantekin EI, Mandel EM, Bluestone CD, Rockette HE, Paradise JL, Stool SE, Fria TJ, Rogers KD. Lack of efficacy of a decongestant-antihistamine combination for otitis media with effusion ("secretory" otitis media) in children. Results of a double-blind, randomized trial. N Engl J Med 1983; 308(6):297–301.
51. Manning S. Surgical intervention for sinusitis in children. Curr All Asthma Rep 2001; 1:289–296.
52. Norante JD. Surgical management of sinusitis. Ear Nose Throat J 1984; 63:155–162.
53. Gross CW, Gurucharri MJ, Lazar RH, Long TE. Functional endonasal sinus surgery (FESS) in the pediatric age group. Laryngoscope 1989; 99(3):272–275.
54. Ramadan HR. Adenoidectomy vs endoscopic sinus surgery for the treatment of pediatric sinusitis. Arch Otolaryngol Head Neck Surg 1999; 125.
55. Lazar RH, Younis RT, Long TE. Functional endonasal sinus surgery in adults and children. Laryngoscope 1993; 103:1–5.
56. Parsons DS, Phillips SE. Functional endoscopic surgery in children: a retrospective analysis of results. Laryngoscope 1993; 103:899–903.
57. Younis RT, Lazar RH. Criteria for success in pediatric functional endonasal sinus surgery. Laryngoscope 1996; 106:869–873.
58. Stankiewicz JA. Pediatric endoscopic nasal and sinus surgery. Otolaryngol Head Neck Surg 1995; 113(3):204–210.
59. Triglia JM, Dessi P, Cannoni M, Pech A. Intranasal ethmoidectomy in nasal polyposis in children. Indications and results. Int J Pediatr Otolaryngol 1992; 23(2):125–131.
60. Wolf G, Greistorfer K, Jebeles JA. The endoscopic endonasal surgical technique in the treatment of chronic recurrent sinusitis in children. Rhinology 1995; 33:97–103.
61. Bolt RJ, de Vries N, Middelweerd. Endoscopic sinus surgery for nasal polyps in children: results. Rhinology 1995; 33:148–151.
62. Lusk RP, Stankiewicz JA. Pediatric rhinosinusitis. Otolaryngol Head Neck Surg 1997; 117(pt 2):S53–S57.
63. Lee D, Rosenfeld RM. Adenoid bacteriology and sinonasal symptoms in children. Otolaryngol Head Neck Surg 1997; 116:301–307.

64. Rosenfeld RM. Pilot study of outcomes in pediatric rhinosinusitis. Arch Otolaryngol Head Neck Surg 1995; 121:729–736.
65. Vandenberg SJ, Heatley DG. Efficacy of adenoidectomy in relieving symptoms of chronic sinusitis in children. Arch Otolaryngol Head Neck Surg 1997; 123:675–678.
66. Don DM, Yellon RF, Casselbrant ML, Bluestone CD. Efficacy of a step-wise protocol that includes intravenous antibiotic antibiotic therapy for the management of chronic sinusitis in children and adolescents. Arch Otolaryngol Head Neck Surg 2001; 127(9):1093–1098.
67. Buchman CA, Yellon RF, Bluestone CD. Alternative to endoscopic sinus surgery in the management of pediatric chronic rhinosinusitis refractory to oral antimicrobial therapy. Otolaryngol Head Neck Surg 1999; 120(2):219–224.
68. Tanner SB, Foeler KC. Intravenous antibiotics for chronic rhinosinusitis: are they effective? Curr Opin Otolaryngol Head Neck Surg 2004; 12(1):3–8.
69. Muntz HR, Lusk RP. Nasal antral windows in children: A retrospective study. Laryngoscope 1990; 100:643–646.
70. Stankiewicz JA, Newell DJ, Park AH. Complications of inflammatory diseases of the sinuses. Otolaryngol Clin North Am 1993; 26:629–655.
71. Pransky SW, Low WS. Pediatric ethmoidectomy. Otolaryngol Clin North Am 1996; 29:131–142.
72. Perko D. Endoscopic surgery of the formal sinus without external approach. Rhinology 1989; 27:119–123.
73. Stankiewicz JA. Complications of sinusitis and sinus surgery. In: Bailey B, ed. Otolaryngology-Head Neck Surgery. New York: Mosby CV, 1993.
74. Messerlinger W. Endoscopy of the Nose. Baltimore: Urban & Schwarszenburg, 1978.
75. Kennedy DW, Zinreich SJ, Rosenbum AE, Johns ME. Functional endoscopic sinus surgery: theory and diagnostic evaluation. Arch Otolaryngol 1985; 111(9): 576–582.
76. Draf W. Endoscopy of the paranasal and sinuses. Berlin: Springer-Verlag, 1983.
77. Mendelsohn MG, Gross CW. Soft-tissue shavers in pediatric sinus surgery. Otolaryngol Clin North Am 1997; 30(3):443–449.
78. Parsons DS. Rhinologic uses of powered instrumentation in children beyond sinus surgery. Otolaryngol Clin North Am 1996; 29:105–114.
79. Setliff RC, Parsons DS. The "Hummer": new instrumentation for functional endoscopic sinus surgery. Am J Rhinol 1994; 8:275–278.
80. Postec F, Bossard D, Disant F, Froehlich P. Computer-assisted navigation system in pediatric intranasal surgery. Arch Otoalryngol Head Neck Surg 2002; 128(7):797–800.
81. Hauser R, Westermann B, Probst R. Non-invasive tracking of patient's head movements during computer-assisted intranasal microscopic surgery. Laryngoscope 1997; 107:491–499.
82. Gunkel AR, Freysinger W, Thumfart WF. Computer-assisted surgery in the frontal maxillary sinus. Laryngoscope 1997; 107:631–633.
83. Fried MP, Kleefield J, Gopal H, Reardon E, Ho BT, Kuhn FA. Image-guided endoscopic surgery. Laryngoscope 1997; 107:594–601.

84. Anon J. Computer-aided endoscopic sinus surgery. Laryngoscope 1998; 108: 949–961.
85. Metson R, Gliklich RE, Cosenza M. A comparison of image guidance systems for sinus surgery. Laryngoscope 1998; 108:1164–1170.
86. Chang PH, Lee LA, Huang CC, Lai CH, Lee TJ. Functional endoscopic sinus surgery in children using a limited approach. Arch Otolaryngol Head Neck Surg 2004; 130(9):1033–1036.
87. Mitchell RB, Pereira KD, Younis RT, Lazar RH. Pediatric functional endoscopic sinus surgery: is a second look necessary? Laryngoscope 1997; 107: 1267–1269.
88. Walner DL, Falciglia M, Willging JP, Myer CM. The role of second-look endoscopy after pediatric functional endoscopic sinus surgery. Arch Otolaryngol Head Neck Surg 1998; 124:425–428.
89. Fakhri S, Manoukian JJ, Souaid JP. Functional endoscopic sinus surgery in the pediatric population: outcome of a conservative approach to postoperative care. J Otolaryngol 2001; 30:15–18.
90. Younis RT. The pros and cons of second-look Sinonasal Endoscopy after endoscopic sinus surgery in children. Arch Otolaryngol Head Neck Surg 2005; 131:1–3.
91. Herbert RL II, Bent JP III. Meta-analysis of outcomes of pediatric functional andoscopic sinus surgery. Laryngoscope 1998; 108(6):796–799.
92. Lusk RP, Muntz HR. Endoscopic sinus surgery in children with chronic sinusitis: a pilot study. Laryngoscope 1990; 100:654–658.
93. Clary RA. Is there a future for pediatric sinus surgery? An American perspective. Int J Pediatr Otorhinolaryngol 2003; 67(suppl 1):S213–S215.
94. Carpenter KM, Graham SM, Smith RJ. Facial skeletal growth after endoscopic sinus surgery in the piglet model. Am J Rhinol 1997; 11(3):211–217.
95. Mair EA, Bolger WE, Breisch EA. Sinus and facial growth after pediatric endoscopic sinus surgery. Arch Otolaryngol Head Neck Surg 1995; 121(5):547–552.
96. Bothwell MR, Piccirillo JF, Lusk RP, Ridenour BD. Long-term outcome of facial growth after functional endoscopic sinus surgery. Otolaryngol Head Neck Surg 2002; 126(6):628–634.
97. Senior B, Wirtschafter A, Mai C, Becker C, Belenky W. Quantative impact of pediatric sinus surgery on facial growth. Laryngoscope 2000; 110(11): 1866–1870.
98. Salvin RG, Cannon RE, Freidman WH, Patitang E, Sundaram M. Sinusitis and bronchial asthma. J All Clin Immunol 1980; 66(3):250–257.
99. Lieser JD, Derkay CS. Pediatric sinusitis: when do we operate? Curr Opin Otolaryngol Head Neck Surg 2005; 13(1):60–66.

12

Image-Guided Pediatric Sinus Surgery

Sam J. Daniel

Department of Otolaryngology, McGill University, Montreal, Quebec, Canada

INTRODUCTION

Image-guided surgery (IGS) is a new technology that has become an important adjunctive tool in sinus and skull-base surgery. Image-guidance systems rely on preoperative CT and MRI data images to provide the surgeon with a real-time 3D visual localization of the surgical instruments relative to the patient's anatomy during surgery. Therefore, movements of the surgical instruments are tracked by the system and projected onto the preoperative dataset displayed on the monitor, providing a precise surgical roadmap. The technology continues to progress at a fast pace with many systems currently available, each with its own benefits and drawbacks.

Image guidance can assist the endoscopic head and neck surgeon by confirming the position within distorted or pathological anatomic fields. It also helps identify anatomy landmarks in difficult cases, thus reducing the stress placed on the surgeon and augmenting patients' safety (1). Undoubtedly, it does not bypass a thorough knowledge of the anatomy and should not confer a false sense of safety. However, it clearly improves surgical accuracy and greatly reduces the risk of major intracranial or intraorbital complications (2). The advantages of IGS are summarized in Table 1 (3).

Table 1 Advantages and Drawbacks of Image-Guided Surgery

Advantages	Drawbacks
Accurate localization of pathology	Longer set-up
Three-dimensional visualization	Danger of relying on equipment
Increased patient safety	Increased radiation exposure with 3D CT scan
Simplified complex procedures	Costly equipment
Surgeon reassurance	Danger of overconfidence
Improved resident teaching	

TECHNOLOGY

Different IGS systems are currently available on the market, each with its own advantages, drawbacks, and limitations. Tracking systems can be classified into two types based on the type of signal they rely on for localization of instruments. These can be either electromagnetic, such as radiofrequency signals, or optical, such as infrared signals. Most currently available systems are optical-based and require that the patients wear special headsets during surgery in order to monitor head position (4). Electromagnetic systems also require headsets to be worn during the preoperative CT scan.

System Components

Standard IGS systems are made-up of a computer workstation, a display monitor, an image-processing software, a localization system, and specialized instrumentation that can be tracked digitally (Fig. 1).

Tracking Systems

Although both optical and electromagnetic image-guidance systems have proven to be valuable, individual preferences vary based on differences in design and operation. The system utilized at the Montreal Children's Hospital is Vector Vision from Brainlab (Fig. 1). It consists of a powerful computer system, a touch screen monitor, and two cameras which emit infrared signals that determine the patient's position in three dimensions as well as the position of the surgical instruments in relation to the patient's preoperative CT or MR images. The image data is typically displayed in multiplanar format with options of videoscopic feeds.

The infrared cameras detect the reflective markers attached to the patient's body and transmit the continuously collected data to the system. The system then calculates a 3D representation of the patient's anatomy based on diagnostic data. During the operation, the surgeon can follow the movements of his or her instruments on the computer screen in real time. Other tracking systems available on the market are listed in Table 2.

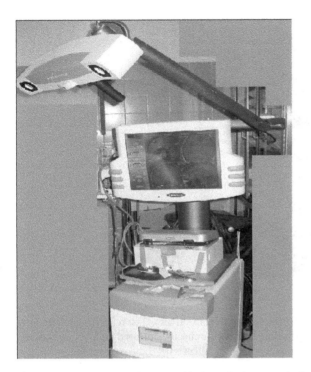

Figure 1 The standard image-guided surgical system includes a computer workstation, a display monitor, and a tracking system. This tracking system utilizes infrared
cameras (Vector Vision, Brainlab).

Optical Systems

Optical-based systems rely on infrared light for the tracking of surgical
instruments. Optical sensors are placed on a headframe worn by the patient
(Fig. 2). There are two types of optical systems, referred to respectively as
active or passive. Active optical systems use a camera to track the position
of flashing light-emitting diodes attached to the instruments and headframe. Passive optical tracking systems detect the reflection of infrared

Table 2 Tracking Systems Most Commonly Utilized in Sinus Surgery

Digitizer	Product's name	Company
Electromagnetic	Insta Trak	GE Medical
Optical	Vector Vision	Brainlab
Optical	LandmarX	Medtronic
Optical	Stryker Navigation	Stryker Corporation

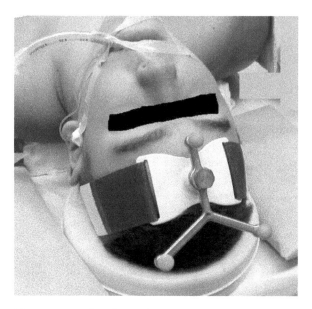

Figure 2 Headband worn by the patient during surgery. The reflective spheres have a known geometric configuration and their reflected infrared light is tracked by cameras, allowing the system to localize the patient's head throughout the procedure.

light from reflective markers placed on cordless instruments (no need for cable attachment). In both types, line-of-sight must be maintained between the system components to allow tracking.

Electromagnetic Systems

Electromagnetic tracking systems use electromagnetic sensors to detect variations in the electromagnetic field caused by instrument or patient movement. They have a transmitter located near the surgical field and a receiver placed on the surgical instrument. A brief comparison between electromagnetic and optical systems is provided in Table 3.

Patient Registration

Registration is the process of matching preoperative images to the 3D space occupied by the patient during surgery. This allows accurate localization of the surgical tools within the surgical volume of interest (3,5). In fact, the registration process is a major factor in the accuracy of image-guided systems. There is a steep learning curve but set up and registration time do decrease over time (4,6). A synopsis of the main types of registration techniques currently in use is presented in Table 4.

Table 3 Comparison of Electromagnetic and Optical Systems

Electromagnetic	Optical
Relatively less expensive	More expensive
Does not require line-of-sight between transmitter and receiver	Requires a clear line-of-sight between transmitter and receiver
Can have signal interference from metallic objects in the operating field	Can have signal interference from the operating room lights
Requires specialized headsets to be worn by patients during surgery	Requires specialized headsets to be worn by patients during surgery

Table 4 Summary of Registration Techniques

Anatomic fiducial registration	Anatomic landmarks such as tragus, nasion, menton, medical, and lateral canthus are selected on the patient.
Extrinsic markers	Skin-affixed fiducial markers are attached before CT scanning and are left until registration is complete.
Surface mapping registration	Multiple surface data points are gathered from the patient's face using a laser device. The computer matches the patient's facial contour to the preoperative image dataset.
Autoregistration	A special headframe provides a fixed arrangement of registration markers relative to the patient's head. The patient must wear this frame at the time of the CT and in the OR during surgery.

USE OF IGS IN PEDIATRIC OTOLARYNGOLOGY

Introduction

Intraoperative use of IGS is *not* considered standard care in all cases of sinus or skull-base surgery. However, it has undeniable value in many selected clinical settings as it assists the surgeon in confirming the position of normal or distorted anatomical structures as well as pathology. The American Academy of Otolaryngology-Head and Neck Surgery (AAO-HNS), in its policy statement on intraoperative use of computer-aided surgery, lists some examples of indications for image-guided sinus surgery; these are summarized in Table 5 (7). While this list is not exhaustive, usefulness of IGS in

Table 5 AAO-HNS Policy on Intraoperative Use of Computer-Aided Surgery

Revision sinus surgery
Distorted sinus anatomy of development, postoperative, or traumatic origin
Extensive sinonasal polyposis
Pathologic conditions involving the frontal, posterior ethmoid, or sphenoid sinuses
Disease abutting the skull base, orbit, optic nerve, or carotid artery
Cerebrospinal fluid rhinorrhea or conditions where there is a skull-base defect
Benign and malignant sinonasal neoplasms

Source: From Ref. 7.

many of the indications listed in the table will be demonstrated in the next section using clinical case scenarios with radiological images.

Revision Sinus Cases

One of the principal uses of image guidance is in revision cases where the landmarks have been altered as in resected middle turbinates or distorted skull-base anatomy. This is particularly true in revision cases with extensive sinonasal polyposis and in children with cystic fibrosis. The following case of a 15-year-old girl with severe cystic fibrosis who has had two previous sinus operations is illustrative. She presented three years following her second operation with severe sinus symptoms and fever unresponsive to antibiotics. Flexible endoscopy and imaging revealed extensive polyposis and inflammation with shifting of the nasal septum and extension of the disease to the skull base. A representative CT scan section is shown below (Fig. 3). IGS was performed with complete eradication of the disease.

Disease Abutting Important Structures

Image guidance can enhance patient's safety when used to confirm the anatomy or disease along risky areas. This includes the skull base, particularly along the superomedial portion of the ethmoid sinus near the cribriform plate attachment. Other problematic areas include the periorbital area and the frontal sinus, since the angles of approach and variability of this sinus can make the surgery very challenging. The sphenoethmoid recess can also be difficult to identify at times (8). Image guidance can be particularly useful in confirming the position of the anterior face of the sphenoid as well as vital structures in close proximity or within the sinus such as the carotid arteries, the cavernous venous sinuses, and the optic nerve. The latter can sometimes be found within an Onodi cell. The 3D orientation with coronal, axial, and sagittal sections simultaneously correlated in real time can be extremely helpful as illustrated in Figure 4.

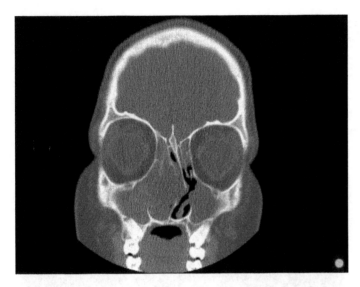

Figure 3 A 15-year-old girl suffering from fibrosis with severe disease recurrence following two previous surgeries. Note the extensive pathology deviating and fracturing the nasal septum.

Figure 5 is the MRI of a 15-year-old boy with pan-sinusitis and sphenoid sinus mucocele abutting the carotid arteries. Notice the compression of the right carotid artery (white arrow) by the mucocele, as well as the dural enhancement on that side. Image guidance was used to confirm the position of the carotid arteries during resection.

Image guidance can also be very helpful in cases of periorbital/orbital abscesses drained endoscopically, as well as in optic nerve decompression (Fig. 6).

Extensive Sinonasal or Skull-base Tumors

Image-guided surgery is extremely useful in extensive sinonasal and skull-base tumors. Again, IGS should be used as an adjunctive tool to confirm anatomy and/or disease, not to seek it. Benign or malignant tumors invading, distorting, or abutting important or vital structures can now be accessible endoscopically in a better and safer way. The following clinical cases are illustrative (Figs. 7–9).

Clinical case 1

An 18-year-old girl presented with acute visual loss and a one-month history of left eye disformat, nasal congestion, and frontal headache. She

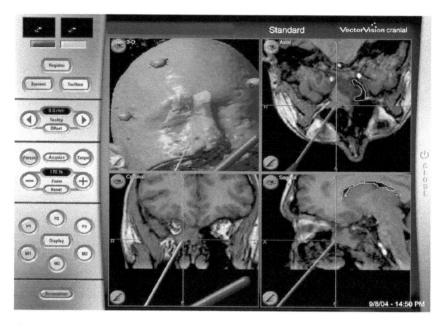

Figure 4 A 16-year-old boy with neurofibroma of the sphenoid sinus resected under image guidance. The white wand represents the surgical instrument pointing to the anterior face of the sphenoid. The usefulness of the 3D orientation with the coronal, axial, and sagittal sections can be appreciated.

was diagnosed with bilateral retinoblastoma as an infant, and was treated with right eye enucleation and left eye radiotherapy. Figure 7 shows representative MRI sections demostrating a large tumor involving the left maxillary sinus and the orbit with skull-base and intracranial invasion. Pathology revealed an aggressive sarcoma.

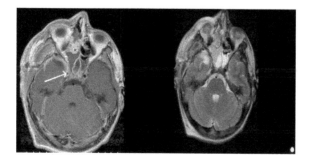

Figure 5 A 15-year-old boy with right pan-sinusitis and sphenoid sinus mucocele. White arrow is pointing to compressed right carotid artery.

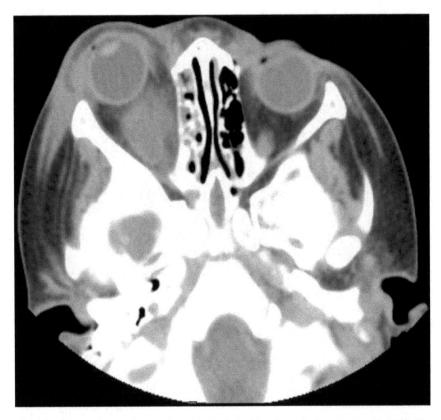

Figure 6 A 4-year-old boy with periorbital and intraconal abscesses on the left side. Notice the impressive proptosis on the same side. The abscess was drained endoscopically.

Clinical case 2

A nine-year-old boy was referred for chronic headache, severe growth delay below the fifth percentile, and chronic nasal obstruction. A CT scan and MRI revealed a suprasellar mass measuring $3.5 \times 3.5 \times 2.5$ cm extending into the sphenoid sinus through a sellar floor defect. There was also displacement of the optic chiasm and peripheral calcification typical of craniopharyngioma. Representative CT scan and MRI cuts are shown in Figure 8.

The current practice at the Montreal Children's Hospital and many tertiary care academic centers is to approach pituitary and other skull-base tumors using an endoscopic transethmosphenoidal approach with a navigation system (9–11). Resection was performed endoscopically using the Brainlab Vector Vision unit, with excellent results. During surgery, the location of the carotid arteries, optic nerves, and floor of sella were confirmed using image guidance. Pathology confirmed the suspected diagnosis.

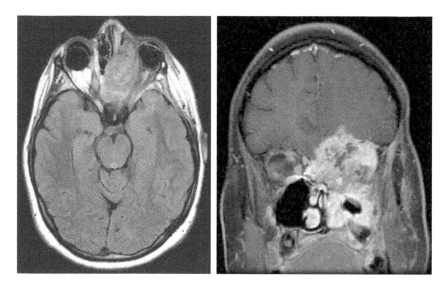

Figure 7 Post-contrast axial and coronal T$_1$-weighted MRI of an 18-year-old girl diagnosed with an aggressive sarcoma invading the orbit and skull-base with intracranial extension.

Clinical case 3

The following case illustrates the usefulness of image guidance in traditionally difficult-to-reach areas such as the pterygomaxillary fossa. A nine-year-old boy with severe intractable epistaxis was referred to pediatric otolaryngology after a CT scan revealed a large mass compatible with juvenile nasopharyngeal angiofibroma. Representative cuts from the MRI are illustrated in Figure 9. This impressive tumor extended from the base of the skull into the palate, displacing the latter inferiorly. It also had pseudopods extending into the pterygomaxillary fossa. The tumor was excised endoscopically after angioembolization.

LIMITATIONS OF IMAGE-GUIDED SURGERY

While IGS is by a useful innovative technology with a growing role in head and neck surgery, surgeons should be cautious when using it. Calibration errors could result in serious injury to the patient if IGS is used to identify rather than confirm anatomical landmarks. It is also important to remember that the CT scan or MRI sections represent a preoperative and not a real-time image. For instance, if the anatomy changes due to hemorrhage in the tumor, necrosis, or tumor growth, the image on the screen will not reflect reality. Furthermore, it is important to remember that the accuracy of currently available systems is up to 2 mm (12–14). Accuracy can even be worse

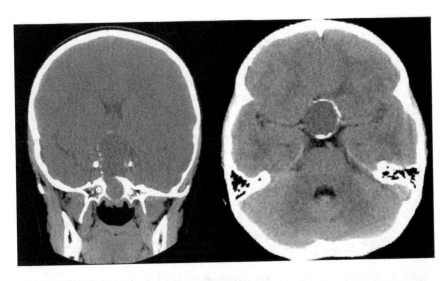

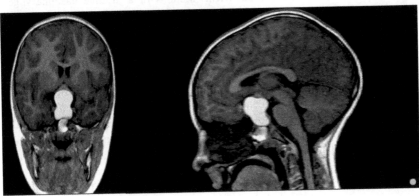

Figure 8 CT and MR images (*above* and *below*, respectively) showing the cranio-pharyngioma abutting the optical chiasm. Note the inferior extension through a defect of the sellar floor into the sphenoid sinus, and the rim of calcification on CT scan typical of these bengin tumors.

in case of headframe movement, poor CT or MRI image acquisition, and unsuccessful registration process. This technology is also very susceptible to computer malfunction and operator error (15). Finally, a major danger of this technology is overreliance on it, as well as surgeon overconfidence.

CONCLUSION

While not yet considered standard care, IGS is extremely useful in pediatric sinus and skull-base surgery. It clearly provides added safety and comfort

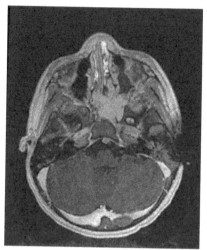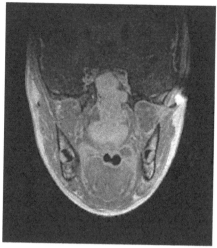

Figure 9 Axial (*left*) and coronal (*right*) sections of a juvenile nasopharyngeal angiofibroma (*JNA*) in a 9-year-old boy resected endoscopically with IGS.

level for the pediatric otolaryngologist working in high-risk areas or with difficult and/or distorted anatomy. The 3D visualization, including the sagittal reconstruction, greatly improves accuracy in many complex areas, and is an enormous asset in any academic residency-training program as it improves teaching and the learning curve of residents (16,17). This said, computer-aided image-guided surgery is not infallible and is not an adequate substitute for surgical experience, solid anatomical knowledge, and clinical judgment.

REFERENCES

1. Caversaccio M, Bachler R, Ladrach K, Schroth G, Nolte LP, Hausler R. Frameless computer-aided surgery system for revision endoscopic sinus surgery. Otol Head Neck Surg 2000; 122(6):808–813.
2. Heermann R, Schwab B, Issing PR, Haupt C, Hempel C, Lenarz T. Image-guided surgery of the anterior skull base. Acta Otolaryngol 2001; 121(8): 973–978.
3. Citardi MJ. Computer-aided frontal sinus surgery. Otolaryngol Clin North Am 2001; 34(1):111–122.
4. Metson RB, Gliklich RE, Cosenza MJ. A comparison of image guidance systems for sinus surgery. Laryngoscope 1998; 108:1164–1170.
5. Kingdom TT, Orlandi RR. Image-guided surgery of the sinuses: current technology and applications. Otolaryngol Clin North Am 2004; 37(2):381–400.
6. Gall RM, Witterick IJ, Hawke M. Image-guided sinus surgery. J Otolaryngol 2004; 33(1):22–25.

7. American Academy of Otolaryngology-Head and Neck Surgery Foundation. Intra-operative use of computer aided surgery: AAO-HNS policy on intra-operative use of computer-aided surgery. September 12, 2002, revised November 4, 2002. Available at: http://www.entlink.net/practice/rules/image-guiding.cfm.
8. Bolger WE, Keyes AS, Lanza DC. Use of the superior meatus and superior turbinate I the endoscopic approach to the sphenoid sinus. Otolaryngol Head Neck Surg 1999; 120(3):308–313.
9. Ohhashi G, Kamio M, Abe T, Otori N, Haruna S. Endoscopic transnasal approach to the pituitary lesions using a navigation system (InstaTrak system): technical note. Minim Invasive Neurosurg 2002; 45(2):120–123.
10. White DR, Sonnenburg RE, Ewend MG, Senior BA. Safety of minimally invasive pituitary surgery (MIPS) compared with a traditional approach. Laryngoscope 2004; 114(11):1945–1948.
11. Thomas RF, Monacci WT, Mair EA. Endoscopic image-guided transethmoid pituitary surgery. Otolaryngol Head Neck Surg 2002; 127(5):409–416.
12. Fried MP, Kleefield J, Gopal H, Reardon E, Ho BT, Kuhn FA. Image-guided endoscopic surgery: results of accuracy and performance in a multicenter clinical study using an electromagnetic tracking system. Laryngoscope 1997; 107:594–601.
13. Metson RB, Cosenza MJ, Cunningham MJ, Randolph GW. Physician experience with an optical based image guided system for sinus surgery. Laryngoscope 2000; 110:972–976.
14. Anon JB. Computer-aided endoscopic sinus surgery. Laryngoscope 1998; 108(7):949–961.
15. Hwang P. Surgical rhinology: recent advances and future directions. Otolaryngol Clin North Am 2004; 37(2):489.
16. Anand VK, Kacker A. Value of radiologic imaging and computer assisted surgery in surgical decisions of the anterior skull base lesions. Rhinology 2000; 38:17–22.
17. Eliashar R, Sichel JY, Gross M, Hocwald E, Dano I, Biron A, Ben-Yaacov A, Goldfarb A, Elidan J. Image guided navigation system-a new technology for complex endoscopic endonasal surgery. Postgrad Med J 2003; 79(938):686–690.

13

A Step-Wise Approach to Endoscopic Surgery for Advanced Sinonasal Disease

Roy R. Casiano

Department of Otolaryngology, University of Miami School of Medicine, Miami, Florida, U.S.A.

INTRODUCTION

Since its introduction into Europe in the late 1970s, endoscopic sinus surgical technique has undergone numerous refinements. Most of these refinements were made to facilitate the localization of the dependent sinuses (especially the sphenoid or maxillary sinus) and to minimize the chance of intraorbital or intracranial complications.

Despite these advances, complications still arise with major orbital and intracranial complications estimated to occur in 0.05 to 2% and 0.32 to 0.9% of cases, respectively (1–3). Inadvertent penetration of the anterior cranial fossa may result in CSF rhinorrhea, meningitis, brain abscess, focal brain hemorrhage, central nervous system deficits, or death. Inadvertent orbital penetration may result in an orbital hematoma, medial or inferior rectus muscle injury, nasolacrimal duct stenosis, or loss of vision. For the most part, these complications arise due to the surgeon's lack of orientation while operating endoscopically around the paranasal sinuses in the presence of anatomical distortion due to prior surgery or inflammatory disease.

The recent introduction of intraoperative image-guidance devices (computer-assisted surgery) may help to reduce some complications by improving the surgeon's orientation. However, the cost of these devices precludes their widespread availability to the average practicing otolaryngologist. Also, with the exception of a few studies regarding their reliability and potential benefits, the value of these devices in actually preventing significant complications or improving clinical outcomes has yet to be determined (4). Failure to properly register or calibrate these instruments combined with overreliance on the information given may result in misleading information with a subsequent error in anatomical localization and a new list of complications. It should be noted that, despite these technological advancements, a thorough knowledge of the complex endoscopic paranasal sinus, orbital, and skull-base anatomy gained through laboratory dissections and surgical experience remains the single most important factor for decreasing operative morbidity.

It is not uncommon for a complication to be blamed on inexperience or inadequate training. However, some responsibilities may rest with the teaching methodology most commonly used today. In the laboratory, surgeons are taught to identify endoscopically critical anatomical landmarks in non-pathologic fresh cadaver specimens. These anatomical reference points, which are vital for maintaining the proper surgical orientation away from critical orbital and skull-base structures, include the uncinate process, ostium of the maxillary sinus, middle and superior turbinate and surrounding recesses, basal lamella of the middle and superior turbinates, the anterior ethmoid artery, and the anterior and posterior ethmoid air cells (5–11). However, in real-life situations, these landmarks often have significant anatomical variations or are obscured by blood, polyps, and/or other inflammatory or postsurgical changes. Failure to correctly identify these landmarks in these unfamiliar circumstances can misdirect the surgeon with disastrous consequences for the patient. This potential for significant morbidity or mortality is further increased with inappropriate utilization of powered instrumentation.

While laboratory training is undisputedly vital for the understanding of normal anatomy, surgeons must also be equipped with the endoscopic anatomical knowledge and surgical skill to safely and precisely navigate through even the most distorted sinus cavities. They must be able to achieve this while maximizing mucosal preservation and maintaining the disease-directed (functional) surgical principles that govern endoscopic sinus surgery.

Accordingly, other more consistent anatomical landmarks are needed to combat these surgical challenges.

The ideal anatomical reference point must be consistent, easily found even in the most distorted sinus cavities, and easily used. It must also provide the surgeon with a sense of direction as one proceeds anteroposteriorly through the complex ethmoid labyrinth into the maxillary, sphenoid, and/or frontal sinuses. The medial orbital floor (MOF) and adjacent bony ridge of the antrostomy, when combined with columnellar measurements, are easily identifiable and consistent anatomical landmarks providing even the most inexperienced surgeon with reliable information to find all of the paranasal sinuses and other critical skull-base and orbital structures (12–15). None of the landmarks is affected by the presence of significant inflammatory disease or prior surgery. The following represents an anatomically based approach to performing ESS for advanced sinonasal disease.

Surgical Technique

In patients with advanced sinus disease (Figs. 1 and 2), the surgical technique proceeds methodically in an inferosuperior and anteroposterior direction, identifying known anatomical reference points or structures along the way. This approach is designed to teach the inexperienced surgeon to identify and use key anatomical landmarks to find the approximate location of the dependent sinuses and critical skull-base structures throughout the course of a typical endoscopic surgical procedure.

The endoscopic dissection technique described here is divided into six steps, which represent increasing levels of surgical difficulty: (i) intranasal exposure and identification of the posterior choanal structures, (ii) identification of the MOF and bony ridge of the antrostomy, (iii) anterior ethmoidectomy, (iv) posterior ethmoidectomy, (v) sphenoid sinusotomy, and (vi) frontal sinusotomy. Clearly, the inexperienced surgeon must master each level before proceeding to the next. Failure to do so may result in incomplete disease removal and inadequate exposure and subsequent improper orientation, as the surgeon proceeds anteroposteriorly into the ethmoid, sphenoid, and/or frontal sinuses.

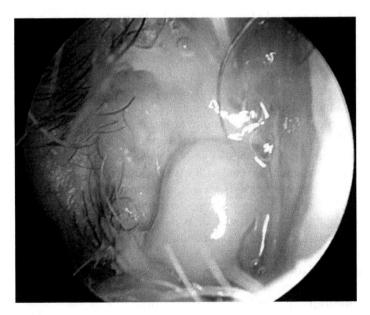

Figure 1 Endoscopic exam of the right nostril, showing extensive nasal polyps filling the vestibule.

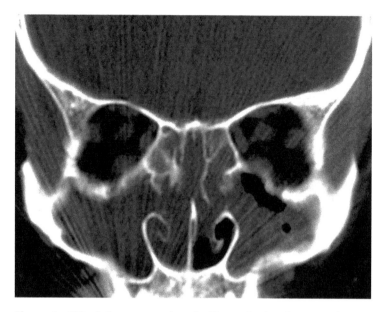

Figure 2 CT of the same patient in Figure 1, showing extensive mucoperiosteal thickening and osteoneogenesis of the maxillary sinus and ethmoid septations bilaterally, worse on the right.

Intranasal Exposure and Identification of the Posterior Choanal Structures

The structures of the posterior nasal choana, i.e., the eustachian tube opening, choanal arch, posterior septum, and posterior nasopharyngeal wall, along with the inferior turbinate, are routinely identified prior to performing a maxillary antrostomy. This immediately establishes the anteroposterior dimensions of the nasal airway, provides a drainage route for blood into the nasopharynx, and facilitates the introduction of sinus telescopes and endoscopic sinus surgery (ESS) instrumentation. Once the nasal airway is established, the nose is topically decongested and infiltrated with vasoconstrictive agents.

When bilateral polyp disease is present, a polypectomy is performed bilaterally first to reestablish the anteroposterior dimensions of the nose as well as to facilitate the placement of a contralateral nasopharyngeal suction (Fig. 3). Separate contralateral suction may be used for the continuous evacuation of accumulated blood or debris in the nasopharynx. Hypertrophied middle and/or inferior turbinates or septal spur/deviations obstructing the nasal airway or limiting endoscopic exposure are addressed at this time prior to proceeding with any sinus work.

Hemostasis and adequate nasal exposure and evacuation of blood are imperative when addressing advanced inflammatory disease of the nose and

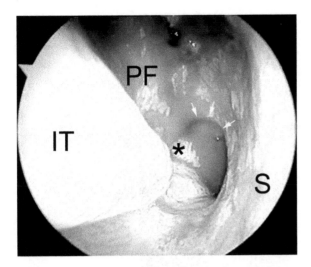

Figure 3 Establishment of a nasal airway to identify all posterior choanal structures and the posterior fontanella area. *Abbreviations*: PF, posterior fontanelle; S, septum; IT, inferior turbinate; asterisk, eustachian tube orifice.

paranasal sinuses. Monopolar or bipolar suction cautery is helpful if discrete bleeding points are encountered during the surgery. However, excessive cauterization should be avoided to minimize crusting and prolonged healing in these areas.

Identification of the Medial Floor of the Orbit and/or Bony Crest of the Antrostomy

For more limited disease of the ostiomeatal complex, an uncinectomy and exposure of the maxillary sinus natural ostium may be all that is necessary. However, if further ethmoidal work is required or if there is significant anatomical distortion or polyp disease, then the medial orbital floor (MOF) should be identified prior to proceeding with an ethmoidectomy. As the surgeon gains more experience, this step may merely require visualizing the superior margin of the maxillary sinus natural ostium (representing the anterior MOF), obviating the need for a wider antrostomy. In patients with more advanced disease and/or anatomical distortion due to prior surgery, a wider antrostomy is performed. This immediately identifies the bony ridge of the antrostomy, the MOF, and the posterior wall of the maxillary sinus.

In the absence of any normal osteomeatal complex references, or when difficulty is experienced identifying the natural ostium of the maxillary sinus, the maxillary sinus should be entered through the posterior fontanelle, superior to the posterior one-third of the inferior turbinate (Fig. 4). This

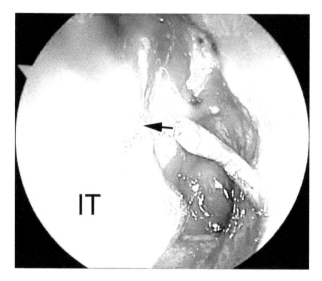

Figure 4 In situations where an uncinate is not readily identified, safe entry through the posterior fontanelle (*arrow*), over the posterior one-third of the IT, is preferred. A frontal curette assures proper penetration through both layers of muscosa (nasal and maxillary sinus) to avoid inadvertent creation of a maxillary sinus mucocele. *Abbreviation*: IT, inferior turbinate.

approach will ensure the surgeon remains a safe distance from the orbit floor, which rises superiorly at this level. Once the posterior wall of the maxillary sinus and MOF are identified by palpation with a probe and endoscopic visualization, a wide antrostomy is created by removing most of the posterior fontanelle (Fig. 5).

The site of the natural ostium is incorporated into the maxillary antrostomy to reduce the chances of circular mucous flow. This is achieved by following the MOF and the horizontal portion of the antrostomy ridge to a point just behind the convexity of nasolacrimal duct where the MOF appears to be approximating the lamella of the inferior turbinate.

When performing an antrostomy through the posterior fontanelle area, care must be taken that the nasal, as well as the medial maxillary sinus mucosa of the fontanelle area, is penetrated. Failure to do so may result in the formation of a maxillary cyst, or mucocele, due to lateral elevation of the medial maxillary sinus mucosa and concomitant disruption of the natural ostium.

The MOF and bony ridge of the antrostomy provide the surgeon with the correct anteroposterior trajectory, as the surgeon dissects posteriorly, starting with the anterior ethmoid and subsequently into the posterior ethmoid and sphenoid sinuses. The MOF must always be kept in view on the

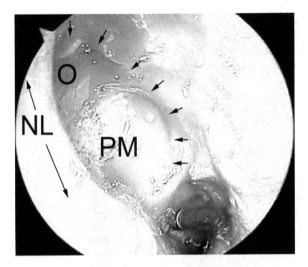

Figure 5 Completion of a wide middle meatal antrostomy with incorporation of the natural osteal area just behind the NL, at the level of the medial O. The PM identifies the approximate level (in the coronal plane) of the anterior wall of the sphenoid, more medially adjacent to the septum, and 7 cm from the columnella. The small arrows identify the bony ridge of the antrostomy (*horizontal portion* superiorly, and the *vertical portion* posteriorly). *Abbreviations*: NL, nasolacrimal duct; O, orbital floor; PM, posterior wall of the maxillary sinus.

video monitor and be constantly referred to throughout the surgery. Failure to visualize the superior margin of the antrostomy alerts the surgeon that he/she is proceeding in a more superior direction towards the skull-base.

The camera alignment on the monitor screen must also be periodically checked to ensure that it has not been inadvertently rotated. The opening of the antrostomy should face medially in the sagital plane, parallel to the nasal septum, with the horizontal portion of the antrostomy ridge projecting in an anteroposterior direction towards the orbital apex. The posterior wall of the maxillary sinus, as seen through the antrostomy, demarcates the approximate level, in the coronal plane, of the anterior wall of the sphenoid sinus, or posterior wall of the posterior ethmoid.

Anterior Ethmoidectomy

The anterior ethmoid cells border the horizontal bony ridge of the antrostomy (Fig. 6). The surgeon first performs an inferior ethmoidectomy (anterior and/or posterior, depending on disease extent) to identify the medial orbital wall inferiorly. At this point, the surgeon must begin regularly palpating the eye prior to exenterating any additional ethmoidal cells. By looking for movement in the orbital wall, any bony dehiscence will be identified. The orbital

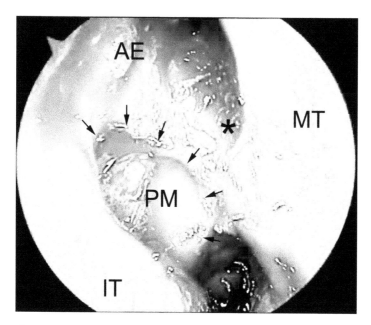

Figure 6 The anterior ethmoid cavity (ethmoid bulla, adjacent wall of the infundibulum, and suprabullar air cells) is found medial to the horizontal portion of the antrostomy ridge (*small arrows*). The PM, IT, and MT are also noted. *Abbreviations*: PM, posterior wall of the maxillary sinus; IT, inferior turbinate; MT, middle turbinate.

wall, once identified, represents the lateral limits of the dissection and is followed posteriorly or superiorly as needed (see posterior ethmoid and sphenoid dissection below).

In advanced disease, the surgeon initially maintains a safe distance of approximately 10 mm as he/she proceeds around the antrostomy ridge posteriorly (Figs. 7 and 8), in an inferomedial direction. The posterior ethmoid and sphenoid are identified as described below. A retrograde dissection of the superior ethmoid cells is later performed, only after the roof and lateral wall of the posterior ethmoid or sphenoid are identified to determine the superior and lateral extent of dissection, respectively.

Posterior Ethmoidectomy

The posterior ethmoid cells may be entered safely through the most horizontal portion of the middle turbinate lamella. Endoscopically, this location is identified by drawing a line from the posterior MOF (adjacent to the bony ridge) to the nasal septum. Another line is drawn along the vertical portion of the antrostomy ridge. A third or optional line is drawn along the free edge of the middle turbinate, or free edge of the basal lamella, if the middle

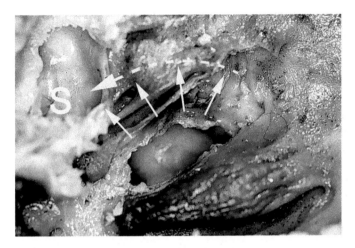

Figure 7 Sagittal dissection after reduction of the middle turbinate head and a wide middle meatal antrostomy, with incorporation of the natural ostium anteriorly. The solid arrows note the superior extent of initial dissection as one proceeds posteriorly through the anterior and posterior ethmoids towards the middle one-third of the S. Dissection follows a parallel course around the antrostomy in an inferomedial direction (*dotted arrow*). *Abbreviation*: S, sphenoid sinus.

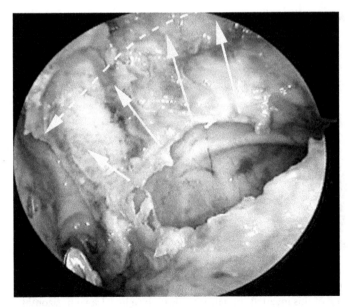

Figure 8 Endoscopic view of the extent of an inferior ethmoidectomy as shown in Figure 7.

turbinate head is removed. The triangle thus formed demarcates the safe entry zone into the inferior aspect of the posterior ethmoid sinus, i.e., through the horizontal portion of its basal lamella (Fig. 9).

Once the lateral or orbital wall of the posterior ethmoid is identified, the surgeon may proceed with the dissection of the superior cells of the posterior ethmoid or suprabullar cells, thus completing a total ethmoidectomy. The remaining portion of the middle turbinate vertical lamella, more anterosuperiorly, or other ethmoid septations are carefully removed in a posteroanterior and superoinferior direction. Initially, the surgeon restricts the dissection to an area adjacent to the orbital wall and lateral ethmoid roof where the bone is the thickest. Additional passes to exenterate more medially located cells are performed once the roof of the ethmoid is identified laterally. The surgeon should observe that the roof of the ethmoid slopes medially by as much as 45°, especially at the anterior ethmoid roof.

Sphenoid Sinusotomy

When significant anatomical distortion exists in the area of the sphenoethmoidal recess and the posterior insertion of the superior turbinate is not clearly visible, then the orbital floor is used to approach the sphenoid sinus, similar to the identification of the posterior ethmoid sinus, but more medially along the horizontal line demarcating the level of the orbital floor (Figs. 10 and 11). The

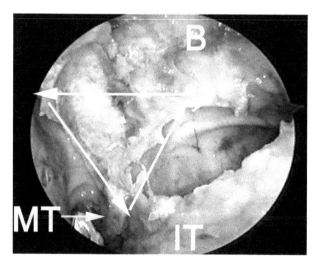

Figure 9 Triangular zone of safe entry into the inferior–posterior ethmoid air cell through the basel lamella of the middle turbinate, approximately 5 cm from the columnella. The base of this inverted triangle is made up by a line drawn horizontally from the posterior MOF to the nasal septum. The MT, IT, and B are identified. *Abbreviations*: MT, middle turbinate; IT, inferior turbinate; B, ethmoid bulla.

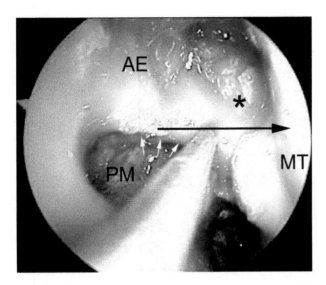

Figure 10 Probe introduced into the inferior aspects of the posterior ethmoid sinus, at the level (*solid black line*), and just medial to the transitional area of the antrostomy ridge (where the *horizontal* and *vertical portions* meet). The AE, MT, and basal lamella of the middle turbinate (*asterisk*) are identified. Columnellar measurement to this area is approximately 5 cm. *Abbreviations*: AE, anterior ethmoids; MT, middle turbinate.

sphenoid sinus is entered and identified medially, adjacent to the nasal septum, approximately 7 cm from the base of the columnella, at the level of the posterior MOF. The sphenoid sinus will be entered consistently in its inferior to middle third, which also corresponds to the location of the sphenoid ostium in most cases (Fig. 12). If the maxillary natural ostium or anterior antrostomy ridge is used as a reference point, then the sphenoid will be entered slightly more inferiorly, where thicker bone may be encountered, and needs to be removed with curettes or thinned with cutting burrs.

Frontal Sinusotomy

The frontal sinus is identified as shown in Figure 13 by drawing a line parallel to the bony nasolacrimal duct and directed superiorly from the anterior border of the antrostomy (i.e., natural ostium area) to a point several millimeters behind the anterior attachment of the middle turbinate. The correct point of entry will be directed superomedially away from the wall of the orbit and anteriorly away from the anterior ethmoid artery.

Palpation is key to identifying the posterior wall of the frontal sinus and opening the frontal sinus ostium, if indicated. The septations that comprise the roof of the suprabullar cells and the agger nasi, or frontal, cells are gently displaced inferoanteriorly to avoid inadvertent penetration

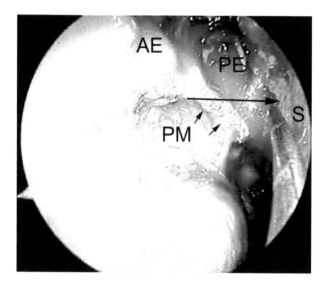

Figure 11   Probe introduced into the sphenoid sinus further along the same line drawn from the posterior MOF to the nasal septum. Entry into the sphenoid is through its natural ostium area, adjacent to the S. A good portion of the middle turbinate basal lamella has been removed to improve visualization of the nasal septum. The AE and the majority of the PE cavities are identified superior to this line. The PM demarcates the coronal plane of the anterior wall of the sphenoid sinus. *Abbreviations*: MOF, medial orbital floor; AE, anterior ethmoid; PE, posterior ethmoid sinus; PM, posterior maxillary sinus; S, septum.

through the anterior skull-base at the level of the anterior ethmoid artery, which represents the transitional area into the frontal recess and ostium. As with the ethmoid, maxillary, and sphenoid sinuses, an attempt is made to preserve as much of the frontal recess and frontal ostium mucosa to diminish the chances of prolonged healing or fibrosis with possible stenosis (Fig. 14).

CONCLUSIONS

The MOF and adjacent bony ridge of the antrostomy, when combined with columnellar measurements, are easily identifiable and consistent anatomical landmarks providing even the most inexperienced surgeon with reliable information to find all of the paranasal sinuses and other critical skull-base and orbital structures. None of the landmarks is affected by the presence of significant inflammatory disease or prior surgery. These reference points may better assist the rhinologic surgeon in determining the correct anteroposterior trajectory during ESS. A step-wise approach to the ethmoid labyrinth and

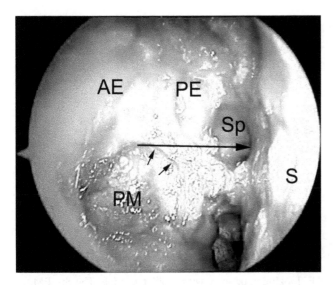

Figure 12 Completed SP. At least one-half of this cavity lies below the level of the MOF (*solid line*), once the anterior face is lowered inferiorly and medially. The transitional area of the antrostomy ridge (*small arrows*), PM, AE, PE, and nasal septum, are identified. *Abbreviations*: Sp, sphenoid sinusotomy; MOF, medial orbital floor; PM, posterior maxillary sinus; AE, anterior ethmoids; PE, posterior ethmoids; S, septum.

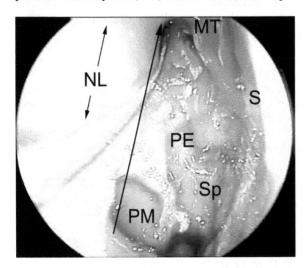

Figure 13 Palpation of the posterior wall of the frontal sinus with an ostium seeker. The level of safe entry is in the direction of line drawn parallel to the NL apparatus and a few millimeters behind the anterior attachment of the middle turbinate, but anterior to the anterior ethmoid artery (if visualized). The PM, Sp, PE, and septum are noted. *Abbreviations*: NL, nasolacrimal; PM, posterior maxillary sinus; Sp, sphenoid; PE, posterior ethmoid; S, septum.

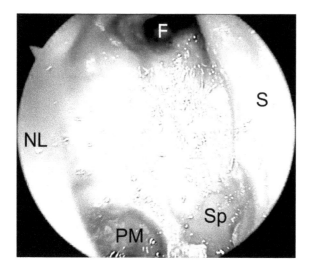

Figure 14   Completed F, looking superiorly with a 30° telescope. The Sp, PM, S, and NL are also seen. *Abbreviations*: F, frontal sinusotomy; Sp, sphenoid; PM, posterior maxillary sinus; S, septum; NL, nasolacrimal duct.

dependent sinuses, utilizing these consistent reference points, may minimize the chance of inadvertent intracranial or intraorbital complications in the face of significant anatomical distortion due to disease or prior surgery.

REFERENCES

1. Vleming M, Middelweerd RJ, DeVries N. Complications of endoscopic sinus surgery. Arch Otolaryngol Head Neck Surg 1992; 118:617–623.
2. May M, Levine HL, Mester SJ, Schaitkin B. Complications of endoscopic sinus surgery: analysis of 2108 patients—incidence and prevention. Laryngoscope 1994; 104:1080–1083.
3. Gross RD, Sheridan MF, Burgess MF. Endoscopic sinus surgery complications in residency. Laryngoscope 1997; 107:1080–1085.
4. Casiano RR. Intraoperative image-guidance technology. Arch Otolaryngol Head Neck Surg 1999; 125(11):1275–1278.
5. Messerklinger W. Uber die drainage der menschlichen nasennebenholen unter normalen und pathologischen bendingungen II: die stirnhole und ihr ausfuh-rungssystem. Monatsschr Ohrenheilkd 1967; 101:313–326.
6. Messerklinger W. Endosckopiche diagnose und chirurgie der rezidivierenden sinusitis. In: Krajina Z, ed. Advances in Nose and Sinus Surgery. Zagreb: Zagreb University, 1985.
7. Naumann H. Pathologische anatomie der chronischen rhinitis und sinusitis. In: Proceedings VIII International Congress of Oto-Rhinolaryngology. Amsterdam: Excerpta Medica, 1965:80.

8. Stamberger H. Endoscopic endonasal surgery—concepts in treatment of recurring rhinosinusitis. Part I. Anatomic and pathophysiologic considerations. Otolaryngol Head Neck Surg 1986; 94:143–147.

9. Stamberger H. Endoscopic endonasal surgery—concepts in treatment of recurring rhinosinusitis. Part II. Surgical technique. Otolaryngol Head Neck Surg 1986; 94:147–156.

10. Draf W. Die chirugische behandlung entzundlicher erkrankungen der nasennebenhohlen. Arch Otorhinoalaryngol 1982; 235:133–305.

11. Kennedy DW, Zinreich SJ, Rosenbaum AE, Johns ME. Functional endoscopic sinus surgery. Theory and diagnostic evaluation. Arch Otolaryngol 1985; 111: 576–582.

12. Schaefer SD. An anatomic approach to endoscopic intranasal ethmoidectomy. Laryngoscope 1998; 108:1628–1634.

13. May M, Schaitkin B, Kay SL. Revision endoscopic sinus surgery: six friendly surgical landmarks. Laryngoscope 1994; 104(6):766–767.

14. May M, Sobol SM, Korzec K. The location of the maxillary os and its importance to the endoscopic sinus surgeon. Laryngoscope 1990; 100(10):1037–1042.

15. Casiano RR. A stepwise surgical technique using the medial orbital floor as the key landmark in performing endoscopic sinus surgery. Laryngoscope 2001; 111(6):964–974.

14

Role of Tonsils and Adenoids in Pediatric Sinusitis

Hassan H. Ramadan

Department of Otolaryngology, West Virginia University, Morgantown, West Virginia, U.S.A.

Pediatric sinusitis is a very common disease that otolaryngologists and primary care physicians see in their offices. The exact incidence of sinusitis is unknown due to lack of precise definition and diagnostic criteria that can give us the appropriate incidence. It is, however, very well known that about 0.5 to 5% of all upper respiratory tract infections (URI) are complicated by sinusitis (1). The average child has between six and eight URIs per year, making sinusitis a common problem in the pediatric population (1). The incidence is on the rise, especially in developed countries, because of the increased incidence of allergic rhinitis. In 1994, Wright estimated that about 42% of children in the United States have allergic rhinitis by the age of six years (2).

The symptoms of chronic sinusitis in children are very similar to and overlap those of tonsil and adenoidal hypertrophy. This promotes confusion on the part of the physician as to whether the child has sinusitis versus tonsilitis and adenoiditis. The most common symptoms of sinusitis in younger children are those of colored discharge and rhinorrhea as well as cough, whereas in the older child they are merely headache with nasal stuffiness and congestion (3). Despite the fact that sinusitis is a very well-known disease, the literature does not provide clear cut indicators to distinguish between symptoms of sinusitis versus tonsil and adenoidal infection or hypertrophy (4–6). Previous investigations, however, suggest that there is a relationship between diseased tonsils and adenoids as well as sinusitis. This evidence is more of a general impression and is not based on objective scientific evidence (7–17).

ADENOIDS AND SINUSITIS

The relationship between tonsils and adenoids as well as sinusitis dates back to 1921 when Cleminson noted that a tonsillectomy and adenoidectomy was not found to consistently correct chronic sinusitis (18). In 1922, Mollison and Kendall found that about 22% of patients who underwent tonsillectomy and adenoidectomy had evidence of maxillary sinus infection as shown by a positive antral puncture through the middle meatus (14). In 1925, Dean was supportive of a tonsillectomy and adenoidectomy as a treatment modality for sinusitis; however, the indications were not clearly defined in the article (19). In 1931, Carmack found that 14.2% of children undergoing routine tonsillectomy and adenoidectomy had a positive finding suggesting sinusitis on antral lavage (17). Similarly, Crooks and Signy in 1936 noted a 24% incidence of sinusitis in children undergoing tonsillectomy and adenoidectomy in 1936 (15). In 1939, Gerrie noted a 9% incidence of sinusitis in those children (16). In 1937, Griffiths thought that the indications for a tonsillectomy and adenoidectomy were ill-founded and that the procedure had not been found to consistently correct chronic sinusitis (20). In 1947, Stevenson stated that he had never seen a case of maxillary sinusitis that did not have an enlarged adenoid present (21). At the same time, however, walker found that the degree of infection of the tonsils was more of a factor than the size of the adenoid pad (22). In 1952, Birrell noted that 27% of patients undergoing adenoidectomy and tonsillectomy had maxillary sinus infection as evidenced by a positive antral puncture (7). In 1955, Preston noted that purulent rhinorrhea was associated with tonsil adenoid hypertrophy in about 65% of the children (8). Similarly in the same year, Wilson found that rhinorrhea was present in 27% of newborns (23).

As noted from all of the above literature that was reviewed between 1921 and 1955, there is some anecdotal evidence that suggests that purulent rhinorrhea as well as findings of sinusitis on antral punctures are associated with tonsil and adenoid hypertrophy. However, tonsillectomy and adenoidectomy were not found to consistently correct chronic sinusitis. In 1974, Hoshaw and Nickman found that a tonsillectomy and adenoidectomy did not consistently correct chronic sinusitis in children (24). In 1981, Paul found that rhinorrhea, which was usually purulent and occurred in 84% of the patients with sinusitis, did not always clear after adenoidectomy and tonsillectomy. His success rate with tonsillectomy and adenoidectomy alone was 36%; however, this study did not specify how long the patients remained asymptomatic after the procedure (25).

ADENOID SIZE AND SINUSITIS

There is little support that the tonsils have any relationship to sinusitis, however, it seems that the relationship between adenoid hypertrophy and sinusitis is not very clear. It would seem that if the adenoids were large and there were stasis of secretions, symptoms of sinusitis could be mimicked. These secretions could also cause inflammation of the sinuses with blockage of the ostia of the sinuses causing sinusitis. In 1988, Fujita et al. examined the effect of adenoidectomy on the cure rate of sinusitis. They found that sinusitis was cured six months after surgery in 56% of 45 children who underwent an adenoidectomy (26). However, 24% of children who had not undergone adenoidectomy, had control of their sinusitis symptoms. The basis of deciding which children received the adenoidectomy was not stated by the authors.

In 1995, Van Cauwenberge et al. in a symposium noted that since the paranasal sinuses lie in close anatomical contact with the adenoids, it is tempting to presume that the pathological process in the nasopharynx will influence the sinuses and that adenoidectomy may help cure sinusitis (27). This influence, however, might work in the other direction in which rhinitis or sinusitis might cause an adenoiditis and/or an adenoid hypertrophy. An infection or hypertrophy of the adenoid caused by this mechanism might then lead to impairment of ventilation or drainage of the nasal and paranasal cavities.

In 1974, Merck divided children with sinusitis into three groups according to the size of their adenoids. He had five children with small adenoids, 17 with medium size adenoids, and 14 with large adenoids. Adenoidectomy improved sinusitis in 20% of the group with the small adenoids, 35% of the group with medium adenoids, and 57% of the children with large adenoids (28).

In an attempt to evaluate adenoid size and symptoms of chronic rhinosinusitis in 1997, Wang et al. investigated the relationship between the size of the adenoid and the upper respiratory symptoms in children by using a fiberoptic examination of the nasal cavity and nasopharynx. This was performed on 817 children and the size of the adenoid was classified into three categories according to the distance between the vomer and the adenoid tissue. They noted a significant relationship between the size of the adenoid and the complaints of nasal obstruction and snoring, but not with the presence of purulent sinusitis (32). In 2001, Tosca et al. evaluated children with asthma with nasal endoscopic examination for rhinosinusitis and adenoiditis. He noted that by using nasal endoscopy, rhinosinusitis as well as adenoiditis could be diagnosed better than by using clinical symptoms alone. Those findings were corroborated in a statistically significant manner with cytology and microbiology (33). In 1992, Bluestone on indications for tonsillectomy and adenoidectomy for paranasal sinusitis, thought that the benefit of adenoidectomy for children with chronic sinusitis is uncertain. Surgery to improve the nasal airway should be considered in a child with moderate to severe nasal obstruction secondary to obstructive adenoids Antimicrobial therapy for children with adenoiditis is indicated in an attempt to reduce the size of the adenoids and relieve the obstruction (34). In 1981, Dharam evaluated 100 children who were suffering from adenoid hypertrophy and sinusitis. They divided the children into two groups of 50; the first group was managed with antibiotics and anti-allergy drugs and the second group had an adenoidectomy as well as tonsillectomy. Of the antimicrobial treatment group, 11 (22%) had relief of their symptoms, whereas 18 (36%) of the adenoidectomy group had relief of their symptoms.

Both groups had to be managed surgically for control of their infections. In 1989, Fukuda et al. studied the relationship of the adenoid size to rhinosinusitis. They obtained lateral radiographic analysis of the nasopharynx on 404 children ages 2 to 14 years. An adenoidal nasopharyngeal (AN) ratio was measured. The results showed that the AN ratio of children with rhinosinusitis was equal to that of normal children. In those children with symptoms of adenoid hypertrophy such as snoring, mouth breathing, and nasal obstruction, the AN ratios were significantly higher than in normal controls (35).

In 1995, Rosenfeld evaluated a step-treatment approach for refractory chronic sinusitis whereby children were initially treated medically, and then those who failed went on to have an adenoidectomy. Those who failed an adenoidectomy went on to receive endoscopic sinus surgery. Adenoidectomy was noted to improve all major symptoms in about 75% of the children (29).

ADENOIDITIS AND SINUSITIS

Another situation facing clinicians is the patient with chronic sinonasal symptoms but without significant adenoid hypertrophy. Some argue that size does not matter and it is the adenoiditis rather than hypertrophy that predisposes to rhinosinusitis. In 1996, Lee and Rosenfeld studied the correlation between sinonasal symptoms in children and the prevalence of bacterial pathogens in the adenoid core. One or more bacterial pathogens were recovered from all samples of adenoids. *Hemophilus influenzae*, Group-A beta hemolytic streptococcus, and *Staphylococcus aureus* were encountered most often. A multivariate analysis revealed a significant correlation of sinonasal infections symptoms scores with colony forming units of adenoid core pathogens. The authors concluded that sinonasal infectious symptoms explain 48% of the variability in a quantitative bacteriology of the adenoid core independent of the adenoid size. Thus, they support a potential role for adenoidectomy in the management of refractory pediatric sinusitis despite the fact that the adenoid size may not be enlarged (30). In 2000, Bernstein et al. evaluated 52 children, who were undergoing an adenoidectomy. Bacterial cultures, were taken from the crypts of the adenoids and from the lateral wall of the nose under endoscopic control during the procedure. Bacterial pathogens were isolated from 79% of the adenoids and 46% of the lateral wall of the nose. Molecular typing revealed that in 16 of 18 pairs (89%) bacterial strains that were present in the adenoids were also present in the lateral wall of the nose. This led him to support the concept that bacterial pathogens that may cause rhinosinusitis are found concurrently in the nasopharynx and lateral wall in the nose and they are usually identical (31).

ADENOIDECTOMY AND SINUSITIS

In 1999, Ramadan performed a prospective nonrandomized study on 66 consecutive children referred for surgery because of chronic sinusitis that was refractory to medical management. He noted that adenoidectomy was successful in 47% of the children compared to a 77% success rate for those who underwent endoscopic sinus surgery (36). Our experience has been that adenoidectomy may be indicated in children who have a low-CT score and are under six years of age. It seems that in this age group, if sinus surgery was performed, revision sinus surgery was high and the success of adenoidectomy was not statistically different than endoscopic sinus surgery alone. However, for those children who are older than six years and have a high-CT score, an endoscopic sinus procedure was statistically better than an adenoidectomy alone. Children with asthma seem to respond better with sinus surgery than adenoidectomy alone (37).

REFERENCES

1. Wald ER. Sinusitis in children. Pediatr Infect Dis J 1988; 7(suppl 11): S150–S153.
2. Wright AL, Holberg CJ, Martinex FD, Halonen M, Morgan W, Taussig LM. Epdiemiology of physician-diagnosed allergic rhinitis in childhood. Pediatrics 1994; 94(6 Pt 1):895–901.
3. Lund VJ, Neijens HJ, Clement PA, Lusk R, Stammberger H. The treatment of chronic sinusitis: a controversial issue. Int J Pediatr Otorhinolaryngol 1995; 32(suppl):S21–S35.
4. Rachelefsky GS. Sinusitis in children-diagnosis and management. Clin Rev All 1984; 2:397.
5. Rachelefsky GS, Goldberg M, Katz RM, Boris G, Gyepes MT, Shapiro MJ, Mickey MR, Finegold SM, Siegel SC. Sinus disease in children with respiratory allergy. J All Clin Immunol 1978; 61:310.
6. Hoshaw TC, Nickman NJ. Sinusitis and otitis in children. Arch Otolaryngol 1974; 100:194.
7. Birrell JF. Chronic maxillary sinusitis in children. Arch Dis Child 1952; 27:1–9.
8. Preston HG. Maxillary sinusitis in children, its relation to coryza, tonsillectomy and adenoidectomy. Va Med Mon 1955; 82:229–232.

9. Shone GR. Maxillary sinus aspiration in children. What are the indications? J Laryngol Otol 1987; 101:461–464.
10. Clark WD, Bailey BJ. Sinusitis in children. Tex Med 1983; 79:44–47.
11. Paul D. Sinus infection and adenotonsillitis in pediatric patients. Laryngoscope 1981; 91:997–1000.
12. Merck W. Relationship between adenoidal enlargement and maxillary sinusitis. HNO 1974; 6:198–199.
13. Nickman NJ. Sinusitis, otitis and adenotonsillitis in children: a retrospective study. Laryngoscope 1978; 88:117–121.
14. Mollison WM, Kendall NE. Frequency of antral infection in children. Guy's Hosp Rep 1922; 72:225–228.
15. Crooks J, Signy AG. Accessory nasal sinusitis in childhood. Arch Dis Child 1936; 11:281–306.
16. Gerrie J. Sinusitis in children. Br Med J 1939; 2:363–364.
17. Carmack JW. Sinusitis in children. Ann Otol Rhinol Laryngol 1931; 40: 515–521.
18. Cleminson FJ. Nasal sinusitis in children. J Laryngol Otol 1921; 36:505–513.
19. Dean LW. Paranasal sinus disease in infants and young children. JAMA 1925; 85:317–321.
20. Griffiths I. Functions of tonsils and their relations to aetiology and treatment of nasal catarrh. Lancet 1937; 2:723–729.
21. Stevenson RS. The treatment of subacute maxillary sinusitis especially in children. Proc R Soc Med 1947; 40:854–858.
22. Walker FM. Tonsillectomy and adenoidectomy: unsatisfactory results due to chronic maxillary sinusitis. Br Med J 1947; II:908–910.
23. Wilson TG. Surgical anatomy of ENT in the newborn. J Laryngol Otol 1955; 69(4):229–254.
24. Hoshaw TC, Nickman NJ. Sinusitis and otitis in children. Arch Otolaryngol 1974; 100:194–195.
25. Paul D. Sinus infection and adenotonsillitis in pediatric patients. Laryngoscope 1981; 91(6):997–1000.
26. Fujita A, Takahashi H, Honjo I. Etiological role of adenoids upon otitis media with effusion. Acta Otolaryngol Suppl 1988; 454:210–213.
27. van Cauwenberge PB, Bellussi L, Naw AR, Maw AR, Paradise JL, Solow B. The adenoid as a key factor in upper airway infections. Int J Pediatr Otorhinolaryngol 1995; 32(suppl):S71–S80.
28. Merck W. Pathogenetic relationship between adenoid vegetations and maxillary sinusitis in children. HNO 1974; 22(6):198–199.
29. Rosenfeld RM. Pilot study of outcomes in pediatric rhinosinusitis. Arch Otolaryngol Head Neck Surg 1995; 121(7):729–736.
30. Lee D, Rosenfeld RM. Adenoid bacteriology and sinonasal symptoms in children. Otolaryngol Head Neck Surg 1997; 116(3):301–307.
31. Bernstein JM, Dryja D, Murphy TF. Molecular typing of paired bacterial isolates from the adenoid and lateral wall of the nose in children undergoing adenoidectomy: implications in acute rhinosinusitis. Otolaryngol Head Neck Surg 2001; 125(6):593–597.

32. Wang DY, Bernheim N, Kaufman L, Clement P. Assessment of adenoid size in children by fibreoptic examination. Clin Otolaryngol 1997; 22(2):172–177.
33. Tosca MA, Riccio AM, Marseglia GL, Caligo G, Pallestrini E, Ameli F, Mira E, Castelnuoro P, Pagella F, Ricci A, Ciprandi G, Canonica GE. Nasal endoscopy in asthmatic children: assessment of rhinosinusitis and adenoiditis incidence,correlations with cytology and microbiology. Clin Exp All 2001; 31(4):609–615.
34. Bluestone CD. Current indications for tonsillectomy and adenoidectomy. Ann Otol Rhinol Laryngol Suppl 1992; 155:58–64.
35. Fukuda K, Matsune S, Ushikai M, Imamura Y, Ohyama M. A study on the relationship between adenoid vegetation and rhinosinusitis. Am J Otolaryngol 1989; 10(3):214–216.
36. Ramadan HH. Adenoidectomy vs. endoscopic sinus surgery for the treatment of pediatric sinusitis. Arch Otolaryngol Head Neck Surg 1999; 125(11):1208–1211.
37. Ramadan HH. Surgical management of chronic sinusitis in children. Laryngoscope 2004; 114(12):2103–2109.

15

Complications of Sphenoid Sinus Surgery

Sarita Kaza

New York, New York, U.S.A.

Ramzi T. Younis

*Department of Pediatrics,
University of Miami, Miami, Florida, U.S.A.*

INTRODUCTION TO SPHENOID SURGERY

The sphenoid sinus in children starts to develop at around the fourth month of life, contrary to the maxillary and ethmoid sinuses, which start developing in utero. The importance of the sphenoid sinus rests on the fact that it is located in close proximity not only to the brain, but also to the other vital anatomical structures, such as the optic nerve and carotid artery. Any disease process, trauma, or surgery needs to be taken with extreme seriousness and delicate attention to the details of those anatomical landmarks. Hence, it is important to give this "special" sinus more attention and meticulous care in our evaluation and treatment.

In early childhood, the sphenoid sinus may not pose a serious concern to us; however, it is always crucial to address it meticulously, especially whenever it is involved in a disease process. Subsequently, we may see more sphenoid sinus in older children (more than 12 years) and adolescents or in unusual cases, such as immune deficiency, cystic fibrosis, allergic fungal or fungal sinusitis, and immotile cilia syndrome. The last few are not only very unique cases with systemic illnesses that require continuous care, but also deserve careful cognizance of full details of the sphenoid sinus anatomy to avoid potential fatal complications. Other conditions that may involve the sphenoid in adolescents are neoplasms such as juvenile nasopharyngeal angiofibroma (JNA).

This chapter stresses the importance of the anatomy and serious complications of sphenoid sinus surgery. The management of these serious complications is detailed.

ANATOMY

The sphenoid sinus is located at the base of the skull, in the midline, and has variable pneumatization. It drains along with the posterior ethmoid cells in the sphenoethmoidal recess, and the body lies below this opening, making it a "dependent" sinus. There are several vital structures in close proximity to the sinus. The carotid artery runs behind the lateral wall and then into the cavernous sinus, which sits superior and lateral to the sphenoid. The optic nerve chiasm sits above the sphenoid sinus and the nerve runs superior and lateral. The vidian nerve and the maxillary branch of the trigeminal nerve run inferior and lateral in the sinus. If a lateral sinus recess is present, the superior lateral border is formed by second branch of trigeminal nerve (V2) and the inferior border by the vidian nerve.

ANATOMIC VARIATIONS

The sphenoid sinus has variable pneumatization and has several well described anatomical variations. The Onodi cell is a posterior ethmoid cell that pneumatizes lateral and/or superior to the sphenoid sinus. Onodi described 38 different cells in 12 groups, so they are sometimes inconsistently described in practice, but all are felt to arise from such posterior ethmoid cells. The incidence has been studied by CT review and in cadavers. Two different Turkish groups [Odabassi et al. and Sirikci et al. (1,2)] studied this on CT review. Odabassi found the presence of Onodi cells in 13% of reviewed scans and Sirikci found 26% of reviewed scans to contain Onodi cells. Zinreich et al. (3) studied 21 cadavers, both by CT and by dissection. He concluded that the incidence was 7% by CT, but much higher by dissection at 39%. This "missed diagnosis" by CT was associated with oblique or horizontal orientation of the sphenoid face.

A dehiscent optic nerve is also well described. The CT scan studies found a range of incidence of 8% (4) to 13% (Odabassi) to 31.5% (2). Authors noted that this finding was consistently associated with pneumatization of the anterior clinoid. Kantaci et al. (5) describe the "sphenomaxillary plate," which is a pneumatized maxillary crest, in about 15% of cases reviewed by CT. This is important in that it not be mistakenly confused for the sphenoid. A dehiscent carotid artery is another known variation. CT study reports vary from 7% to 26%, again correlating with the presence of anterior clinoid aeration. Kantaci (5) noted this to be a bilateral finding in

16% of CT scans reviewed. Fujji et al. (6) performed a cadaver study, demonstrating that 88% had less than 0.5 mm of bony covering over the carotid canal, and 8% had true dehiscence. Kennedy (7) performed a cadaver study, which identified dehiscence in 20% of specimens.

PRESENTATION/PATHOPHYSIOLOGY

Ear, nose, and throat (ENT) physicians perform sphenoidotomy for a variety of reasons. Acute and chronic sinusitis are common referrals for the ENT physician. In addition to polyps, mucoceles form necessitating sphenoidotomy and drainage. Fungal sinusitis, both invasive and allergic, can present as isolated sphenoid disease. Tumors can also develop in the sinus. Presenting in the sphenoid, the most common primary sinonasal tumor is inverted papilloma, and the most common tumor of intracranial origin is pituitary adenoma. Both are most often benign, but due to their location in the sinus adjacent to critical structures, they necessitate surgery, as do the infectious processes. Entry into the sphenoid sinus is also encountered in endoscopic vidian neurectomy for vasomotor rhinitis and V2 nerve block for unremitting facial pain, recently described in patients with head and neck cancer. The petrous apex is also accessible from the posterior wall of the sphenoid sinus, and drainage of cholesterol granuloma via endoscopic sphenoidotomy has been described.

The presentation of disease is intimately associated with its location. Lawson and Reino (8) reviewed 132 cases of isolated sphenoid disease, and their findings are similar to those of some smaller studies. In this series, the most common presenting symptom was headache, usually retro-orbital and then vertex. The second most common finding on presentation was visual change. The next most common was cranial nerve palsy. In this group, cranial neuropathy was a presenting sign in 60% of benign tumors, 52% of malignancies, and 12% of inflammatory conditions. The etiologies in this group of patients were as follows: 60% inflammatory, 29% neoplastic, 3% fibro-osseus, and 8% traumatic or developmental. If bony erosion is present or a neoplasm or a vascular lesion is suspected then the work-up should include both computed tomography (CT) and magnetic resonance imaging (MRI).

COMPLICATIONS AND MANAGEMENT

Maniglia (9) reviewed a series of 40 cases of complications arising from sphenoid sinus surgery. In this group there were 13 intracranial injuries, four of which resulted in death. There were 10 cases of blindness, two of which were bilateral. Three fatalities occurred from carotid injury, and of four major anesthesia-related complications, three resulted in death. He concluded that while some injuries were preventable, sphenoid sinus surgery carries a risk of major complication even in the hands of experienced surgeons.

Hudgins et al. (10) identified a series of 10 complications at their own institution, consisting of eight intracranial injuries and two vascular injuries. All were identified in the postoperative period. There were six patients that presented with meningitis (one meningocele), and two patients with mental status change as a result of pneumocephalus. The vascular injuries presented as subarachnoid hemorrhage from anterior cerebral artery aneurysm and epistaxis from pseudoaneurysm of cavernous carotid. All injuries were managed without death.

Of the intracranial complications, cerebral spinal fluid (CSF) leak is the most common and can be estimated at 1 to 3%. One risk factor for postoperative leak is bony erosion, which may lead to inadvertent removal of dura and brain tissue through the preexisting defect. Patients with increased intracranial pressure are also more likely to develop a postoperative CSF leak. A newer issue is the use of powered instrumentation. Church et al. (11) performed a chart review of the last four years and looked for all cases of iatrogenic skull-base injury resulting in skull-base defects greater than 2 cm. Three cases were identified, all with removal of brain tissue, none of which were recognized at the time of surgery. In all cases, review of the operative report showed that a microdebrider was used at the fovea and heavy bleeding was encountered. All cases were noted postoperatively, presenting with either profuse bleeding after pack removal, headache, or pneumocephalus. Once identified, all cases were repaired endoscopically and the patients did not experience further sequelae.

The endoscopic management of CSF leak has been well described. Zweig et al. (12) reviewed a series of 53 patients that underwent such repair. The locations of the leaks are as follows: 37% sphenoid, 35% cribriform, and 28% ethmoid. The overall success rate was high (94%) and was found to be independent of the choice of graft material, glue or packing materials, onlay or underlay technique, or the size of the defect. A postoperative lumbar drain was used in 57% of patients. Graft materials used included mucoperichondrial graft, pedicled septal flap, alloderm, and fat. Glue and packing materials included gelfoam, fibrin glue, and surgical and nasal tampons. Also included were defects greater than 2 cm. All three failures were later found, at the time of revision surgery with lumbar drain placement, to have an elevated intracranial pressure. Ventricular peritoneal (VP) shunts were placed at the time of revision surgery, and all three revision surgeries had successful outcomes. Casiano and Jsaair (13) reviewed 33 cases of endoscopic CSF leak repair with a success rate of 97%. This was independent of the size of the defect (<1 mm up to 3 cm defects were included). In addition, this study demonstrated that, a lumbar drain is not required in primary cases. The failures were all noted to have high intracranial pressure and this was addressed in the revision surgery.

Tension pneumocephalus is also a known but rare intracranial complication. This occurs from packing in the sinus that is loose enough to allow air to escape around it. This occurs from a defective ball valve mechanism and is aggravated by coughing. This may present as blindness (suprasellar air), but may also present with more global symptoms of altered mental status, headaches, seizures, hypertension, bradycardia, or cranial nerve palsy. Low intracranial pressure is a significant risk factor, typically from CSF leak or lumbar drain. This allows penetration of air into the subdural, subarachnoid, or even intraventricular space. Forced air or coughing aggravates this problem. Patients with obstructive sleep apnea are at higher risk, and this may be secondary to habitually forceful airflow from anatomic differences or a central component. The management of pneumocephalus begins with CT scan and MRI (MRI will be used to follow the resolution of air) and a neurosurgical consult to evaluate for possible evacuation of the air and repair of the dural defect. At the time of repair, special attention should be paid to packing the sinus to avoid a recurrence.

Blindness can also occur following sphenoid sinus surgery. Although this can occur from pneumocephalus as described above, the primary differential is optic nerve injury versus retrobulbar hematoma. Optic nerve injury classically presents immediately postoperatively with an afferent pupillary defect (Marcus Gunn pupil). Retrobulbar hematoma initially presents with ecchymosis, chemosis, and subconjunctival hemorrhage. Later the patient may develop restricted gaze, a firm globe, and proptosis. This develops over 30 to 60 minutes, and after 90 minutes an afferent pupillary deficit may occur from secondary compressive injury to the optic nerve. More injuries occur on the right side.

Optic nerve injury can occur from an unrecognized dehiscent nerve in the lateral wall of the sinus. This is most frequently associated with the presence of an Onodi cell. The management is immediate postoperative identification and ophthalmology consult to measure pressure and help distinguish this from retrobulbar hematoma. If optic nerve injury has occurred, nothing can be done and there is a poor prognosis. If nerve injury presents in a delayed fashion in the postoperative period, this may be due to edema or hematoma along the nerve, and optic nerve decompression should be considered.

Intraorbital injury can take the form of intraorbital emphysema, injury to the extraocular muscles, or intraorbital bleeding. Muscle injury typically occurs to the medial rectus or inferior oblique and presents as gaze restriction. This can be direct muscle injury, which requires surgical exploration by ophthalmology. This may also be due to a small confined hematoma or secondary edema resulting in a transient paresis, which can be observed. This distinction is made by exam and, if needed, CT scan. Risk factors include thin or absent lamina papyrecea from revision surgery, hypertension, nasal packing, and powered instrumentation. The absence of a normal lamina eases entry into the orbit. Hypertension increases the risk of bleeding from exposed orbital fat, and nasal packing eliminates the ability of the blood to drain, promoting hematoma and compression of the globe. Graham and Nerad (14) reviewed the use of powered instrumentation and orbital complications in their institution and identified four patients with muscular injury, one with hemorrhage, and one with blindness. All patients had permanent deficits.

Once retrobulbar hematoma is suspected, immediate ophthalmologic consult should be obtained to measure intraocular pressures. In the first 30 to 60 minutes, conservative measures should be taken, including eye massage to encourage egress of the blood and diuresis. Mannitol can be given at 1–2 g/kg as 20% infusion over 30 to 60 minutes; it acts rapidly and the effect lasts 6 to 8 hours. Acetazolamide can also be given 500 mg IV every 2 to 4 hours, but it has later onset of action (hours), and electrolytes need to be followed. If conservative measures fail, surgical decompression should be considered. The quickest, easiest approach is lateral canthotomy. If this is insufficient, medial decompression can be performed, either through an external (Lynch) incision or endoscopically. The source of the bleeding may be an ethmoid artery that has retracted into the globe or a transected vessel within the orbital fat, and both can be controlled with bipolar cautery.

Vascular injury during sphenoid surgery has been described involving the cavernous carotid, posterior septal, anterior and posterior ethmoid, and anterior cerebral arteries. This occurs more commonly when there is dehiscence or an aberrant course of the carotid, or during pituitary surgery when the suprasellar bone is removed. Management consists of immediate packing of the sinus and ipsilateral compression of the carotid in the neck. If necessary, surgical control of the carotid may be obtained in the neck. Neurosurgical and neuroradiological consultation should be obtained immediately. Intraoperative angiography is performed with a balloon occlusion test paired with EEG. If the patient has electroencephalography (EEG) changes with occlusion, emergent carotid bypass may be indicated. If the patient tolerates balloon occlusion, there are several interventional techniques to control the vessel. Coil embolization, release of the balloon for permanent occlusion, and stenting of the vessel have all been described. Coil embolization has a reported risk of 12% transient and 5% permanent neuropathy.

ENDOSCOPIC SURGICAL APPROACHES

Numerous endoscopic surgical approaches have been described for the sphenoid sinus, and each tries to utilize known surgical landmarks. Parsons (15) describes a modification of the anterior–posterior (A–P) approach, beginning with anterior and posterior ethmoidectomy. The natural ostium of the sphenoid sinus is visualized medial to the superior turbinate (ridge) and measured. The distance to the posterior-most ethmoid cell is then measured and compared. If the distance to the natural ostium of the sphenoid is farther than the limit of posterior ethmoid dissection, the surgeon may then fracture the septation between the two-sinus inferomedially, toward the septum.

Bolger et al. (16) describe an approach to the sphenoid without performing ethmoidectomy. The surgeon resects 2–3 mm of the medial and inferior portion of middle turbinate basal lamella to visualize the superior turbinate. Using the superior turbinate as landmark for natural ostium, a "parallelogram" is described with the inferior and medial borders as the superior turbinate attachments, the lateral border as the lamina, and the superior border as the skull base. Entering in the inferomedial half of this area will enter into the sphenoid sinus. Wigand and Hoseman (17) describe entry next to the nasal septum and medial to the superior turbinate. The ostium is 10–12 mm above the arch of the choanae, and this corresponds to the middle 13 of the sinus in 88% of patients. For adequate visualization, a limited posterior ethmoidectomy is performed and identified as the boundary, and the sinus is entered with a suction tip.

Casiano (18) describes an approach combining the landmarks described above and related it spatially with a view of the nasal septum and medial orbital floor and using standardized columnellar measurements. From the columnella, the following structures are noted in a range and mean value: the posterior maxillary wall is 5–8 cm (9), anterior face of the sphenoid 6–9 cm (11), and posterior wall of the sphenoid is 9–10 cm (13); the optic nerve is 6–10 cm (12), carotid atery 6–10 cm (12), and anterior ethmoid artery 5–7 cm (10) from the columnella; from the antrostomy ridge, the optic nerve is 12–20 mm, and the carotid artery 10–25 mm. The most reliable identification of the sphenoid sinus should result from combining as many landmars, visual cases, and measurements as are known.

APPLICATION OF IMAGE-GUIDED SURGERY

At present, there are two types of image-guided systems on the market, based on different technologies. The stealth is based on an optical (infrared) signal system. The CT scan is loaded into the computer, and the headset is introduced when the patient is in the OR. The fiducials are then recorded, and since many points are required to assure accuracy, this can take some time. Since the system is optically based, the overhead receiver piece has to be in direct line of site with the instrument at all times. Any equipment that blocks the line of site will interfere with the functioning of the system. Fiducials may need to be verified at different points in the case. The Instatrak system is electromagnetically (radiofrequency) based. The headset is registered to the patient during the initial CT scan and is brought with the patient to the OR. Only a few points are needed to verify the headset registration at the start of the case, but the patient and staff need to make sure it is the correct headset for that patient. Metal objects interfere with tracking in this system, and should be kept at a minimum around the workstation.

Both systems have been shown to have an accuracy of 2 mm when properly registered and verified. Citardi et al. in 2000 used the stealth system on 62 patients and looked at where the device was most helpful (19). In his review, he noted that it was used mostly in the frontal and spheno-ethmoidal recess. It was also used to identify the face of the sphenoid, the limits of the maxiallary sinus, and residual ethmoid cells. Casiano and Numa (20) looked at the application of the Instatrak system in training residents. Using cadavers, four second year otolaryngology residency (PGY 2) residents were divided into two groups and used a total of eight heads (two heads per resident). None had previously performed sinus surgery. The CAS, or computer assisted, group was found to be significantly better at identifying critical landmarks: 97% successful in the CAS group, 77% in the non-CAS group. The CAS group took longer to do the surgery but had no complications, while the non-CAS group had three major complications. In the clinical setting, image guidance is most useful in revision surgery, massive disease, sphenoid surgery, frontal surgery, or the presence of Onodi cells or other anatomic variations on CT. In those situations, image guidance should improve accuracy and speed during the surgery, though the overall time, especially in the first series of cases, may be longer. Hwang et al. (21) reported six cases of transient neuropathy from headset use: five sensory and one motor (buccal branch of facial nerve) from pressure at the points where the headset was secured. Vendors have been working on advances to address the current system constraints. The software is improving to reduce registration time. More instruments have been created with tracking devices in the tip to improve speed and accuracy. "Wireless" workstations are being developed to simplify the system and reduce issues of interference. Finally, the cost of these systems is decreasing. Now an older model can be bought for $80,000, while the originals could not be purchased for under $150,000.

CONCLUSION

Sphenoid sinus surgery is frequently encountered by the otolaryngologist. The anatomy is highly variable, and surgery can carry a significant risk of major complications. If recognized intraoperatively, these can sometimes be managed without long-term sequelae. The risk of complications can be reduced with a careful review of preoperative imaging, proven anatomical approaches to surgery, and assistance with image-guided technology in select patients.

REFERENCES

1. Basak S, Karaman CZ, Akdilli A, Mutlu C, Odabasi O, Erpek G. Evaluation of some important anatomical variations and dangerous areas of the paranasal sinus by CT for safer endonasal surgery.

2. Sirikci A, Bayazit YA, Bayram M, Mumbuc S, Gungor K, Kanlikama M. Variations of sphenoid and related structures. Eur Radiol 2000; 10(5):844–848

3. Zinreich SJ. Functional anatomy and computed tomography imaging of the paranasal sinuses. AM J Med Sci 1998; 316(1):2–12.

4. Dessi P, Moulin G, Castro F, Chagnaud C, Cannoni M. Protrusion of the optic nerve into the ethmoid and sphenoid sinus: prospective study of 150 CT studies. Neuroradiology 1994; 36(7):515–516.

5. Kentarci M, Karasen RM, Alper F, Onbas O, Okur A, Karaman A. Remarkable anatomic variations in paranasal sinus region and their clinical importance. Eur J Radiol 2004; 50(3):296–302. Review.

6. Fujii K, Chambers SM, Rhoton AL Jr. Neurovascular relationships of the sphenoid sinus. A microsurgical study. J Neurosurg 1979; 50(1)31–39.

7. Kennedy DW. Diseases of the paranasal sinuses. 2000.

8. Lawson W, Reino AJ. Isolated sphenoid sinus disease: an analysis of 132 cases. Laryngoscope 1997; 107(12 pt 1):1590–1595.

9. Maniglia AJ. Fatal and major complications secondary to nasal and sinus surgery. Laryngoscope 1991; 101(4 pt 1):349–354.

10. Hudgins PA, Browning DG, Gallups J, Gussack GS, Peterman SB, Davis PC, Silverstein AM, Beckett WW, Hoffman JC Jr. Endoscopic paranasal sinus surgery: radiographic evaluation of severe complications. AJNR Am J Neuroradiol 1992; 13(4):1161–1167.

11. Church CA, Chiu AG, Vaughan WC. Endoscopic repair of large skull base defects after powered sinus surgery. Otolaryngol Head Neck Surg 2003; 129(3):204–209.

12. Zweig JL, Carrau RL, Celin SE, Schaitkin BM, Pollice PA, Snyderman CH, Kassam A, Hegazy H. Endoscopic repair of cerebrospinal fluid leaks to the sinonasal tract: predictors of success. Otolaryngol Head Neck Surg 2000; 123(3):195–201.

13. Casiano RR, Jassir D. Endoscopic cerebrospinal fluid rhinorrhea repair: is a lumbar drain necessary? Otolaryngol Head Neck Surg 1999; 121(6):745–750.

14. Graham SM, Nerad JA. Orbital complications in endoscopic sinus surgery using powered instrumentation. Laryngoscope 2003; 113(5):874–878.

15. Smith WC, Boyd EM, Parsons DS. Pediatric sphenoidotomy. Otolaryngol Clin North America 1996; 29(1):159–167.

16. Bolger WE, Keyes AS, Lanza DC. Use of the superior meatus and superior turbinate in the endoscopic approach to the sphenoid sinus. Otolaryngol Head Neck Surg 199; 120(3):308–313.

17. Wigand ME, Hoseman W. Microsurgical treatment of recurrent nasal polyposis. Rhinol Suppl 1989; 8:25–29.

18. Casiano RR. A stepwise surgical technisuw using the medial orbital floor as the key landmark in performing endoscopic sinus surgery. Laryngoscope 2001; 111(6):964–974.

19. Citardi MJ, Cox AJ 3rd, Bucholz RD. Acellular dermal allograft for sellar reconstruction after transsphenoid hypophysectomy. Am J Rhinol 2000; 14(1)69–73.

20. Casiano RR, Numa WA Jr. Efficacy of computed tomographic image-guided endoscopic sinus surgery in residency training programs. Laryngoscope 2000; 110(8):1277–1282.

21. Hwang PH, Maccabee M, Lingren JA. Headset-related sensory and motor neuropathies in image guided sinus surgery. Arch Otolaryngol Head Neck Surg 2002; 128(5):589–591.

16

How to Set Up a Sinus Center

Michael Setzen

Department of Otolaryngology, North Shore University Hospital, Manhasset, New York, U.S.A.

Gavin Setzen

Department of Surgery and Albany ENT and Allergy Services, Albany Medical College, Albany, New York, U.S.A.

Mary LeGrand

KarenZupko & Associates Inc., Chicago, Illinois, U.S.A.

INTRODUCTION

Contemporary otolaryngology surgery has evolved over time to include the practice of pediatric otolaryngology and rhinology in an office setting, incorporating in-office diagnostic as well as therapeutic interventions including surgery. Other options that have become increasingly popular during the past decade include freestanding surgical centers as a mechanism for increasing patient access to health care, as well as enhancing practice viability through an alternative revenue stream in the form of physician participation in facility-fee reimbursement. These settings can either be incorporated into one's immediate office environment or represent a separate freestanding surgical location depending on the nature of one's practice. The concept of a sinus center alludes to a facility where an otolaryngologist is able to comprehensively evaluate and manage the pediatric sinus patient, both medically and surgically. The development of minimally invasive surgical techniques, together with enhanced anesthesia options, makes the potential for office-based surgery, distinct from hospital-based surgery, a much more attractive alternative for both the practicing otolaryngologist and the patient.

Most outpatient surgical procedures in the United States are performed in office-based surgical facilities and freestanding ambulatory surgical centers. This represents a convenient form of practice for both the patient and the physician. The insurance industry has also evolved to the point where many procedures are only reimbursed when performed on an outpatient basis, and several procedures are no longer covered if performed in a hospital setting. As demand for hospital operating room time and the complexity of in-hospital surgery increase, there has been a commensurate increase in demand for outpatient surgical treatment options. Single specialty and multispecialty group practices have become increasingly popular and blend well with the concept of out-of-hospital treatment, including surgical therapy. As otolaryngologists, we have had to contend with declining reimbursement, increasing overhead, and increased medical liability. Otolaryngologists have had to become far more savvy with respect to the commercialization of medical practice in order to remain economically viable while providing quality medical care.

The discussion that follows details how one might set up a sinus center that includes both the medical and surgical management of pediatric sinus patients. This will include a discussion about physical planning, management, medical and legal requirements, certification, insurance, and other socioeconomic issues.

ORGANIZATIONAL CONSIDERATIONS

In developing a "*Center of Excellence*," consideration must be given to organizational structure and business functions to ensure ease of access, quality patient care, and optimal reimbursement for the center's ongoing success.

To ensure operational efficiency and maximize the patient experience, it is necessary to understand how patients access the physician's office in addition to how patients and information flow. The goal is streamlined operational processes that minimize the need for rework and give the practice control over both patient and information progression.

Most likely, the receptionist is the first person with whom a patient will have contact via phone call(s) to the practice or center. The communication skills and professionalism of this person are critical to ensure the caller has an initial positive experience.

Understanding the functional tasks or assignments throughout reimbursement process helps sort out the various functions and key positions in the center. This process stretches across the boundaries of all departments within a medical practice. It begins when a patient makes contact with the practice for an appointment, and ends at the point when all services provided have been paid for. Key functional areas include appointment scheduling, preregistration and insurance verification, check-in/check-out, clinical services by all providers (physicians, non-physician providers, allergy nurses, technicians, etc.), presurgical financial counseling, precertification, proper claim submission, payment posting, appeals, and account follow-up. Table 1 reflects key components of each of the functional responsibilities.

A key component of successful scheduling is to define key physician preferences as to how patients will access his/her practice. Poor access to the clinical practice site will create barriers to building a successful practice. Understanding the patient's and physician's expectations related to patient's access (personal visits and phone calls) and aligning these expectations is critical.

Special consideration must be given to patient flow and appointment schedules for any types of services. Preset appointment times provide the greatest efficiency for the staff, as referrals may be checked in advance of the appointment, medical records may be pulled, and the staff is not hurried in preparing the patients. Job descriptions are key to creating the successful team and assigning responsibilities.

Table 1 Reimbursement Process: Key Function

Functional area	Tasks/activities
Appointment scheduling	Make appointment and collect basic demographic information
Preregistration and insurance verification	Collect remainder of patient demographic information
	Verify insurance eligibility and benefits; check for deductible, coinsurance, copay
	Obtain managed care referral or authorization for visit
Check-in/check-out	Verify patient registration information
	Collect co-pays, deductibles
	Enter and post charges during check-out process
Clinical services	Providers see patient; document services
Presurgical counseling	Discuss with patient any financial concerns
	Collect surgical deposits as appropriate
Precertification	Verify eligibility
Proper claim submission	Enter charges and ensure all information is accurate for clean claim submission
Payment posting	Post payments and rejections/denials
Appeals	Initiate the appeal process on all rejected claims or claims inappropriate denials
Account follow-up	Follow up, at regular intervals, on all outstanding accounts

TELEPHONE TRIAGE

In any practice, triage services provide quality patient care, improve the quality of work life for the physician, assist in managing patient's information, and allow for a dedicated person to ensure the patients' needs are addressed in a timely manner. Similarly, in a sinus/allergy center, triage services are extremely important to ensure patients have access to clinical staff with questions regarding immunotherapy plans of care, preoperative and postoperative surgical issues, or other medical and related questions.

Telephone triage allows a staff member to assess a patient's health concern using interviewing skills, assessment skills, and clinical knowledge. An essential triage skill is the ability to listen and assess the clues the caller is providing (those clues that you cannot see because you are on the telephone), while at the same time comforting the patient without creating a sense of fear or panic.

Patients typically call into the physician's office to discuss their symptoms, ask questions regarding medications, or to follow up after surgical or medical interventions. The triage person determines whether the patient needs to be seen immediately, needs to be referred to the emergency room, or if the patient's questions can be answered via the telephone. Typical triage questions in an otolaryngology practice are medically based, so the need for clinical expertise is critical. Patients may call with symptoms of an acute sinus infection, signs and symptoms related to runny noses, headaches, potential life-threatening nosebleeds, or allergy reactions.

Because of the clinical conditions listed above, triage by a qualified individual in the physician office supports good quality patient care and decreases the number of delayed or unreturned phone calls. Otolaryngologists with busy surgical practices spend more time away from the office, with fewer hours to return patient calls or for add-on appointments that could be handled by answering patients' questions on the telephone.

The best way to manage triage functions is to formalize the position and create standard protocols for the center.

Ask the following questions to begin to create the triage position

1. What are the common calls coming into the office?
2. Who currently handles phone calls? What are the credentials for these persons? Are they trained in otolaryngology?
3. How many calls are handled on the typical day? How many of those calls turn into same day appointments, no appointments, or appointments sent to emergency room?
4. What is the "typical" response to the questions? (There may already be unwritten and informal protocols in place that merely need formalizing.)
5. Is there a confidential workspace from which to call patients?

6. Will the telephone system allow for voicemail for the triage nurse?
7. How are medical records managed? Electronic? Paper?
8. How are notes currently taken? Are staff members already recording all phone messages and responses?
9. Does a protocol exist for taking information—what's important, what's not?
10. How quickly are phone calls returned?
11. Is there a physician dedicated as the contact person for the day or specific week? Or, do the calls go to each individual physician/provider?

Are protocols necessary?

To ensure accurate, consistent information and to allow the nurses to use their assessment skills, protocols are essential in a successful triage program. Nurses who are not advanced practice nurses cannot make a diagnosis; instead they use their clinical and interviewing skills to obtain a complete history and may then use protocols for the "normal range of questions." Protocols act as a guide and are always subject to change dependent on patient condition.

EMBRYOLOGY OF A SINUS CENTER

It has become increasingly clear that in order to develop a sinus center or other *"Center of Excellence"* where one can comprehensively evaluate and treat a particular patient, one should have extensive training, experience, and expertise in that particular field. It is also important to have established a broad-based referral network to ensure that one's patient volume is sustained in order to allow the facility to thrive and be able to maintain one's skill level in that particular field. In this case, for an otolaryngologist practicing pediatric otolaryngology as part of a general otolaryngology practice, or for a fellowship-trained pediatric otolaryngologist, the basic premise remains the same. In order to set up a sinus center, one needs not only manage pediatric patients well, but should ensure that the physical plant and associated diagnostic and therapeutic interventions appropriately cater to the needs of all of the patients. For the purposes of this discussion, we will assume that the sinus center will cater to both children and adults.

The physical space and location of the facility should include office space in which the otolaryngologist can provide a pleasant and safe environment for patient interaction. This should include optimal physical access and adequate parking and access to the facility. In planning the facility, consideration must be given to the Americans with Disabilities Act (ADA). Typically, it has been suggested that each physician in a practice requires approximately 1500 to 2000 square feet, together with approximately four full time equivalent staff persons to sustain a workable office environment. Today, most single or multispecialty office groups are located near a facility that provides a freestanding surgical center or have a surgical center within the office itself.

Physical planning of the office and surgical suite should be individualized and tailored to the specific requirements of each otolaryngologist, while meeting the overall needs of the group in general. This requires planning with an architect who has experience in developing medical and surgical facilities. Important considerations include access, physical layout, electrical planning, heating, lighting, air conditioning, medical gases, and several other aspects which require specific consideration.

In general, an adequately sized waiting room, reception area, secretary's office, internal corridors, nursing stations, and diagnostic and treatment rooms should be available. Attention must also be given when planning space needs and adequate storage space, clean and soiled utility rooms, and a conference or "break" room should also be available. Generally, three examination rooms are optimal per physician, and planning should include optimizing ergonomics with respect to patient examination, including nasal evaluation and, in particular, flexible or rigid nasal endoscopy. Ideally, in a contemporary facility visual monitors should be positioned in each examination room, together with equipment that would allow for accurate photo-documentation of anatomical findings at each visit. It is also useful to be able to view sinus CT scans, MRI scans and other imaging studies in the examination room with the patient. A recessed X-ray viewing station should be present in each examination room. This can easily be facilitated by having a wall, mounted television monitor, together with a digital video recorder or digital camera, to allow for patient demonstrations and photo-documentation. This allows for improved patient understanding of a particular problem and facilitates surgical planning. Medicolegally, this can be very beneficial in terms of preoperative informed consent and demonstrating abnormalities requiring intervention. Depending on the nature of one's practice and preference with respect to leasing or purchasing equipment to facilitate such an examination, one might choose to use a mobile video endoscopy cart which could be used in different examination rooms by different individuals, thereby limiting the cost of providing such a service. Data archiving should be well managed to ensure patients' confidentiality, accessibility, and accuracy. The examination room might need to be slightly larger than the standard 8 ft × 8 ft or 9 ft × 9 ft exam room to accommodate additional equipment including a fiberoptic light source and endoscopes.

Treatment rooms for minor surgical procedures, microscopic examinations of the ears, nasal endoscopy, and debridement can be helpful as well. These are generally larger than the typical examination rooms and might facilitate limited interventions, including sinonasal debridement and poly-pectomy as well as flexible and rigid endoscopy.

At this point in the planning and development phase, one has to determine whether to proceed with an in-office operating room suite versus a freestanding ambulatory surgical center within the same building that can be utilized by other individuals as well. Otolaryngologists can usually set up a center based on a single-specialty model because the reimbursement for these cases tends to be higher than for other surgical fields, including urology, ophthalmology, and gastroenterology. In setting up a sinus center, both of these models are appropriate. The term "sinus center" inherently implies a certain level of excellence and skill in approaching the patient with sinus and nasal pathology from a diagnostic perspective as well as being able to intervene therapeutically to address the particular problem.

In-office surgery continues to grow in popularity, especially as issues relating to patient's access, convenience, and reimbursement become more prevalent. While costly to establish, in-office surgical suites have an excellent return on investment by virtue of the fact that the physician is able to participate in the facility expense component of the reimbursed procedure, as opposed to automatically being excluded from this process in a typical hospital-based surgical facility model. In developing a sinus center with in-office operating rooms, one is able to perform minor procedures, including endoscopic débridements in postoperative pediatric patients using topical or intravenous anesthesia or intravenous sedation. This also facilitates polypectomy, closed-reduction of nasal fractures, and other limited procedures. When using intravenous sedation, it is important to have an anesthesiologist available. Several areas use both anesthesiologists and certified nurse anesthetists working together in one or more surgical suites. One also requires a recovery area for patients requiring intravenous sedation and general anesthesia.

When planning the office surgical suite, it is usually optimal to develop two or more suites simultaneously, given the inherent cost in the physical construction and requirements for medical gases, high-grade lighting, ventilation, and electrical formatting. It is also useful to integrate computer accessibility and photo documentation in the operating room that can interface with the operating facility as well as the office facility. This is particularly useful for teaching purposes and possibly to obtain an intraoperative opinion from a colleague regarding a particular clinical problem.

An office-based surgery center certainly can be a financially attractive investment opportunity and provides a unique chance to become involved in the "surgery center business," either on an individual or group basis, or as part of a multispecialty group with ownership potential at a fraction of the cost normally associated with such projects. Physician syndication is also an attractive mechanism for acquiring such a facility, and allows otolaryngologists to realize a significant return on their original investments, with limited initial financial impact and exposure.

The legal structure most often used is that of a limited liability company (LLC). One has the option of out-sourcing the management of the surgery center in partnership with the otolaryngologist. Management issues can be quite significant and include financial functions and accounts payable, financial statements, billing, and collections, as well as quality management programs combining all national and state requirements, along with compliance programs including the Occupational Safety and Health Administration (OSHA) and Health Insurance Portability and Accountability Act (HIPPA).

In determining the viability of a surgery center, either in-office or free-standing, it is critical to accurately calculate one's case volume by evaluating Current Procedural Terminology (CPT) codes and the volume of each code performed annually by the otolaryngologist and any other physicians participating in the facility. Based on this information, one can establish a financial feasibility study to determine the viability and potential profitability of such a center. A typical pro forma income statement will usually be based on the volume of cases during an anticipated three-year period looking at net revenue as a function of wages, benefits, drugs, and medical supplies. Other direct expenses include billing and collection, loan and interest, lease and rentals, as well as general management and administrative expenses. One also has to keep in mind depreciation and amortization in order to determine net income. Cash available for distribution can be determined on this basis with one-, two-, and three-year projections. The capital required for setting up a sinus center or other freestanding surgical center is usually realized with most current models demonstrating 100 units for sale as shares, representing 1% of the total investment.

Any partnership agreement will require due diligence with respect to both financial accountability and legal issues as these differ on a state-by-state basis. The center must also comply with federal health care requirements.

The greater the number of practicing surgeons with an ownership interest in the facility, the greater the volume of cases performed, and the greater the likelihood of successfully maintaining the surgery center and ensuring an economically viable undertaking. Any office-based surgery center or freestanding surgical center requires certification by various certifying agencies, and in many different areas one still requires a Certificate of Need (CON) application.

REIMBURSEMENT AND INSURANCE ISSUES

As mentioned previously, one of the advantages of maintaining an in-office surgical facility or freestanding surgery center is that most insurance companies, both federal, state, and third-party insurers, will pay a facility fee to the surgery center given the fact that this represents a cost-savings to the reimbursing organization. In most cases, the surgical procedure being performed can be carried out more cost-effectively at a surgery center than in a hospital. The facility fee is usually predetermined and, in terms of cost-benefit analysis, most surgery centers can provide the same service more cost-effectively. Depending on the type of facility that one is able to establish and the nature of the health care environment in which one practices, it is also possible to negotiate on an individual basis with a particular carrier to provide certain CPT codes at a particular rate, incorporating the global fee for such a procedure, including the facility fee. This should be addressed on an individual and local basis, and in most instances precertification should be obtained when such contracts have been negotiated. As a general rule, each contract should specify that the facility fee will be paid and precertification will likely lessen the risk and exposure on the part of the surgery center since claim denials will be greatly reduced.

Most cost-accounting structures are based on the resource based relative value scale (RBRVS) and relative value unit (RVU). While not perfect, these two measures determine presumed direct and indirect costs that are used to calculate overall reimbursement for a particular CPT code. The cost-accounting measures take into consideration both direct and indirect costs and might include disposable and durable equipment and personnel. Indirect costs are usually attributable to rent, information technology maintenance, utilities, and other infrastructure requirements. In cost-accounting, one can usually determine a standard percentage of the direct costs, usually 30–40%, that is considered, an indirect cost added to the total cost in determining a particular fee when negotiating "carve-outs" or specialized contracts for specific procedures.

Most insurers use the RBRVS model used by Medicare, and a predetermined profit margin is agreed upon and added to the cost of a particular procedure. Usually that profit margin incorporates direct and indirect costs, which are then applied to the particular procedure. In order to insure the financial success of the sinus center, one has to be meticulous in determining what the level of reimbursement will be for each procedure, and financial planning and cost analysis must be carried out on an ongoing basis, either in-house or by using an external management company. Medicare Part B reimburses a certified ambulatory surgery center (ASC) a facility payment for services covered under their ASC coverage list. The ASC must be a distinct entity for the purpose of providing outpatient surgical services, and must be approved by Medicare as such. Medicare will not reimburse the ASC a facility payment if the procedure is not listed on the approved list of ASC-covered services.

The facility payment does not cover physician billing as the physician submits his/her own surgical fees. The facility payment is expected to cover administrative costs such as space (operative and recovery), anesthesia supplies, drugs, surgical dressings, supplies, appliances, equipment, clinical staffing, and housekeeping staffing.

The ASC payment rates vary according to the procedure type to cover the ASCs incurred costs. Medicare has nine payment groups as of October 2004. A review of the ASC Medicare facility group lists found the sinus endoscopy procedures in a variety of groups. For example, diagnostic nasal endoscopy, CPT 31231, is not on the list of covered services in an ASC. Endoscopic maxillary, frontal, sphenoid, and anterior ethmoid procedures are assigned to group 3, while endoscopic total ethmoid procedures are in group 5. In 2005, group 3 payment is $510 and group 5 payment rates are $717 for the primary procedure.

Medicare reimburses at the same multiple-procedure payment formula for groups as for physicians. A bilateral procedure in the ASC reported as two procedures is subject to the multiple-procedure payment formula. This means that if the physician performs a bilateral endoscopic maxillary antrostomy, expected reimbursement is 100% of the wage-adjusted group 3 rate for the first procedure and 50% of the wage-adjusted group rate for the second procedure. The staff must keep a close eye on the explanation of benefits form (EOBs) to ensure proper reimbursement, especially when multiple procedures are performed.

Key to the success of the practice is accurate and timely account follow-up. Avoid a common misconception that the "billing staff" can be pulled to staff any area of the practice, as shortages or staff absences occur. Treat the billing office with the same attitude you treat the clinical area. Keep staff in all areas aligned with their job duties.

CORRECT CODING

Coding has a tremendous impact on collections and comes under the scrupulous eyes of all payors, who are monitoring for adherence to CPT coding rules. With the Office of Inspector General focus on coding and billing (visit their website by typing in "office of inspector general"), physician practices should establish, at a minimum, some of the elements of the government's compliance plan recommendations with an emphasis on coding and documentation, to ensure accurate coding.

Resources available to assist with accurate coding include, but are not limited to:

1. AMA CPT manual for procedural/office coding (updated annually)
2. Subscription to the AMA CPT assistant publication
3. Medicare website

4. American Academy of Otolaryngology Head–Neck Surgery practice management resources, including www.ENTcodingtoday. com
5. E-subscriptions to payor websites including Medicare
6. International Classification of Diseases, 9th Revision, Clinical Modification (ICD-9-CM)for diagnosis coding (updated annually)

Many of these resources are available through electronic means. In fact, Medicare no longer publishes paper monthly manuals.

To ensure accurate reporting of services, use the appropriate charge capture tools. The goal is timely capture of charges for office services, any ancillary-owned services, and surgery center or hospital services including any emergency room consultations, in-hospital consultations, and subsequent hospital visit services.

The AMA CPT manual contains all the CPT codes for reporting office and surgical services. The manual is broken down into sections: evaluation and management, anesthesia, surgical, medicine, radiology, pathology/laboratory, and category-III codes.

The key sections of the CPT manual for a sinus practice/sinus center specifically include the evaluation and management section, the surgical section for reporting surgical sinus procedures, the medicine section for allergy-related services, pathology/laboratory for any RAST testing or other related services, and radiology for sinus X-rays, CT scans, and other radiology services.

CODING OFFICE-BASED PROCEDURES

If the physician sees a new patient in the office and performs a diagnostic nasal endoscopy, the physician may report both the new patient's visit and the endoscopy if the documentation supports both services.

According to the AMA CPT rules, the physician may report both the new patient's visit and the endoscopy if the evaluation and management (E&M) service is a significant separate service. Table 2 shows how the physician reports this service according to the 2005 AMA CPT rules.

The CPT rules state it is not necessary to have two separate diagnoses to report the E&M service and the endoscopy. The E&M service is considered as

Table 2 Office Coding

CPT code/ modifier	Description	ICD-9-CM
9920x–25	Office or other outpatient service for a new patient	473.0 (chronic maxillary sinusitis)
31231	Nasal endoscopy, diagnostic, unilateral, or bilateral (separate procedure)	473.0 (chronic maxillary sinusitis)

a significant, separate service, because this is a new patient the physician never examined in the past. Assuming the documentation requirements are met, the physician reports both services and appends modifer-25.

Modifier-25 indicates to the payor that the E&M is a significant separate service on the same day as a minor procedure. This modifier tells the payor it was necessary to do the E&M, and reimbursement is expected on both services.

CODING SURGICAL SINUS PROCEDURES

To accurately report sinus surgical procedures, the physician will choose a code based on:

- Surgical approach, i.e., open versus endoscopic
- Unilateral or bilateral procedures
- Sinus procedures with or without removal of tissue

Additionally, the physician will indicate if additional procedures were performed at the same operative session, such as:

- Turbinate surgery (document location of turbinates)
- Septal surgery

Each service performed and reported to the payor must include a diagnosis code to support the medical necessity of the service.

For example, according to the 2005 AMA CPT rules, the physician reports the following procedure accordingly in Table 3.

Pre-Op Diagnosis:

- Chronic ethmoid sinusitis
- Chronic maxillary sinusitis

Post-Op Diagnosis:

- Chronic ethmoid sinusitis
- Chronic maxillary sinusitis
- Sinus polpys

Procedure:

- Bilateral endoscopic total ethmoidectomy
- Bilateral endoscopic maxillary antrostomy with removal of sinus polyps.

Key coding and documentation and reimbursement considerations in the above example include:

- Reporting services using the CPT appropriate code (i.e., specific sinus with or without tissue removal)
- Documentation of procedure as endoscopic (approach)
- Dictation of procedure as bilateral
- Identification of specific sinuses and inclusion of tissue removal in the maxillary sinus
- List CPT codes in descending value order
- Appropriate use of modifier-50 (bilateral procedures on second CPT codes 31255 and 31267)
- Appropriate use of modifier-51 (multiple procedure) on CPT code 31267 (first time it is listed)
- Link procedures to specific diagnosis code avoiding the use of a "pansinusitis" diagnosis
- Document removal of polyps in procedure dictation (operative note detail will also include the removal of polyps in the maxillary sinus)

Key reimbursement consideration for this case as submitted (Table 4):

1. List procedures in descending value order and ensure the Explanation of Benefts (EOB) form is returned with the same CPT codes and modifiers.
2. Post the surgical cases by line item into the computer system. (See table that follows to show line item posting.)
3. Obtain the payor's fee schedule and put the fee schedules into the computer system. This will allow you to detect any payments not made at the expected rate.
4. Watch EOBs closely to ensure proper payment is received. Independent of how the codes are submitted (line item vs. linear), expect payment to be made according to the multiple procedure payment formula. Currently, Medicare reimburses:

   - 100% for the first procedure
   - 50% for the second procedure
   - 50% for the third procedure
   - 50% for the fourth procedure
   - 50% for the fifth procedure
   - after the fifth procedure, reimbursement is at payor discretion

Post all payments and non-payments received. For any non-payments, post zero dollars and leave the line item open. Post the denial reason, and then begin the appeal/account-follow-up process.

- For any non-payments, ensure the case was coded correctly, modifiers placed appropriately, and the diagnosis supports the medical

Table 3 Surgical Sinus Coding and Line Item Reporting

CPT code/modifier	Description	ICD-9-CM	2005 RVUs (Medicare)	Expected reimbursement RVUs
31255	Nasal/sinus endoscopy, surgical; with ethmoidectomy, total (anterior and posterior)	473.2	11.79	11.79
31255-50	Nasal/sinus endoscopy, surgical; with ethmoidectomy, total (anterior and posterior)	473.2	11.79	5.90
31267-51	Nasal/sinus endoscopy, surgical, with maxillary antrostomy; with removal of tissue from maxillary sinus	473.0	9.29	4.65
31267-50	Nasal/sinus endoscopy, surgical, with maxillary antrostomy; with removal of tissue from maxillary sinus	473.0	9.29	4.65

Note: This example uses RVUs to demonstrate fees. The physician practice and surgical center will report actual fees.

Table 4 Surgical Sinus Coding and Linear Posting (Medicare Preferred Method)

CPT code/modifier	Description	ICD-9-CM	2005 RVUs (Medicare)*	Expected reimbursement RVUs
31255-50	Nasal/sinus endoscopy, surgical; with ethmoidectomy, total (anterior and posterior)	473.2	11.79 or 23.58	17.69 (150%) total both procedures
31267-50	Nasal/sinus endoscopy, surgical, with maxillary antrostomy; with removal of tissue from maxillary sinus	473.0	9.29 or 18.58	9.29 (100%) total for both procedures (the second set of code assumes payor reimburses 100%–50%–50%–50%).

Note: This illustration uses RVUs to demonstrate fees. The physician practice and surgical center will report actual fees.
*Determine if payor wants fee submitted at one time normal fee or double fee for both procedures. Medicare will apply a double adjudication to second 31267-50 and pay at 75%.

necessity of the service. If the answer to any of these three factors is no, correct the claim prior to appealing.

Sample: Linear Posting

NOTE: When payors instruct you to submit your services linear, ask them the following questions:

1. How many units go in the unit box, i.e., one or two?
2. Do I submit my fee one time, or do I double my fee?

These questions can only be answered by the payor.

CHARGE ENTRY AND ACCOUNT FOLLOW-UP

Time of Service (TOS) Charge Entry and Payment Posting

Ideally, charge entry for physician offices occurs at the end of the patient visit at checkout. Timely posting of charges is essential as payors are decreasing their filing deadlines and appeal deadlines.

Post all charges at the time of service, as well as collecting and posting of any payments due from the patients. The TOS payments include, but are not limited to, co-pays, deductibles, self-pay responsibilities, and outstanding patient balances.

At the end of each day, a "daily close" is performed to ensure charges are captured for all patients seen that day.

Charge posting for surgical cases should occur within 24 to 48 hours of the surgical case. In today's market, practices have to provide CPT codes and diagnosis codes when precertifying a case. If the physician provides the CPT codes to precertify the case, coding the case after surgery requires the physician to review the precertified codes and modify any surgical CPT codes provided on the front end to the actual surgical procedure performed.

Any delay in charge entry places the practice or center at risk for delayed reimbursement or denied reimbursement if filing deadline dates are passed.

CLAIM SUBMISSION

All claims that can be sent electronically should be sent immediately after the posting session. Verify that payors have received the claims and that the information provided is "clean."

Posting Payments, Appeals, and Account Follow-Up

Ideally, all charges and payments are entered into the computer system in line item format, which allows the staff to post all payments or non-payments directly against the service posted.

If a payor's EOB form identifies the reason for a rejection or denial, post this into the system so that you may trend payor activity regarding reasons for non-payment.

WATCHING REIMBURSEMENT

As demonstrated in the previous clinical examples (Tables 1–3), monitoring coding and documentation is critical to ensuring accurate reimbursement.

In the office examples, payors will frequently "bundle" the E&M service into the surgical procedure as part of the surgical package and only reimburse the surgical procedure.

Astute billing office staff will detect this when posting the services and begin the appeal process. Action steps for the appeal will include:

1. review the reason for denial to begin the appeal process
2. check the diagnosis code to ensure the diagnosis supports the medical necessity of both services
3. review the E&M for documentation requirements
4. ensure the nasal endoscopy procedure and findings are documented
5. make sure modifier-25 was appended to the E&M when the claim was submitted
6. review the reason for denial

Table 5 Sinus Surgery Procedure Codes and RVUs

CPT code/ modifier	Description	2005 RVUs (Medicare)	Expected reimbursement RVUs (2005)
31255	Nasal/sinus endoscopy, surgical; with ethmoidectomy, total (anterior and posterior)	11.79	11.79 (100%)
31255-50	Nasal/sinus endoscopy, surgical; with ethmoidectomy, total (anterior and posterior)	11.79	5.73 (50%)
31267-51	Nasal/sinus endoscopy, surgical, with maxillary antrostomy; with removal of tissue from maxillary sinus	9.29	4.50 (50%)
31267-50	Nasal/sinus endoscopy, surgical, with maxillary antrostomy; with removal of tissue from maxillary sinus	9.29	4.50 (50%) (see note)

Note: This illustration uses RVUs to demonstrate fees. The physician practice and surgical center will report actual fees. Medicare will apply a double adjudication to a CPT code 31267-50 and pay at 25% for second bilateral procedure.

If the claim is clean and documentation supports the services, the staff contacts the payor via telephone as the first line of appeal. The goal is to overturn the denial via the telephone versus a written appeal. If this is not successful, the staff writes a formal appeal letter.

The major concern with the surgical example is ensuring the payors reimburse appropriately on the multiple sinus procedures. Currently, many payors reimburse according to Medicare's multiple procedure payment formula, but may develop their own payment formula. Assuming Medicare's 100%, 50%, 50%, 50%, and 50% formula previously outlined, we expect to see the surgical procedures reimbursed as follows in Table 5, unless they apply for double adjudication on the 4th procedure.

INFORMED CONSENT/MEDICOLEGAL ISSUES

In order to maintain a high standard of practice, one should familiarize oneself with the American Academy of Otolaryngology-Head and Neck Surgery guidelines for management of sinus and nasal disease. The otolaryngologist and/or other surgeons involved in the facility, as well as the nursing staff and anesthesia staff, must be appropriately licensed to perform the various procedures incorporated into the surgical facility. Optimal medical documentation of procedures must be developed, including those addressing medical necessity and comprehensive informed consent. In particular, informed consent must be obtained preoperatively and must be incorporated into the record. Sinonasal surgery represents a high risk for potential medicolegal action. Informed consent can be obtained by various methods although a comprehensive discussion with the patient together with signing a document affirming this usually serves the physician well. Figure 1 is an example of a comprehensive review of the risks associated with sinonasal surgery. This consent form, modified to suit your practice, will provide excellent documentation for an informed consent discussion (Fig. 1).

By signing this document, the patient agrees that informed consent has been obtained and that the patient fully understands the risks, benefits, and reasonable alternatives to the proposed surgical procedure. Also, postoperative documentation, including the operative procedure, should be dictated immediately following the surgery, and should be complete and accurate.

In addition, from a medicolegal perspective, the operating suite should be safe, well-equipped, and fully functional to deal with all possible emergencies including resuscitation, if needed. Training and certification for staff need to be current.

Business property and liability insurance are mandatory and coverage should include loss or damage to business-owned property, equipment, infrastructure, and other associated potential losses. In addition, medical malpractice and professional liability insurance is required prior to initiating any services in the sinus center. For the most part, one million dollars per

---

Informed Consent For
Endoscopic Sinus Surgery, Septoplasty & and Other Nasal Surgeries

The risks, benefits and alternatives to endoscopic sinus surgery, image-guided sinus surgery, septoplasty and other nasal surgeries were discussed with me and reviewed in detail.

Possible complications of endoscopic sinus surgery, septoplasty and other nasal surgeries include though are not limited to:

- Nasal complications including nasal bleeding (possibly requiring blood transfusion), infection, toxic shock, synechiae, nasal lacrimal duct injury, mucocele formation, change in sense of smell, neuroma, septal perforation, atrophic rhinitis, nasal sensitivity, subjective sensation of nasal blockage, alteration of sensation with numbness of the lips, gums and teeth and requirement for further nasal packing and further surgery.

- Orbital complications, including periorbital ecchymosis (bruising), periorbital emphysema (swelling due to air accumulation), extraocular muscle injury, diplopia (double vision), other visual disturbances, orbital cellulitis and abscess, intraorbital or retroorbital hematoma, optic nerve injury and neuritis, blindness (temporary or permanent) and the possible need for further surgery.

- Intracranial complications, including cerebral spinal fluid leak, meningitis, brain injury, pneumocephalus, vascular injury, encephalocele and the possible need for further surgery.

- Revision sinus surgery has a higher risk for the aforementioned complications since the usual landmarks and other intranasal and sinus structures might be surgically altered or absent, or they may be altered by polyps and other chronic inflammatory and sinonasal diseases.

If the surgery is performed on both the left and right hand sides, the risks outlined above apply to each side separately.

If you take any medication, in particular pain medication or cold preparations which contain aspirin, Motrin, Advil, etc. or a combination of medications, please **discontinue its' use 7 days prior to surgery.** Tylenol may be taken. Continued use of these medications could impair your body's ability to stop bleeding. This may result in your surgery having to be rescheduled. Consult the Doctor if this will be a problem.

I have read the above and am willing to accept the risks of surgery and believe that the potential benefits outweigh the potential risks.
Patient Signature/Date: _____
Physician Signature/Date _____

Figure 1 Informed consent for endoscopic sinus surgery, septoplasty, and other nasal surgeries.

Accreditation Association for Ambulatory Health Care, Inc.
9933 Lawler Avenue, Skokie, IL 60077-3702
Telephone: 708-676-9610

Joint Commission on Accreditation of Healthcare Organizations
One Renaissance Boulevard, Oak Brook Terrace, IL 60181
Telephone: 708-916-5600

Occupational Health and Safety Administration (OSHA) Guidelines
Room N3101, 200 Constitution Avenue, NW, Washington D.C. 20210
Telephone Number: 202-523-9667

Clinical Laboratory Improvement Amendments of 1988 Federal Register
February 28, 1992. May be obtained in your local library.

The Americans With Disabilities Act (ADA) Guidelines.
For copies of the ADA guidelines for new construction and alterations to existing buildings,
visit their web site at www.ccoc.gov. or call the Department of Justice at 202-514-0301
or 1-800-USA-ABLE.

For state and local guidelines, rules, and regulations, contact the state's
Department of Public Health.

Figure 2 Credentialing organizations.

occurrence and three million dollars aggregate coverage is an average used by most physicians. The otolaryngologist and all levels of support personnel should obtain malpractice coverage in addition to coverage offered by the physician's malpractice policy.

CREDENTIALING

Office-based and freestanding surgical facilities require credentialing by one or more organizations. Usually a Certificate of Need (CON) application is required for more than one operating room in an outpatient facility; however, these regulations are becoming less stringent in many states, especially as patient access improves and the safety and viability of alternative surgical facilities continue to grow. Credentialing occurs at both the federal and state level and varies from state to state. In order to operate, most surgery centers require credentialing from the Center for Medicare and Medicaid Services (CMS). This ensures payment from the Health Care Finance Administration (HCFA). With Medicaid credentialing in place, most state and local third party insurers will follow suit, although this is not universal.

Two voluntary accrediting organizations, namely the Joint Commission on the Accreditation of Health Care Organizations (JCAHO) and the Accreditation Association for Ambulatory Health Care (AAAHC), have also been approved to accredit Medicare facilities. In general, accreditation is a lengthy, detailed process that requires extensive planning and preparation and may require 6 to 12 months or longer to complete. Each of the credentialing organizations has specific criteria and requirements that are clearly documented and which need to be adhered to completely to facilitate accreditation. Both the facility and any physician using the facility must be credentialed and a detailed policy and procedures manual needs to be maintained reflecting, among other things, credentialing by the facility, physician, and supporting staff. Contact information for AAAHC and JCAHO is provided (Fig. 2).

OCCUPATIONAL SAFETY AND HEALTH ADMINISTRATION

The Occupational Safety and Health Administration (OSHA) is a division of the Department of Labor which has a critical oversight role in reference to the "blood–borne pathogen standards" to insure workers' safety with minimization of exposure to HIV, hepatitis, and other blood–borne pathogens transmitted in job-related tasks. Each facility has to have a well-documented workable exposure control plan (ECP) and the plan must be comprehensive and readily available to employees. OSHA has strict requirements with respect to annual updates, and periodic site visits may be performed. Detailed protocols are available from OSHA regarding the various categories for employees with different likelihood of exposure. Documentation of training is an important part of OSHA requirements.

Hazards in the workplace including scalpels and needles need to be appropriately disposed of in SHARPS containers, scalpel and needle dispensers, and soiled linen receptacles. Noxious or toxic chemicals also need to be appropriately removed.

Personal protective clothing and equipment (PPCE) must be readily available to employees. One must provide gloves, gowns, and laboratory coats as well as face shields and other eye protection as well as caps and masks especially when a recognized risk level for contamination is present. One has to cater to the specific requirements of the employee, for example, hypoallergenic and latex free gloves.

Engineering and work practice controls are also mandated by OSHA to limit employee exposure to blood–borne pathogens.

Universal precautions should be practiced as a matter of routine. Hepatitis B vaccines should be provided to all office staff, especially in the clinical realm where exposure might be anticipated. Appropriate documentation of OSHA issues must be maintained.

The OSHA requirements are quite extensive and additional material is available directly from OSHA as well as the AMA. The OSHA web site address is http://www.osha.gov.

ANCILLARY SERVICES

In general, whether onsite or contracted out, ancillary services including laboratory, radiology, pathology, and pharmaceutical services should be made available in accordance with the patient's needs and the types and volume of procedures and surgery performed in the sinus center. The services provided should be supervised by personnel qualified in these respective areas. If the supervisor is the otolaryngologist, he or she should be qualified to assume the professional, organizational, and administrative responsibility for the quality of the service rendered.

All ancillary services located in the sinus center must meet the standards issued by the Occupational Safety and Health Administration (OSHA) and promulgated under the Clinical Laboratory Improvement Act (CLIA), as well as other applicable state and federal standards. Ancillary services can be an integral part of the sinus center.

Allergy Testing and Treatment

Allergy testing and treatment are excellent ancillary services which dovetail very well with sinonasal disease. In vivo and in vitro allergy testing may be a part of the sinus and rhinology practice, in both pediatric and adult settings. Allergy skin testing is a valuable diagnostic tool, the results of which can facilitate enhanced environmental avoidance techniques as well as immunotherapy if indicated for a particular patient. In addition, the rationale for otolaryngologists playing a more active role in allergy care cannot be understated given the atopic associations in otitis media, otitis externa, Ménière's disease, recurrent upper respiratory tract infections, rhinosinusitis, and asthma.

Generally screening can be accomplished with 10 to 15 allergens; full testing usually requires 40 or more antigens. The Academy of Otolaryngic Allergy is an excellent resource for training and certification in order to provide optimal and comprehensive allergy care for your patient. Diagnosis and management of allergy is an integral part of managing children, especially with sinonasal and other pathology.

Diagnostic Imaging Services

Diagnostic imaging services include, but are not limited, to radiography, fluoroscopy, CAT scans, MRI, ultrasound, and nuclear medicine. The sinus center will likely utilize CAT scanning more than any other modality, including its use as it relates to image-guided sinus surgery, and should be an integral part of the sinus center. Diagnostic imaging should be performed by qualified, certified staff and interpreted by a qualified practitioner. Complete patient records should be maintained in a readily accessible location in the sinus center. This allows for comprehensive patient evaluation and enhances the patient experience by providing an effective onsite radiographic test eliminating the need to go to another radiology facility or hospital. In addition, one is able to obtain the CT scan at any time for immediate review in determining whether or not further antibiotic treatment or other management is indicated. Having a CAT scanner onsite makes for a more complete, convenient, and efficient patient experience. In addition, this is a favorable ancillary revenue source where one can be reimbursed for performing the technical component of the study. Depending on the medicolegal environment where one practices, one might choose to interpret one's own CAT scans and obtain reimbursement for both the technical and diagnostic component, or one might outsource the interpretation of the CAT scan to a radiology practice. In addition, given the fact that sinus disease and rhinology often represent a large portion of one's practice, the CAT scanner can be well-utilized and supported by two or more otolaryngologists. Other studies including non-contrast head, temporal bone, and soft tissue studies of the head and neck are also frequently necessary, thereby maintaining efficiency of the scanner.

Laboratory and Pathology

Other ancillary services that might be considered in the setting of a sinus center or ambulatory surgery facility include chemical pathology and histopathology testing. Practices should comply with federal and state regulations. Routine laboratory testing, cytology, and histopathology are usually contracted out based on the patient's insurance obligations.

OFFICE ADMINISTRATION

Policies and Procedures

Develop simple written policies and procedures to ensure the provision of safe and quality medical and surgical care. One must be able to inform patients, respond to their needs, and assure consistent personnel performance to maintain a high quality sinus center. The policies and procedures should include an emergency care and transfer plan, medical record maintenance and security, surgical services and invasive procedures, maintenance of surgical and anesthesia equipment as well as a structured infection control policy, organizational structure and job description and a clear delineation of patient rights.

Performance Improvement Program

The sinus center should establish and maintain a performance improvement program, which should assess both process and clinical outcomes of the practice to improve the quality of care. This typically includes peer review.

The scope and breadth of the program should reflect the size of the practice and the sinus center as well as the level of anesthesia used and the complexity of services performed.

CONCLUSION

The creation of a sinus center with the understanding that it will function as a "center of excellence" requires much preparation. The organizational requirements are listed in detail in the chapter. A thorough understanding of the issues pertaining to coding and reimbursement are critical to the success of the center. Credentialing, satisfying OSHA requirements, and knowledge of the legal ramifications including malpractice issues are essential requirements for a successful **"Sinus Center of Excellence."**

Index